Breast Reconstruction

Editor

NEIL TANNA

CLINICS IN PLASTIC SURGERY

www.plasticsurgery.theclinics.com

April 2023 • Volume 50 • Number 2

ELSEVIER

1600 John F. Kennedy Boulevard ● Suite 1800 ● Philadelphia, Pennsylvania, 19103-2899

http://www.theclinics.com

CLINICS IN PLASTIC SURGERY Volume 50, Number 2
April 2023 ISSN 0094-1298, ISBN-13: 978-0-323-93971-3

Editor: Stacy Eastman
Developmental Editor: Jessica Nicole B. Cañaberal

Clinics in Plastic Surgery (ISSN 0094-1298) is published quarterly by Elsevier Inc., 360 Park Avenue South, New York, NY 10010-1710. Months of issue are January, April, July, and October. Business and Editorial Offices: 1600 John F. Kennedy Blvd., Suite 1800, Philadelphia, PA 19103-2899. Periodicals postage paid at New York, NY and additional mailing offices. Subscription prices are $559.00 per year for US individuals, $1024.00 per year for US institutions, $100.00 per year for US students and residents, $625.00 per year for Canadian individuals, $1218.00 per year for Canadian institutions, $696.00 per year for international individuals, $1218.00 per year for international institutions, $100.00 per year for Canadian Students and $305.00 per year for international students/residents. To receive student/resident rate, orders must be accompanied by name of affiliated institution, date of term, and the *signature* of program/residency coordinator on institution letterhead. Orders will be billed at individual rate until proof of status is received. Foreign air speed delivery is included in all *Clinics* subscription prices. All prices are subject to change without notice. **POSTMASTER:** Send address changes to *Clinics in Plastic Surgery*, Elsevier Health Sciences Division, Subscription Customer Service, 3251 Riverport Lane, Maryland Heights, MO 63043. **Customer Service: 1-800-654-2452 (US and Canada). From outside of the United States and Canada, call 314-447-8871. Fax: 314-447-8029. E-mail: JournalsCustomerService-usa@elsevier.com (for print support); JournalsOnlineSupport-usa@elsevier.com (for online support).**

Reprints. For copies of 100 or more of articles in this publication, please contact the Commercial Reprints Department, Elsevier Inc., 360 Park Avenue South, New York, New York 10010-1710. Tel.: +1-212-633-3874; Fax: +1-212-633-3820; E-mail: reprints@elsevier.com.

Clinics in Plastic Surgery is covered in *Current Contents, EMBASE/Excerpta Medica, Science Citation Index, MEDLINE/PubMed (Index Medicus), ASCA,* and *ISI/BIOMED*.

Contributors

EDITOR

NEIL TANNA, MD, MBA, FACS
Professor of Plastic Surgery, Donald and Barbara Zucker School of Medicine at Hofstra/ Northwell, Vice President of Women's Surgical Services, Northwell Health, Great Neck, New York

AUTHORS

SALMA A. ABDOU, MD
Department of Plastic Surgery, MedStar Plastic and Reconstructive Surgery, Washington, DC

ROBERT ALLEN, MD
Clinical Professor of Plastic Surgery, Plastic and Reconstructive Surgery, Department of Surgery, Louisiana State University, New Orleans, Louisiana

ROBERT J. ALLEN Jr, MD
Plastic and Reconstructive Surgery Service, Memorial Sloan Kettering Cancer Center, New York, New York

SAÏD C. AZOURY, MD
Plastic and Reconstructive Surgery Service, Memorial Sloan Kettering Cancer Center, New York, New York

SARAH L. BARNETT, BA
Division of Plastic and Reconstructive Surgery, Northwell Health, Great Neck, New York

JORDAN T. BLOUGH, MD
Division of Plastic and Reconstructive Surgery, Department of Surgery, Baylor Scott and White Health, Texas A&M College of Medicine, Temple, Texas

MICHAEL BORRERO, MD
Resident, Plastic and Reconstructive Surgery, Department of Surgery, Louisiana State University, New Orleans, Louisiana

KARINA CHARIPOVA, MD
Department of Plastic Surgery, MedStar Plastic and Reconstructive Surgery, Washington, DC

MINAS T. CHRYSOPOULO, MD
PRMA Plastic Surgery, San Antonio, Texas

MARK W. CLEMENS, MD, MBA, FACS
Department of Plastic Surgery, The University of Texas MD Anderson Cancer Center, Houston, Texas

ZACK COHEN, MD
Plastic and Reconstructive Surgery Service, Memorial Sloan Kettering Cancer Center, New York, New York

KATIE G. EGAN, MD
Microvascular Reconstructive Surgery Fellow, Clinical Specialist, The University of Texas MD Anderson Cancer Center, Houston, Texas

HEATHER R. FAULKNER, MD, MPH
Emory Division of Plastic and Reconstructive Surgery, Atlanta, Georgia

MEGAN E. FRACOL, MD
Department of Plastic Surgery, The University of Texas MD Anderson Cancer Center, Houston, Texas

FRANCIS D. GRAZIANO, MD
Division of Plastic and Reconstructive Surgery, Department of Surgery, Icahn School of Medicine at Mount Sinai, New York, New York

DAVID T. GREENSPUN, MD, MSc, FACS
Diplomate, American Board of Plastic Surgery;
Plastic, Reconstructive and Microvascular
Surgery, Greenwich, Connecticut

NICHOLAS T. HADDOCK, MD
Associate Professor, Vice Chair Business
Affairs, Department of Plastic Surgery,
University of Texas Southwestern, Dallas,
Texas

HUGO ST. HILAIRE, MD
Division Chairman, Plastic and Reconstructive
Surgery, Department of Surgery, Louisiana
State University, New Orleans, Louisiana

JORDAN M.S. JACOBS, MD
Assistant Professor of Surgery, Icahn School of
Medicine at Mount Sinai, Mount Sinai Hospital,
New York, New York

NOLAN S. KARP, MD
Hansjörg Wyss Department of Plastic Surgery,
NYU Langone Health, New York, New York

ALBERT LOSKEN, MD
Emory Division of Plastic and Reconstructive
Surgery, Atlanta, Georgia

JOCELYN LU, MD
Division of Plastic and Reconstructive Surgery,
Department of Surgery, Icahn School of
Medicine at Mount Sinai, New York, New York

EVAN MATROS, MD, MMSc
Plastic and Reconstructive Surgery Service,
Memorial Sloan Kettering Cancer Center, New
York, New York

JONAS A. NELSON, MD, MPH
Plastic and Reconstructive Surgery Service,
Memorial Sloan Kettering Cancer Center, New
York, New York

REBECCA C. O'NEILL, MD
Division of Plastic and Reconstructive Surgery,
Baylor College of Medicine, Houston, Texas

OSCAR OCHOA, MD
PRMA Plastic Surgery, San Antonio, Texas

EMMA L. ROBINSON, BS
Division of Plastic and Reconstructive Surgery,
Donald and Barbara Zucker School of
Medicine at Hofstra/Northwell, Hempstead,
New York

MEGAN M. RODRIGUEZ, BS
Department of Plastic Surgery, The University
of Texas MD Anderson Cancer Center,
Houston School of Medicine, Houston, Texas

MICHEL H. SAINT-CYR, MD, MBA, FRCSC
Plastic and Reconstructive Surgery, Banner
MD Anderson Cancer Center, Gilbert, Arizona

ARA A. SALIBIAN, MD
Division of Plastic and Reconstructive Surgery,
University of California, Davis, Sacramento,
California

CHARLES ANDREW SALZBERG, MD
Professor of Surgery, Cleveland Clinic Florida,
Vero Beach, Florida

HANI SBITANY, MD
Chief, Division of Plastic and Reconstructive
Surgery, Professor, Department of Surgery,
Icahn School of Medicine at Mount Sinai, New
York, New York

JESSE C. SELBER, MD, MPH, MHCM, FACS
Professor, Vice Chair Department of Plastic
Surgery, The University of Texas MD Anderson
Cancer Center, Houston, Texas

MARK L. SMITH, MD, FACS
Division of Plastic and Reconstructive Surgery,
Northwell Health, Great Neck, New York;
Division of Plastic and Reconstructive Surgery,
Donald and Barbara Zucker School of
Medicine at Hofstra/Northwell, Hempstead,
New York

DAVID H. SONG, MD, MBA, FACS
Department of Plastic Surgery, MedStar Plastic
and Reconstructive Surgery, Washington, DC

ALDONA J. SPIEGEL, MD
Institute for Reconstructive Surgery, Houston
Methodist Hospital, Houston, Texas

SNEHA SUBRAMANIAM, MD
Surgical Resident, Northwell Health,
Department of Surgery, Northwell Health, New
York, New York

STEVEN M. SULTAN, MD
Assistant Professor of Surgery, Mount Sinai
Hospital, New York, New York

NEIL TANNA, MD, MBA, FACS
Professor of Plastic Surgery, Donald and
Barbara Zucker School of Medicine at Hofstra/
Northwell, Vice President of Women's Surgical
Services, Northwell Health, Great Neck, New
York

SUMEET S. TEOTIA, MD
Professor, Department of Plastic Surgery,
University of Texas Southwestern, Dallas,
Texas

Contents

Through a multidisciplinary approach, as well as, a nuanced appreciation of patient goals and setting appropriate expectations, breast reconstruction can significantly improve the quality of life following mastectomy. A thorough review of the patient medical and surgical history in addition to oncologic treatments will facilitate discussion and recommendations for an individualized shared decision-making reconstructive process. Alloplastic reconstruction, although a highly popular modality, has important limitations. On the contrary, autologous reconstruction is more flexible but requires more thorough consideration.

Partial breast reconstruction using oncoplastic techniques is performed at the time of lumpectomy and includes volume replacement techniques such as flaps and volume displacement techniques such as reduction and mastopexy. These techniques are used to preserve breast shape, contour, size, symmetry, inframammary fold position, and position of the nipple-areolar complex. Newer techniques such as auto-augmentation flaps and perforator flaps continue to broaden options and newer radiation therapy protocols will hopefully reduce side effects. Options for the oncoplastic approach now include higher risk patients as there is a larger repository of data on the safety and efficacy of this technique.

The modern approach to implant-based breast reconstruction encompasses an evolution in surgical techniques, patient selection, implant technology, and use of support materials. Successful outcomes are defined by teamwork throughout the ablative and reconstructive processes as well as appropriate and evidence-based utilization of modern material technologies. Patient education, focus on patient-reported outcomes, and informed and shared decision-making are the key to all steps of these procedures.

Prepectoral breast reconstruction has gained popularity due to numerous benefits in properly selected patients. Compared with subpectoral implant reconstruction, prepectoral reconstruction offers preservation of the pectoralis major muscle in its native position, resulting in decreased pain, no animation deformity, and improved arm range of motion/strength. Although prepectoral reconstruction is safe and effective, the implant sits closer to the mastectomy skin flap. Acellular dermal matrices play a critical role, allowing for precise control of the breast envelope and providing long-term implant support. Careful patient selection and intraoperative mastectomy flap evaluation are critical to obtaining optimal results with prepectoral breast reconstruction.

Implant-based breast reconstruction remains the most commonly performed type of restorative surgery after mastectomy for breast cancer. Placement of a tissue expander at the time of mastectomy allows gradual skin envelope expansion but requires additional surgery and time to completion of a patient's reconstruction. Direct-to-implant reconstruction provides a one-stage, final implant insertion, thereby bypassing the need for serial tissue expansion. With proper patient selection, successful preservation of the breast skin envelope, and accurate implant size and placement, direct-to-implant reconstruction has a very high rate of success and patient satisfaction.

Breast implant associated anaplastic large cell lymphoma (BIA-ALCL) is an uncommon and emerging malignancy caused by textured breast implants. The most common patient presentation is delayed seromas, other presentations include breast asymmetry, overlying skin rashes, palpable masses, lymphadenopathy, and capsular contracture. Confirmed diagnoses should receive lymphoma oncology consultation, multidisciplinary evaluation, and PET-CT or CT scan evaluation prior to surgical treatment. Disease confined to the capsule is curable in the majority of patients with complete surgical resection. BIA-ALCL is now recognized as one disease among a spectrum of inflammatory mediated malignancies which include implant-associated squamous cell carcinoma and B cell lymphoma.

The latissimus dorsi flap with immediate fat transfer is a viable option for fully autologous breast reconstruction in patients who are not candidates for free flap reconstruction. Technical modifications described in this article allow for high-volume and efficient fat grafting at the time of reconstruction to augment the flap and mitigate complications associated with the use of an implant.

Modern approaches to abdominal-based breast reconstruction have evolved since the introduction of the transverse musculocutaneous flap by Dr Carl Hartrampf in the 1980s. The natural evolution of this flap is the deep inferior epigastric perforator (DIEP) flap, as well as the superficial inferior epigastric artery flap. As breast reconstruction has advanced, so too has the utility and nuances of abdominal-based flaps, including the deep circumflex iliac artery flap, extended flaps, stacked flaps; neurotization; and perforator exchange techniques. Even the delay phenomenon has been successfully applied to DIEP and SIEA flaps to augment flap perfusion.

The deep inferior epigastric perforator flap has become one of the most popular approaches for autologous breast reconstruction after mastectomy. As much of health care has moved to a value-based approach, reducing complications, operative time, and length of stay in deep inferior flap reconstruction is becoming increasingly important. In this article, we discuss important preoperative, intraoperative, and postoperative considerations to maximize efficiency when performing autologous breast reconstruction and offer tips on how to handle certain challenges.

 Video content accompanies this article at http://www.plasticsurgery.theclinics.com.

Autologous free flap breast reconstruction allows for natural-appearing breasts, while avoiding the risks associated with implants, including exposure, rupture, and capsular contracture. However, this is offset by a much higher technical challenge. The abdomen remains the most common tissue source for autologous breast reconstruction. However, in patients with scant abdominal tissue, prior abdominal surgery, or a desire to avoid scarring in this region, thigh-based flaps remain a viable alternative. The profunda artery perforator (PAP) flap has emerged as a preferred alternative tissue source, due to excellent esthetic outcomes and low donor-site morbidity.

The lumbar artery perforator (LAP) flap should be considered for autologous breast reconstruction when a patient's abdomen is unavailable as a donor site. The LAP flap can be harvested with dimensions and volume of distribution that facilitate the restoration of a naturally shaped breast with a sloping upper pole and maximal projection in the lower one-third. Harvest of LAP flaps lifts the buttocks and narrows the waist and, consequently, aesthetic improvement in body contour is generally achieved with these procedures. Although technically challenging, the LAP flap is a valuable tool in the practice of autologous breast reconstruction.

The transverse upper/myocutaneous gracilis is a medial thigh-based flap primarily reserved as a secondary choice for autologous reconstruction of small to moderate-sized breasts in women without a suitable abdominal donor site. Its consistent and reliable anatomy based on the medial circumflex femoral artery permits expedient flap harvest with relatively low donor site morbidity. The primary disadvantage is the limited achievable volume, often necessitating augmentation such as extended flap modifications, autologous fat grafting, flap stacking, or even implant placement.

Total breast reconstruction following mastectomy requires multiple components to achieve an aesthetic result. In some situations, significant skin is required to provide the needed surface area to allow breast projection and breast ptosis. Additionally, ample volume is required to reconstruct all breast quadrants and provide sufficient projection. All aspects of the breast base must be filled to achieve total breast reconstruction. In very specific circumstances, multiple flaps are employed to accomplish this level of uncompromised aesthetic breast reconstruction. The abdomen, thigh, lumbar region, and buttock can all be used in some combination, as needed, to perform both unilateral and bilateral breast reconstruction. The ultimate goal is to provide superior aesthetic results in both the recipient breast and the donor site while maintaining a very low level of long-term morbidity.

There are numerous indications for hybrid breast reconstruction, with the most common being patients who have inadequate donor site volume to achieve the desired breast volume. This article reviews all aspects of hybrid breast reconstruction, including preoperative and assessment, operative technique and considerations, and postoperative management.

Absent or diminished breast sensation is a persistent problem for many postmastectomy patients. Breast neurotization is an opportunity to improve sensory outcomes, which are poor and unpredictable if left to chance. Several techniques for autologous and implant reconstruction have been described with successful clinical and patient-reported outcomes. Neurotization is a safe procedure with minimal risk for morbidity and it presents a fantastic avenue for future research.

Robotic surgery has a history of applications in multiple surgical areas and has been applied in plastic surgery over the past decade. Robotic surgery allows for minimal access incisions and decreased donor site morbidity in breast extirpative surgery, breast reconstruction, and lymphedema surgery. Although a learning curve exists for the use of this technology, it can be safely applied with careful preoperative planning. Robotic nipple-sparing mastectomy may be combined with either robotic alloplastic or robotic autologous reconstruction in the appropriate patient.

CLINICS IN PLASTIC SURGERY

SERIES OF RELATED INTEREST

Facial Plastic Surgery Clinics
https://www.facialplastic.theclinics.com/
Otolaryngologic Clinics
https://www.oto.theclinics.com/

THE CLINICS ARE AVAILABLE ONLINE!
Access your subscription at:
www.theclinics.com

Preface

Contemporary Breast Reconstruction: Optimizing Aesthetics, Efficiency, and Outcomes

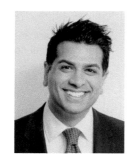

Neil Tanna, MD, MBA, FACS
Editor

Breast reconstruction has evolved significantly in the past generation. Historically, postmastectomy breast reconstruction was largely limited to subpectoral two-staged prosthetic reconstruction and autologous abdominal flap-based reconstruction. Today, the armamentarium of breast reconstruction methods is enhanced with options such as direct-to-implant reconstruction, prepectoral implant reconstruction, alternative flap reconstruction, hybrid breast reconstruction, and breast neurotization, to name a few.

With limited breast reconstruction options in the past, patients and surgeons were restricted in their choice of procedure. As such, patients were previously managed with a cookie-cutter approach, rather than surgical plans uniquely tailored to individuals. With advancements in the field, an individualized approach can now be performed to best complement breast anatomy, body habitus, and patient preference. Furthermore, surgical techniques can be executed to optimize aesthetic, satisfaction, efficiency, and safety outcomes.

The strength of this issue of *Clinics in Plastic Surgery* is in the collective surgical talent of the contributing authors. These experts in breast reconstruction have collaborated to put forth the latest options and techniques of reconstructive breast surgery. Each author, a subspecialist in their assigned topic, discusses their specific approach with a background of the full spectrum of current surgical options. These experts couple anecdotal experience with scientific evidence to justify their approaches.

The issue begins with an overview of the assessment and evaluation of a breast reconstruction patient. For patients with partial mastectomy defects, oncoplastic surgical approaches are offered. This is followed by a series of articles

Clin Plastic Surg 50 (2023) xiii–xiv
https://doi.org/10.1016/j.cps.2022.12.016
0094-1298/23/© 2022 Published by Elsevier Inc.

plasticsurgery.theclinics.com

on modern-day considerations in implant-based breast reconstruction. The full gamut of microsurgical breast reconstruction options is provided, including the deep inferior epigastric artery perforator (DIEP) flap, profunda artery perforator (PAP) flap, transverse upper gracilis (TUG) flap, lumbar artery perforator (LAP) flap, and stacked flaps. Finally, innovations in reconstructive breast surgery, including hybrid reconstruction, breast neurotization, and robotic breast surgery, are presented.

It is our humble belief that this issue will serve as an everyday reference to practicing surgeons, helping them deliver the highest-quality breast reconstruction to women. In the same spirit, we are hopeful that what follows will also inspire passion, ingenuity, and innovation in breast reconstruction.

Neil Tanna, MD, MBA, FACS
Zucker School of Medicine at Hofstra/Northwell
Northwell Health
600 Northern Boulevard
Suite 310
Great Neck, NY 11021, USA

E-mail address:
ntanna@gmail.com

Preoperative Assessment of the Breast Reconstruction Patient

Oscar Ochoa, MD*, Minas T. Chrysopoulo, MD

KEYWORDS

- Preoperative assessment • Breast reconstruction • Autologous reconstruction
- Implant reconstruction • Adjuvant therapy • Shared decision-making

KEY POINTS

- Breast reconstruction must be performed in a multidisciplinary environment.
- Optimal patient satisfaction is achieved by aligning patient goals and expectations with likely outcomes given present risk factors.
- Thorough patient assessment will facilitate individualized counseling and selection of appropriate reconstructive options using a shared decision-making approach.

BACKGROUND

It is estimated that more than 300,000 women are diagnosed with breast cancer in the United States every year.[1] Risk factors associated with the development of breast cancer are both environmental and hereditable with an estimated 5% to 10% of all breast cancers attributed to germline mutations in breast cancer-associated genes such as BRCA.[2] A breast cancer diagnosis can be not only life-altering but also has profound and long-lasting emotional sequela.[3] In addition, for patients who forego or are not candidates for breast conservation therapy (BCT), mastectomy may represent a daunting challenge to their feminine self-image and psychosocial well-being.[4–8] On the contrary, breast reconstruction has been associated with improved quality of life following mastectomy in both the immediate and delayed setting.[9–13]

When breast reconstruction is considered, it must be approached in a thoughtful and deliberate manner. Fundamentally, to optimize therapeutic outcomes, from an oncologic and reconstructive standpoint, a multidisciplinary approach with effective collaboration is paramount.[11,14] Medical, surgical, and radiation oncologists, as well as reconstructive surgeons, anesthesiologists, diagnostic radiologists, and physical therapists form the essential components of a well-staffed breast cancer care team. Although outcomes germane to health-related metrics such as overall and disease-free survival must be rigorously pursued and maximized, quality-of-life measures play an equally valuable role in a comprehensive therapeutic framework. Facilitated by widely accepted and used patient-reported outcome measures such as the BREAST-Q,[15,16] the reconstructive surgeon is uniquely positioned to guide patients through a shared decision-making process[17] for selecting the optimal reconstructive modality founded on evidence-based patient satisfaction and quality of life.

To properly counsel a patient through an individualized reconstructive algorithm, not only is an accurate assessment of their previous and/or anticipated oncologic treatments critical, but also an understanding of the patient's preferences, values, and reconstructive goals. Based on this information, a more productive and educated discussion can take place in an effort to identify the reconstructive modality that most

PRMA Plastic Surgery, 9635 Huebner Road, San Antonio, TX 78240, USA
* Corresponding author.
E-mail address: dr.ochoa@prmaplasticsurgery.com

Clin Plastic Surg 50 (2023) 201–210
https://doi.org/10.1016/j.cps.2022.10.002

safely and effectively achieves these goals. For example, a woman with early-stage breast cancer and an active, supportive family, and a strong desire to minimize the possibility of repeated surgeries throughout her survivorship period would be guided toward autologous reconstruction. Alternatively, a busy professional with a thin body habitus and a history of augmentation mammoplasty may be better suited for alloplastic reconstruction.

Although patient satisfaction is closely associated with surgical outcomes,[18–21] setting appropriate expectations is key to properly frame the patient's perspective throughout their reconstructive experience. In addition, aligning expectations between the patient and potential immediate and long-term reconstructive outcomes will promote the maintenance of productive communication between the patient and reconstructive team, especially if complications arise along the reconstructive journey. With a more thorough and granular mutual understanding of expectations following breast reconstruction, patient satisfaction and perception of outcomes are maximized.

Shared Decision-Making

Shared decision-making occurs when the health care professional and patient work *together* to make a health care decision that is best for the patient. The optimal decision takes into account evidence-based information about the available treatment options, the provider's knowledge and experience, and patient factors including their values and preferences.

The "information exchange"[22] that occurs between the patient and physician is very different to the paternalistic approach traditionally witnessed during surgical training. The "Informative" approach to decision-making provides the patient with comprehensive information, but, unlike shared decision-making, does not consider the patient's values or preferences (**Fig. 1**). Shared decision-making also incorporates the biological, sociologic, and psychological factors the patient brings to the table.

Access to the health information on the Internet and via social media is changing the patient's role in health care. Patients are increasingly advocating for themselves and seeking to become more involved in their health care decisions, and to some extent even experts in their own care. Less than half of patients undergoing mastectomy make a high-quality breast reconstruction decision based on their self-reported desires.[23] "High quality" is defined as "having knowledge of at least 50% of the important facts and undergoing

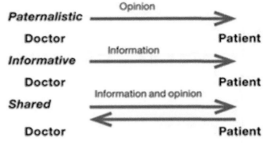

Fig. 1. Types of decision-making. (*From* Dinwoodie M. Consent and shared decision making. 2014. Accessed June 1, 2022. https://www.medicalprotection.org/newzealand/casebook/casebook-january-2014/consent-and-shared-decision-making.)

treatment concordant with one's personal preferences."

Studies across several medical and surgical specialties show shared decision-making offers several benefits:

- Improves patient education
- Decreases patient anxiety
- Decreases decisional conflict
- Helps set appropriate patient expectations
- Improves patient buy-in and satisfaction
- Improves patient outcomes

In addition to being a very effective and ethical approach to patient interaction and treatment planning, shared decision-making also facilitates the delivery of high-quality, patient-centered care. Improving patient outcomes and satisfaction can also create extremely positive secondary effects on the surgeon's practice from a marketing perspective. Happy patients can be very effective advocates for a specific procedure and the whole practice.

The SHARE approach (**Fig. 2**) breaks down shared decision-making into a simple five-step process[24]: Patient-focused, evidence-based decision aids (eg, Breast Advocate® App) can greatly facilitate the shared decision-making process and provide the opportunity for patients to research their options at their own pace, including before the initial consultation. This arms the patient with comprehensive baseline knowledge and allows for more of the consultation time to be allocated toward addressing specific concerns and customizing the treatment plan, rather than reviewing basic information. Digital aids also allow patients to review relevant information repeatedly outside of the clinic setting.

Decision aids improve decision-related outcomes for many breast cancer treatment decisions including surgery, radiotherapy, endocrine

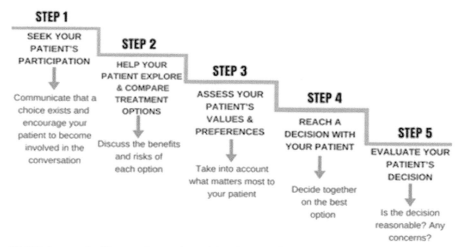

STEP 1

SEEK YOUR PATIENT'S PARTICIPATION

↓

Communicate that a choice exists and encourage your patient to become involved in the conversation

STEP 2

HELP YOUR PATIENT EXPLORE & COMPARE TREATMENT OPTIONS

↓

Discuss the benefits and risks of each option

STEP 3

ASSESS YOUR PATIENT'S VALUES & PREFERENCES

↓

Take into account what matters most to your patient

STEP 4

REACH A DECISION WITH YOUR PATIENT

↓

Decide together on the best option

STEP 5

EVALUATE YOUR PATIENT'S DECISION

↓

Is the decision reasonable? Any concerns?

Fig. 2. The SHARE Approach. (Content last reviewed October 2020). Agency for Healthcare Research and Quality, Rockville, MD. https://www.ahrq.gov/health-literacy/professional-training/shared-decision/index.htm.

therapy, and chemotherapy.[25] Specifically for women considering breast reconstruction, decisional aids also improve patient satisfaction with information and perceived involvement in the decision-making process, and reduce patient-reported decisional conflict.[26]

Patient Preoperative Assessment

General health and medical conditions

A thorough preoperative assessment should begin with an evaluation of the patient's general health and medical conditions. In our practice and supported by previous data,[27,28] breast reconstruction is offered to patients regardless of chronologic age. Although there is no consensus on best practices to assess health fitness or frailty in more senior populations, scoring tools have been developed and are best used in collaboration with a proper anesthesia assessment.[28] Presence of cardiac comorbidities and diabetes should be determined, severity assessed, and optimized through appropriate referrals. Women with diabetes are more likely to experience higher overall complications, surgical complications, and a prolonged hospital stay following breast reconstruction.[29] In our practice, based on previous studies,[30] a hemoglobin A1C of 7% represents the upper acceptable limit for patients to undergo any breast reconstruction procedure. History of deep venous thrombosis, pulmonary embolism, spontaneous abortions/miscarriages, or familial bleeding tendencies warrants referral for coagulopathy evaluation. If present, free flap breast reconstruction should be strongly reconsidered[31] and only performed if the patient truly understands and accepts the increased risk of flap loss. In the

presence of coagulopathy, in collaboration with Hematology consultants, an anticoagulation protocol beyond standard peri-operative prophylaxis should be incorporated to mitigate the thrombotic risk. History of or symptoms consistent with autoimmune connective tissue disease should be determined. Although the association between silicone breast implants and connective tissue disease has been unfounded by large-scale clinical studies, debate is ongoing regarding the possible development of a broader symptom complex referred to as "breast implant illness."[32,33] Although patients with connective tissue disease may be better served with autologous reconstruction, increased risk of wound and pulmonary complications, as well as, venous thromboembolism have been reported.[34]

Active tobacco use should be assessed and immediate cessation encouraged. In our practice, tobacco abstinence of at least 6 weeks is required before any form of breast reconstruction is undertaken, as previous studies have reported a clear association between tobacco use and operative complications.[35,36] Body habitus should be assessed and stratification of surgical risk communicated to patients clearly.[36] Based on previous studies, there is a linear correlation of surgical morbidity to increasing body mass index (BMI).[36] In light of this, in our practice, a BMI of 40 is the absolute upper acceptable limit for candidacy for all breast reconstruction, including deep inferior epigastric perforator (DIEP) flaps. Nevertheless, all patients are encouraged to make appropriate diet and life-style changes to minimize their surgical risk based on body habitus.

Multidisciplinary Oncologic Considerations

Accurate assessment of the patient's tumor and nodal status is critical in determining, not only potentially appropriate reconstructive modalities, but possibly also the sequence of reconstructive procedures. Close communication with other members of the multi-disciplinary team is critical at this point to ensure a thorough diagnostic workup that enables proper patient assessment from a reconstructive perspective. For example, percutaneous axillary lymph node biopsy should be advocated for patients with questionable lymph node enlargement on diagnostic imaging to more accurately determine the existence of nodal metastasis neoadjuvantly which would influence recommendations for postmastectomy radiation (PMRT) using current national comprehensive cancer network (NCCN) guidelines.[37] Although some centers have reported excellent outcomes following PMRT in the setting of immediate autologous reconstruction,[38] for patients with inflammatory, locally advanced (T3) cancers, and/or metastatic nodal disease at the time of diagnosis, delayed reconstruction following PMRT is routinely advised.

Skin/nipple-sparing mastectomy promotes optimal cosmetic outcomes due to the preservation of the native skin envelope.[39] As such, tumor location plays a critical role in determining the possible location of mastectomy incisions as well as candidacy for nipple preservation.[37] Strategic planning of mastectomy incision location will ensure optimal cosmetic outcome (and nipple neurovascular function,[40] if applicable) while providing the breast surgeon with adequate exposure for glandular resection. In addition, adequate exposure will facilitate visualization of the glandular-subcutaneous plane promoting appropriate and uniform mastectomy flap thickness.

Prior history of partial mastectomy (lumpectomy) as a component of BCT needs to be determined. The location of a prior lumpectomy incision will also determine the most appropriate completion mastectomy incision to be used to mitigate perfusion disturbances to the residual mastectomy flaps. If immediate free flap reconstruction is undertaken with internal mammary vessel exposure in the setting of previous BCT, due to observed disruption of normal breast lymphatic drainage to the axilla, internal mammary lymph node biopsy should be performed to more comprehensively assess surgical staging.[41–43]

As an integral component of systemic oncologic treatment, cytotoxic chemotherapy may be administered before or after surgical extirpation with similar oncologic outcomes. If chemotherapy is administered neoadjuvantly, mastectomy and immediate breast reconstruction can be performed safely[44] and is recommended within 4 to 6 weeks of chemotherapy completion, barring prolonged hematologic suppression, to prevent decreased overall, and possibly, disease-free survival.[45–48] If need for adjuvant chemotherapy is anticipated, due to its myelosuppressive effects, probability of surgical complications such as infection and delayed wound healing should be considered. Although episodes of infection or delayed wound healing in the setting of autologous reconstruction are undesirable, most can be managed conservatively without need for delays in adjuvant treatments. On the contrary, in alloplastic reconstruction, adjuvant chemotherapy has been associated with unplanned surgical intervention in approximately 30% of cases with reconstructive failure as high as 22% in the form of implant/tissue expander loss.[49,50]

As approximately 25% of women diagnosed with breast cancer possess the HER-2 + subtype,[51] HER-2-directed monoclonal antibody therapy, as a relatively recent advancement in systemic adjuvant treatment, may also impact the timing of reconstruction. HER-2 + patients with breast cancer are unique in their continued need for targeted antineoplastic therapy after conventional cytotoxic chemotherapy has been completed. Typically, these patients received HER-2 directed therapy for up to 12 months.[52] Although increases in breast reconstruction complications have not been associated with ongoing use of Trastuzumab (Herceptin, Genentech Inc.) alone, increased risk of wound breakdown and infection has been reported with concurrent use of Pertuzumab (Perjeta, Genentech Inc.).[52] As newer therapies become more common in clinical use combining HER-2-directed immunotherapy with cytotoxic agents, such as TDM-1 (Kadcyla, Genentech Inc.), close communication with medical oncology is critical to adequately assess potential reconstructive risk.

Similar to HER-2-directed therapy, adjuvant hormonal therapy is prolonged and typically overlaps with reconstructive procedures. Owing to the increased risk of venous thromboembolism and reported microvascular flap complications,[53] estrogen receptor antagonists (ie, Tamoxifen) should be withheld for 2 weeks before and after surgery if free flap reconstruction is undertaken. On the contrary, aromatase inhibitors can be safely continued peri-operatively during reconstruction.[54]

History of or anticipated need for adjuvant radiation plays a critical role in determining reconstructive options. Radiation exposure produces fibrosis, elastosis, and vascular intimal thickening impacting reconstructive outcomes. Certainly, in patients with loss of the skin envelope from the previous mastectomy without reconstruction and PMRT, re-establishing an adequate skin envelope via tissue expansion is fraught with limitations. In such cases, previous studies have reported 50% overall complication rates with tissue expander or implant loss in 40% of patients.[55] Further underscoring the prolonged effects of radiation, patients requiring salvage/completion mastectomy due to local recurrence or newly diagnosed genetic predisposition for breast cancer in the setting of the previous BCT, alloplastic reconstruction overall complications are only slightly better, ranging between 35% and 70% with 13% reconstructive failure.[55,56] On the contrary, replacement of the absent skin envelope and breast mound with autologous tissue in patients with a previous history of radiation is a more viable and durable option.[57,58] There is currently no consensus as to the optimal timing of free flap reconstruction after radiation.[59,60] In our practice, free flap reconstruction has been safely undertaken any time after resolution of the acute phase of radiation injury,[61] generally coinciding with 3 months following completion of radiation.

In cases where the need for PMRT is preemptively known, the traditional and most evidence-based safe approach has been to offer reconstruction in a delayed fashion. Although patients undergoing delayed reconstruction may suffer from temporary loss of an integral component of perceived femininity, recent patient-reported outcome studies supporting this approach have shown the similar health-related quality of life and satisfaction between delayed and immediate reconstruction patients once autologous reconstruction is ultimately completed.[13] Nevertheless, a shifting emphasis toward offering immediate reconstruction despite a known need for PMRT is evolving. Contrary to traditional standards, in a recent series from 2000 to 2010, immediate implant reconstruction with PMRT increased from 27% to 52%[62] despite well-documented high complication rates.[63,64] Alternatively, with state-of-the-art radiation regimens, recent studies have reported acceptable outcomes after immediate autologous reconstruction followed by PMRT.[38,65,66] Certainly, close collaboration with radiation oncology is imperative in this setting, especially if PMRT is necessary soon after reconstruction (<3 months) or directed at the internal mammary nodal chain.[67]

Although initially conceived as a method to offer immediate reconstruction for patients where the need for PMRT was unknown, a delayed-immediate approach[68] where the immediate placement of a tissue expander followed by PMRT is ultimately converted to autologous reconstruction may be an attractive option for some patients. This approach maintains the skin envelope while eliminating the long-term potential for implant malposition and capsular contracture associated with alloplastic reconstruction and may reverse radiation-induced changes to the skin envelope and chest wall through a well-vascularized autologous flap.[69]

Alloplastic Reconstruction

Implant-based reconstructive techniques are a highly popular method of breast reconstruction[70] due to multiple factors including technical simplicity, short convalescence, and elimination of donor sites. In addition, the development and availability of biologic and prosthetic scaffolds as adjuncts to implant-based reconstruction have facilitated improved cosmetic outcomes[71] with decreased pain while potentially mitigating capsular contracture.[72] Proper patient selection is imperative in alloplastic reconstruction with recognition of systemic risk factors such as high BMI, poorly controlled diabetes mellitus, and active tobacco use as mentioned previously. Ideal candidates are women with a paucity of available autologous tissue undergoing immediate reconstruction with small to moderate-size breasts with good skin quality following bilateral mastectomies without the need for PMRT. Breast dimensions especially breast diameter, breast height, and inframammary fold (IMF)-nipple distance are used to determine optimal tissue expander/implant sizes. Preoperative asymmetry in breast size, shape, footprint, IMF, and nipple position are critically important to assess and document with open patient discussion regarding limitations of cosmetic outcomes based on present asymmetries. Correction of nipple malposition following nipple-sparing mastectomy and implant reconstruction may be challenging but feasible with acceptable outcomes.[73,74]

The decision of whether to perform subpectoral versus prepectoral implant reconstruction may be influenced by individual patient characteristics. In patients who engage their pectoralis muscles frequently through vigorous exercise or occupation, prepectoral tissue expander/implant placement should be strongly considered to eliminate distressing animation deformities and muscle spasms seen with subpectoral implant position. However, if skin quality or anticipated mastectomy flap thickness is suboptimal or irregular, a subpectoral plane may mitigate, to some degree, contour irregularities. In addition, in the subpectoral plane, an underlying implant is better protected, minimizing exposure risk if wound dehiscence occurs at the mastectomy incision due to poor perfusion. If mastectomy flap perfusion is significantly compromised, avoiding implant placement altogether is strongly advised. A preoperative discussion with the patient in preparation of this possibility is highly critical to avoid patient-developed resentment due to an unanticipated setback. Delayed placement of a tissue expander or implant may be subsequently undertaken once mastectomy flap perfusion is reestablished through delayed conditioning.

Oncologically, if close proximity or involvement of the pectoralis is suspected preoperatively, prepectoral implant placement should be avoided so as to not obscure surveillance physical examinations or imaging over a high-risk area.[75] If the possibility of PMRT has not been eliminated and implant reconstruction is undertaken definitively, pre-pectoral tissue expander/implant placement has shown promising results in the setting of post-reconstruction radiation[76] with the theoretic advantage of eliminating implant displacement due to pectoralis contracture.

Single-stage direct-to-implant (DTI) reconstruction has evolved into a viable alternative to a traditional two-stage (tissue expander followed by a permanent implant) approach. Facilitated by the use of acellular dermal matrices, DTI reconstruction may be performed in either the subpectoral or prepectoral plane. If DTI reconstruction is being considered, the mastectomy surgeon must reliably deliver well-perfused mastectomy flaps of consistent thickness. Equally important, achieving a hand-in-glove relationship between the implant construct and overlying mastectomy flaps is essential for the optimal cosmetic outcome and elimination of dead space potentiating seroma formation and infection.[77] In patients where these two requirements are not certain, a traditional two-stage approach is preferential. Patients undergoing mastectomy with a history of subpectoral augmentation mammoplasty with a relatively small amount of breast parenchyma may be ideal candidates for DTI reconstruction in the subpectoral plane if no or only minor changes in net breast volume are desired.

Autologous Reconstruction

Autologous, especially abdominal-based, reconstruction is widely considered "the gold standard" providing a soft, warm, and enduring breast mound with high patient satisfaction. If selected at the conclusion of a shared decision-making process, breast-specific physical assessment is identical as previously mentioned for immediate reconstruction candidates. For patients undergoing delayed reconstruction, location of the mastectomy scar, quality of the residual mastectomy skin including possible radiation changes, presence of any skin lesions, chest wall, or axillary masses concerning cancer recurrence must be assessed. Although irregularities in skin quality are more readily obscured with an underlying autologous tissue flap compared with a prosthetic device, replacement of damaged or poor quality residual mastectomy skin with the cutaneous portion of the autologous flap should be considered. Similarly, underscoring the flexibility of an underlying autologous flap in relation to the native breast skin envelope optimizing cosmetic outcome, nipple-areolar complex ptosis can be reliably corrected following nipple-sparing mastectomy.[78]

The preferred donor site for autologous reconstruction is the infraumbilical abdomen due to the close resemblance of tissue consistency relative to the breast, the volume of harvestable soft-tissue, length and size of the pedicle vessels, subsequent improved abdominal contour, and low donor-site morbidity when performed as a perforator (DIEP) flap.[79] When evaluating the abdomen, skin quality, abdominal soft-tissue excess, and previous abdominal incisions are inspected in relation to the anticipated flap borders and volume needs. In patients with breast volume or skin needs beyond a hemiabdominal flap, stacked flaps must be considered.[80,81] Lower midline and/or Pfannenstiel incisions are commonly encountered in the typical breast cancer patient population and do not usually preclude successful flap harvest. Similarly, suction-assisted lipectomy is common in this patient population and is considered a relative contraindication for abdominal-based reconstruction. In our practice in general, preoperative abdominal CT angiogram is used selectively but required in patients with multiple open abdominal surgeries, a history of infraumbilical suction-assisted lipectomy, and/or laparoscopic bladder suspension or inguinal hernia repair. Although operative times have not been decreased in our practice and others[82] by the use of preoperative computer-assisted tomography angiogram (CTA), valuable anatomic data beyond presence and location of perforators can be assessed.[83] Certainly, MR angiogram is an acceptable alternative imaging modality for the assessment of relevant anatomic features. Presence of rectus diastasis, as well as incisional and umbilical hernias requires assessment and repair integrated into abdominal donor-site closure. The anticipated final location of the abdominal scar upon closure is reviewed with the patient to set appropriate expectations related to improvement in abdominal aesthetics.

In patients where abdominal soft-tissue is not sufficient or harvestable due to low BMI or a prohibitive surgical history such as previous abdominoplasty, respectively, alternative donor sites require assessment. Gluteal (gluteal artery perforator [GAP] flap), flank (lumbar artery perforator [LAP] flap), medial (transverse upper gracilis/ vertical upper gracilis [TUG/VUG] flap), posterior (profunda artery perforator [PAP] flap), and lateral (lateral thigh perforator [LTP] flap) thigh-based donor sites are selected based on location of relative soft-tissue excess, prior incisions, or suction-assisted lipectomy. Owing to the anatomic variability of vasculature in these alternative donor sites, preoperative CTA or MRA is necessary. In patients where thoracodorsal vessel-based reconstruction is being considered on the side of previous mastectomy with axillary lymph node sampling, not only is posterior trunk soft-tissue excess assessed but also latissimus function determined by voluntary contraction. If the latissimus does not contract on command, thoracodorsal nerve injury is suspected and patency to the thoracodorsal vessels requires assessment with CTA.

For patients undergoing free flap breast reconstruction, the internal mammary vessels are the preferred recipient vessels due to ease of exposure and optimal flap positioning. Although the right internal mammary vein is invariably of sufficient caliber for primary venous outflow, the left internal vein is significantly smaller[84] and may be unusable in up to 20% of cases,[85] especially if left-sided radiation has been delivered. Consideration for alternative venous outflow channels must take place preoperatively. The thoracodorsal vein is readily accessible within the same operative field; however, sacrifice eliminates the potential use of the latissimus as a backup flap if free flap failure occurs. Alternatively, the cephalic and external jugular veins are viable and reliable options if the internal mammary veins are inadequate.[86]

SUMMARY

Breast reconstruction plays a vital role in improving the quality of life following mastectomy. Through a multidisciplinary approach, optimal oncologic and reconstructive outcomes are promoted. A thorough review of the patient's preferences, reconstructive goals, medical and surgical history, as well as oncologic treatments will facilitate a shared decision-making process optimizing perceived outcomes. Both alloplastic and autologous reconstruction require thorough evaluation and consideration.

CLINICS CARE POINTS

- Breast reconstruction should take place in a multidisciplinary environment.
- Patient preferences and goals must be assessed and considered, and appropriate expectations established.
- Relevant medical and surgical history must be assessed.
- Previous or anticipated oncologic treatments must be considered.
- Implant-based reconstruction has meaningful benefits, but important limitations.
- Autologous reconstruction is considered the "gold standard" but requires thorough consideration.

DISCLOSURE

Dr M.T. Chrysopoulo is the founder of Toliman Health, creators of the Breast Advocate ® App.

REFERENCES

1. American Cancer Society. Breast cancer facts & figures 2017–2018. Available at: https://www.cancer.org/content/dam/cancer-org/research/cancer-facts-and-statistics/breast-cancer-facts-and-figures/breast-cancer-facts-and-figures-2017-2018.pdf. Accessed Oct 17,2019.
2. Wendt C, Margolin S. Identifying breast cancer susceptibility genes – a review of the genetic background in familial breast cancer. Acta Oncol 2019; 58(2):135.
3. Avis NE, Crawford S, Manuel J. Quality of life among younger women with breast cancer. J Clin Oncol 2005;23:3322.
4. Nissen MJ, Swensin KK, Ritz LJ, et al. Quality of life after breast carcinoma surgery: a comparison of three surgical procedures. Cancer 2001;91:1238.
5. Weitzner MA, Meyers CA, Stuebing KK, et al. Relationship between quality of life and mood in long-term survivors of breast cancer treated with mastectomy. Support Care Cancer 1997;5:241.
6. Ray C. Psychological implications of mastectomy. Br J Soc Clin Psychol 1977;16:373.
7. Türk KE, Yilmaz M. The effect on quality of life and body image of mastectomy among breast cancer survivors. Eur J Breast Health 2018;14:205.
8. Neto MS, de Aguiar Menezes MV, Moreira JR, et al. Sexuality after breast reconstruction post mastectomy. Aesthetic Plast Surg 2013;37:643.

9. Metcalfe KA, Semple J, Quan ML, et al. Changes in psychosocial functioning 1 year after mastectomy alone, delayed breast reconstruction, or immediate breast reconstruction. Ann Surg Oncol 2012;19:233.

10. Al-Ghazal SK, Sully L, Fallowfield L, et al. The psychological impact of immediate rather than delayed breast reconstruction. Eur J Surg Oncol 2000;26:17.

11. Wilkins EG, Cederna PS, Lowery JC, et al. Prospective analysis of psychological outcomes in breast reconstruction: one-year postoperative results from the Michigan Breast Reconstruction Outcome Study. Plast Reconstr Surg 2000;106:1014.

12. Elder EE, Branberg Y, Björklund T, et al. Quality of life and patient satisfaction in breast cancer patients after immediate breast reconstruction: a prospective study. Breast 2005;14:201.

13. Ochoa O, Garza R III, Pisano S, et al. Prospective longitudinal patient reported satisfaction and health-related quality of life following DIEP flap breast reconstruction: effects of reconstruction timing. Plast Reconstr Surg 2022;149(5):848e.

14. Kesson EM, Allardice GM, George WD, et al. Effects of multidisciplinary team working on breast cancer survival: retrospective, comparative, interventional cohort study of 13,722 women. BMJ 2012;344:e2718.

15. Pusic AL, Klassen AF, Scott AM, et al. Development of a new patient-reported outcome measure for breast surgery: the Breast-Q. Plast Reconstr Surg 2009;124:345.

16. Cohen WA, Mundy LR, Ballard TN, et al. The Breast-Q in surgical research: a review of the literature 2009-2015. J Plast Reconstr Aesthet Surg 2016;69:149.

17. Shinkunas LA, Klipowicz CJ, Carlisle EM. Shared decision-making in surgery: a scoping review of patient and surgeon preferences. BMC Med Inform Decis Mak 2020;20(1):190.

18. Zhong T, McCrathy C, Min S, et al. Patient satisfaction and health-related quality of life after autologous tissue breast reconstruction: a prospective analysis of early postoperative outcomes. Cancer 2012;118:1701.

19. Andrade WN, Baxter N, Semple JL. Clinical determinants of patient satisfaction with breast reconstruction. Plast Reconstr Surg 2001;107:46.

20. Colakoglu S, Khansa I, Curtis MS, et al. Impact of complications on patient satisfaction in breast reconstruction. Plast Reconstr Surg 2011;127:1428.

21. Gopie JP, Timman R, Hilhorst MT, et al. The short-term psychological impact of complications after breast reconstruction. Psychooncology 2013;22:290.

22. Dinwoodie M. Consent and shared decision-making. 2014. Available at: https://www.medicalprotection.org/newzealand/casebook/casebook-january-2014/consent-and-shared-decision-making. Accessed June 1, 2022.

23. Lee CN, Deal AM, Huh R, et al. Quality of patient decisions about breast reconstruction after mastectomy. JAMA Surg 2017;152(8):741.

24. The SHARE approach. In: Agency for Health care research and quality, Rockville, MD. 2020. Available at: https://www.ahrq.gov/health-literacy/professional-training/shared-decision/index.html. Accessed June 1, 2022.

25. Zdenkowski N, Butow P, Tesson S, et al. A systematic review of decision aids for patients making a decision about treatment for early breast cancer. Breast 2016;26:31.

26. Berlin NL, Tandon VJ, Hawley ST, et al. Feasibility and efficacy of decision aids to improve decision-making for postmastectomy breast reconstruction: a systematic review and meta-analysis. Med Decis Making 2019;39(1):5.

27. Torabi R, Stalder MW, Tessler O, et al. Assessing age as a risk factor for complications in autologous breast reconstruction. Plast Reconstr Surg 2018;142:840e.

28. Hamnett KE, Subramanian A. Breast reconstruction in older patients: a literature review of the decision-making process. J Plast Reconstr Aesthet Surg 2016;69:1325.

29. Liu Q, Aggarwal A, Wu M, et al. Impact of diabetes on outcomes in breast reconstruction: a systematic review and meta-analysis. J Plast Reconstr Aesthet Surg 2022;15:29.

30. Avci BS, Saler T, Avci A, et al. Relationship between morbidity and mortality and HbA1c levels in diabetic patients undergoing major surgery. J Coll Physicians Surg Pak 2019;29(11):1043.

31. Wang TY, Serletti JM, Cuker A, et al. Free tissue transfer in the hypercoagulable patient: a review of 58 flaps. Plast Reconstr Surg 2012;129:443.

32. Rohrich RJ, Kaplan J, Dayan E. Silicone implant illness: science versus myth? Plast Reconstr Surg 2019;144:98.

33. Magnusson MR, Cooter RD, Rakhorst H, et al. Breast implant illness: a way forward. Plast Reconstr Surg 2019;143:74S.

34. Rubio GA, McGee CS, Thaller SR. Autologous breast reconstruction outcomes in patients with autoimmune connective tissue disease. J Plast Reconstr Aesthet Surg 2019;72:848.

35. O'Neill AC, Haykal S, Bagher S, et al. Predictors and consequences of intraoperative microvascular problems in autologous breast reconstruction. J Plast Reconstr Aesthet Surg 2016;69:1349.

36. Ochoa O, Chrysopoulo M, Nastala C, et al. Abdominal wall stability and flap complications after deep inferior epigastric perforator flap breast reconstruction: does body mass index make a difference? Analysis of 418 patients and 639 flaps. Plast Reconstr Surg 2012;130:21e.

37. NCCN. NCCN (clinical practice guidelines in oncology: breast cancer) version 3.2022. 2022. Available at: http://www.nccn.org. Accessed May 11, 2022.

38. Cooke AL, Diaz-Abele J, Hayakawa T, et al. Radiation therapy versus No radiation therapy to the neo-breast following skin-sparing mastectomy and immediate autologous free flap reconstruction for breast cancer: patient-reported and surgical outcomes at 1 Year-A mastectomy reconstruction outcomes consortium (MROC) substudy. Int J Radiat Oncol Biol Phys 2017;99(1):165.

39. Jabor MA, Shayani P, Collins DR Jr, et al. Nipple-areola reconstruction: satisfaction and clinical determinants. Plast Reconstr Surg 2002;110:457.

40. Daar DA, Abdou SA, Rosario L, et al. Is there a preferred incision location for nipple-sparing mastectomy? A systematic review and meta-analysis. Plast Reconstr Surg 2019;143:906e.

41. Ochoa O, Azouz V, Santillan A, et al. Internal mammary lymph node biopsy during free-flap breast reconstruction: optimizing adjuvant breast cancer treatment through comprehensive staging. Ann Surg Oncol 2018;25(5):1322.

42. Schultz BD, Sultan D, Ha G, et al. Internal mammary lymph node biopsy during microsurgical breast reconstruction: a prospective study. J Reconstr Microsurg 2022. https://doi.org/10.1055/s-0042-1744503.

43. Karanetz I, Jin M, Nguyen K, et al. Evaluation of internal mammary lymph node biopsy during microsurgical breast reconstruction: an analysis of 230 consecutive patients. Breast J 2021;27(1):7.

44. Varghese J, Gohari SS, Rizki H, et al. A systematic review and meta-analysis on the effects of neoadjuvant chemotherapy on complications following immediate breast reconstruction. Breast 2021;55:55.

45. Yoo T, Moon H, Han W, et al. Time interval of neoadjuvant chemotherapy to surgery in breast cancer: how long is acceptable? Gland Surg 2017;6(1):1.

46. Sanford RA, Lei X, Barcenas CH, et al. Impact of time from completion of neoadjuvant chemotherapy to surgery on survival outcomes in breast cancer patients. Ann Surg Oncol 2016;23:1515.

47. Al-Masri M, Aljalabneh B, Al-Najjar H, et al. Effect of time to breast cancer surgery after neoadjuvant chemotherapy on survival outcomes. Breast Cancer Res Treat 2021;186(1):7.

48. Suleman K, Almalik O, Haque E, al at. Does the timing of breast surgery after neoadjuvant chemotherapy in breast cancer patients affect outcomes? Oncology 2020;98:168.

49. Kooijman MM, Hage JJ, Oldenberg HAS, et al. Surgical complications of skin-sparing mastectomy and immediate implant-based reconstruction in women concurrently treated with adjuvant chemotherapy for breast cancer. Ann Plast Surg 2021;86:146.

50. Jimenez-Puente A, Prieto-Lara E, Rueda-Dominguez A, et al. Complications in immediate breast reconstruction after mastectomy. Int J Technol Assess Health Care 2011;27(4):298.

51. Ravdin PM, Chamness GC. The c-erbb-2 proto-oncogene as a prognostic and predictive marker in breast cancer: a paradigm for the development of other macromolecular markers – a review. Gene 1995;159:19.

52. Shammas RL, Cho EH, Glener AD, et al. Association between targeted HER-2 therapy and breast reconstruction outcomes: a propensity score-matched analysis. J Am Coll Surg 2017;225:731.

53. Kelley BP, Valero V, Yi M, et al. Tamoxifen increases the risk of microvascular flap complications in patients undergoing microvascular breast reconstruction. Plast Reconstr Surg 2012;129:305.

54. Mirzabeigi MN, Nelson JA, Fischer JP, et al. Tamoxifen (selective estrogen-receptor modulators) and aromatase inhibitors as potential perioperative thrombotic risk factors in free flap breast reconstruction. Plast Reconstr Surg 2015;135:670e.

55. Hirsch EM, Seth AK, Dumanian GA, et al. Outcomes of tissue expander/implant breast reconstruction in the setting of prereconstruction radiation. Plast Reconstr Surg 2012;129:354.

56. Olinger TA, Berlin NL, Qi J, et al. Outcomes of immediate implant-based mastectomy reconstruction in women with previous breast radiotherapy. Plast Reconstr Surg 2020;145:1029e.

57. Jo T, Hur K, Min K, et al. Immediate breast reconstruction after salvage mastectomy: case control outcome comparisons of DIEP flap and DTI reconstruction. J Plast Reconstr Aesthet Surg 2021;74:1495.

58. Khajuria A, Charles WN, Prokopenko M, et al. Immediate and delayed autologous abdominal microvascular flap breast reconstruction in patients receiving adjuvant, neoadjuvant, or no radiotherapy: a meta-analysis of clinical and quality of life outcomes. BJS Open 2020;4(2):182.

59. Momoh AO, Colakoglu S, De blacam C, et al. Delayed autologous breast reconstruction after postmastectomy radiation: is there an optimal time? Ann Plast Surg 2012;69:14.

60. Baumann DP, Crosby MA, Selber JC, et al. Optimal timing of delayed free lower abdominal flap breast reconstruction after postmastectomy radiation therapy. Plast Reconstr Surg 2011;127:1100.

61. Ryan JL. Ionizing radiation: the good, the bad, and the ugly. J Invest Dermatol 2012;132:985.

62. Agarwal S, Kidwell KM, Farberg A, et al. Immediate reconstruction of the radiated breast – recent trends contrary to traditional standards. Ann Surg Oncol 2015;22(8):2551.

63. Kronowitz SJ, Robb GL. Radiation therapy and breast reconstruction: a critical review of the literature. Plast Reconstr Surg 2009;124:395.

64. Fowble B, Park C, Wang F, et al. Rates of reconstructive failure in patients undergoing immediate reconstruction with tissue expanders and/or implants and postmastectomy radiation therapy. Int J Radiat Oncol Biol Phys 2015;92:634.

65. Billig J, Jagsi R, Qi J, et al. Should immediate autologous breast reconstruction considered in women who require post-mastectomy radiation therapy? A prospective analysis of outcomes. Plast Reconstr Surg 2017;139:1279.

66. Anderson PR, Hanlon AL, Fowble BL, et al. Low complication rates are achievable after postmastectomy breast reconstruction and radiation therapy. Int J Radiat Oncol Biol Phys 2004;59:1080.

67. Heller DR, Zhuo H, Zhang Y, et al. Surgical outcomes of mastectomy with immediate autologous reconstruction followed by radiation. Ann Surg Oncol 2021;28:2169.

68. Kronowitz SJ, Hunt KK, Kuerer HM, et al. Delayed-immediate breast reconstruction. Plast Reconstr Surg 2004;113:1617.

69. Terao Y, Taniguchi K, Fugii M, et al. Postmastectomy radiation therapy and breast reconstruction with autologous tissue. Breast Cancer 2017;24:505.

70. American Society of Plastic Surgeons. 2019 plastic surgery statistics report. Arlington Heights (IL): American Society of Plastic Surgeons; 2019. Available at: https://www.plasticsur-gery.org/documents/News/Statistics/2018/plastic-surgery- statistics-full-report-2018.pdf. Accessed May 22, 2022.

71. Sbitany H, Sandeen SN, Amalfi AN, et al. Acellular dermis-assisted prosthetic breast reconstruction versus complete submuscular coverage: a head-to-head comparison of outcomes. Plast Reconstr Surg 2009;124(6):1735.

72. Leong M, Basu B, Hicks MJ. Further evidence that human acellular matrix decreases inflammatory markers of capsule formation in implant-based breast reconstruction. Aesthet Surg J 2015;35:40.

73. Yazar S, Bengur FB, Altinkaya A, et al. Nipple-sparing mastectomy and immediate implant-based reconstruction with or without skin reduction in patients with large ptotic breasts: a case matched analysis. Aesthetic Plast Surg 2021;45:956.

74. Salibian AH, Harness JK, Mowlds DS. Secondary mastopexy after nipple-sparing mastectomy and staged subcutaneous expander/implant reconstruction. Ann Plast Surg 2018;80:475.

75. Sbitany H. Important considerations for performing prepectoral breast reconstruction. Plast Reconstr Surg 2017;140:7S.

76. Elswick SM, Harless CA, Bishop SN, et al. Prepectoral implant-based breast reconstruction with postmastectomy radiation therapy. Plast Reconstr Surg 2018;142:1.

77. Safran T, Al-Badarin F, Al-Halabi B, et al. Aesthetic limitations in direct-to-implant prepectoral implant reconstruction. Plast Reconstr Surg 2022. https://doi.org/10.1097/PRS.0000000000009189.

78. DellaCroce FJ, Blum CA, Sullivan SK, et al. Nipple-sparing mastectomy and ptosis: perforator flap breast reconstruction allows full secondary mastopexy with complete nipple areolar repositioning. Plast Reconstr Surg 2015;136:1e.

79. Allen RJ, Treece P. Deep inferior epigastric perforator flap for breast reconstruction. Ann Plast Surg 1994;32:32.

80. Haddock NT, Cho M, Teotia SS. Comparative analysis of single versus stacked free flap breast reconstruction: a single-center experience. Plast Reconstr Surg 2019;144:369e.

81. DellaCroce FJ, Sullivan SK, Trahan C. Stacked deep inferior epigastric perforator flap breast reconstruction: a review of 110 flaps in 55 cases over 3 years. Plast Reconstr Surg 2011;127:1093.

82. Daly LT, Doval AF, Lin SJ, et al. Role of CTA in women with abdominal scars undergoing DIEP breast reconstruction: review of 1,187 flaps. J Reconstr Microsurg 2020;36:294.

83. Rozen WM, Bhullar HK, Hunter-Smith D. How to assess a CTA of the abdomen to plan an autologous breast reconstruction. Gland Surg 2019;8(Suppl 4):S291.

84. Mauch JT, Rhemtulla IA, Katzel EB, et al. Does size matter: evaluating the difference between right and left internal mammary veins in free flap breast reconstruction. J Reconstr Microsurg 2019;35:677.

85. Moran SL, Nava G, Benham AH, et al. An outcome analysis comparing the thoracodorsal and internal mammary vessels as recipient sites for microvascular breast reconstruction: a prospective study of 100 patients. Plast Reconstr Surg 2003;111:1876.

86. Casey WJ, Rebecca AM, Smith AA, et al. The cephalic and external jugular veins: important alternative recipient vessels in left-sided microvascular breast reconstruction. Microsurgery 2007;27:465.

Modern Approaches to Oncoplastic Surgical Treatment

Heather R. Faulkner, MD, MPH, Albert Losken, MD*

KEYWORDS

- Aesthetics • Breast cancer • Breast conserving treatment • Breast deformity • Oncoplastic
- Lumpectomy • Partial mastectomy • Radiation

KEY POINTS

- Reconstruction of the partial mastectomy defect has many benefits over lumpectomy alone for patients with breast cancer.
- The indications continue to expand and include patients with large breasts, large tumors, greater than 15% tumor to breast volume ratio, or patients where poor cosmesis is anticipated with lumpectomy alone.
- The most common technique is using the principles of breast reduction or mastopexy and involves rearranging breast tissue to fill the defect while improving cosmesis.
- Although the initial driving force was to prevent poor cosmetic results, the benefits are now known to include wider margins, larger resections, fewer re-excisions, and broadening the indications for breast-conserving therapy.
- Modern approaches include the use of auto-augmentation flaps to fill remote defects and intraoperative radiation therapy to minimize long-term fibrosis and the benefit of new data on the topic.

INTRODUCTION

Oncoplastic surgery (OPS) refers to the surgical management of breast cancer which combines breast-conserving therapy (BCT) with plastic surgical techniques to optimize outcomes. The goals include (1) oncologic efficacy, (2) improved breast cosmesis, (3) a favorable safety profile, and (4) improved overall patient satisfaction compared with partial mastectomy alone. OPS has also been shown to have increased satisfaction compared with total mastectomy with immediate reconstruction.[1]

Oncoplastic techniques are relatively new and although initially more popular in the United Kingdom and Europe, they have recently gained traction worldwide. Werner Audretsch is credited for coining the term "oncoplastic" in the 1980s.[2] Indications were initially limited, with some oncologic breast surgeons having reservations about reconstructing a partial defect. As we learn more about the safety and efficacy of this approach, partial breast reconstruction today has become an important part of our reconstructive practices. A recent retrospective cohort analysis of data from the ACS-NSQIP database demonstrated an increase in the use of oncoplastic breast reconstruction of 241% from 2008 to 2016, a rate of increase of 11% per year, whereas the rate of partial mastectomy without reconstruction has remained relatively constant.[3]

OPS is now considered by many to be the "gold standard" following partial mastectomy.[4,5] Reduction and flap techniques have been around for a while and are still used in the oncoplastic approach. Innovations have brought refinements in technique, streamlined modalities to deliver radiation therapy, tumor biology testing to determine

Emory Division of Plastic and Reconstructive Surgery, 550 Peachtree Street Northeast, Suite 9000, Atlanta GA 30308, USA
* Corresponding author.
E-mail address: alosken@emory.edu

Clin Plastic Surg 50 (2023) 211–221
https://doi.org/10.1016/j.cps.2022.10.005
0094-1298/23/© 2022 Elsevier Inc. All rights reserved.

the value of adjuvant treatment, and more importantly a better understanding of outcomes and patient satisfaction as more evidence becomes available.

DEFINITION AND CLASSIFICATION

A recent consensus defined OPS as "a form of breast-conservation surgery that includes onco-logic resection with a partial mastectomy, ipsilateral reconstruction using volume displacement, or volume replacement techniques with possible contralateral symmetry surgery when appropriate."[6] Although some surgeons still consider OPS to include any method of breast reconstruction after partial or total mastectomy, others (particularly in the United States) use the terms "oncoplastic surgery" in how it relates to partial breast reconstruction.[7,8]

Most classifications differentiate OPS into volume displacement and volume replacement techniques.[6,9] A level 1 volume displacement oncoplastic operation involves less than 20% of the breast tissue removed in the partial mastectomy and then reconstruction with local tissue rearrangement such as a doughnut mastopexy or crescent mastopexy.[6] A Level 2 volume displacement oncoplastic operation involves 20% to 50% of the breast tissue removed in the partial mastectomy followed by reconstruction typically using mastopexy or reduction patterns. Last, a volume replacement oncoplastic operation occurs when greater than 50% of breast tissue is removed in the partial mastectomy followed by reconstruction using local/regional flaps or implants. Most of the oncoplastic operations use this classification system as a useful algorithm for guiding selection of surgical technique.

Surgical Approach to Optimize Esthetics

The original driving force behind the popularity of the oncoplastic approach was preservation of esthetic results. A recent focus on esthetics has once again stressed the importance of this as a desired and valid outcome. In a recent series, the revision rate following oncoplastic reduction procedures with a follow-up of 3.8 years was 21%, with esthetic improvement as the most common reason for revision being performed in 13% of patients.[10] The surgeon needs refined techniques in their armamentarium to address shape, contour, symmetry, size, and nipple position in attempts to improve cosmesis and subsequently patient satisfaction. **Table 1** shows techniques that can be used to address esthetic concerns in OPS.

Breast shape is affected by both volume loss following tumor resection and radiation (XRT).

XRT will often exaggerate a deformity, which is typically more pronounced when lumpectomy is performed without OPS.[11] Even with oncoplastic techniques, the potentially adverse esthetic effects of XRT are unpredictable. Regarding volume loss in a smaller breast, the easiest way to correct the defect is to fill it with equivalent local tissue. If the volume can be replaced, the shape and contour are more likely to be preserved, even after XRT. Overcorrection can be considered with a slightly larger volume flap than the actual defect to account for tissue contraction after XRT.

In women with larger or ptotic breasts, the oncoplastic reduction or mastopexy options have become an invaluable tool for many reasons.[12] The shape is dictated by reducing the breast size and incorporating the defect into a smaller, lifted breast. In these cases, although the original shape is not preserved, it is often improved. Contour is addressed by filling the defect with surrounding breast tissue and removing additional skin so that the skin/volume discrepancy with lumpectomy alone is corrected, thus additionally improving shape and contour.

Larger, more remote defects and defects in smaller breasts can be reconstructed using auto-augmentation flaps during oncoplastic reduction or mastopexy procedures.[13] This allows the rotation of tissue to fill the defect to preserve the contour in places where surrounding breast tissue is insufficient to reconstruct the defect (**Fig. 1**). Auto-augmentation options include extending the primary pedicle to rotate into a defect or creating a secondary dermoglandular pedicle to move independent to the pedicle containing the nipple-areolar complex. These options further extend the oncoplastic approach to patients who otherwise would not have good esthetic outcomes using regular oncoplastic procedures. In our recent series examining oncoplastic outcomes, auto-augmentation flaps were used 33% of the time with superomedial being the most common extended primary pedicle and lateral being the most common tumor location.[13] Inferolateral was the most common secondary pedicle used for lateral or upper outer defects. There were no significant differences in the overall complication rate with 15.5% in the regular oncoplastic group, 19.6% in the extended pedicle group, and 20% in the secondary pedicle group. **Fig. 2** depicts an algorithm demonstrating oncoplastic techniques based on breast size, defect size, and defect location.[13]

The timing of oncoplastic reconstruction deserves consideration. The advantage of performing a reduction or mastopexy as OPS are that this is done as a single operation which may

Table 1
Esthetic concerns that can be addressed through immediate oncoplastic procedures[10]

Esthetic Concern	Potential Oncoplastic Tools in Women with Small Breasts	Potential Oncoplastic Tools in Women with Larger Breasts
Shape Contour Size Symmetry IMF retraction NAC malposition	Regional autologous flaps, local tissue flaps, breast advancement flaps, periareolar of batwing mastopexy, distant flaps, fat grafting	Oncoplastic reduction, mastopexy, autoaugmentaion techniques, local and distant autologous flaps, local breast flaps, contralateral reduction, or mastopexy

Abbreviations: IMF, inframammary fold; NAC, nipple-areola complex.
From Losken A, Brown CA. How to Optimize Aesthetics for the Partial Mastectomy Patient. Aesthet Surg J. 2020;40(Suppl 2):S55-S65.

improve patient satisfaction and outcome, but if a healing complication should occur, this may delay the receipt of radiation. In addition, performing OPS as a single operation is preferable to performing a reduction on a breast that has already received radiation due to the risk of unpredictable healing and complications such as fat necrosis and seroma secondary to radiation.

Esthetics and Oncoplastic Breast Surgery

Objective data on oncoplastic breast esthetics are limited. Two large systematic reviews of oncoplastic breast procedures claim good cosmetic outcomes in 84% to 90% of patients.[14,15] In a prospective study of patients who underwent oncoplastic breast surgery (OBS), 94% of patients were "very satisfied" or "satisfied" with their cosmetic outcome, and 85% of patients rated their breasts as "nearly identical" or "slightly different," at 1 to 3 months postoperatively. Surgeon evaluation similarly categorized 89% of results as "good" or "excellent."[16] This work suggests good esthetic outcomes in the early postoperative period; however, long-term follow-up is lacking. Clough and colleagues used a three-member panel to evaluate results following OBS and reported good cosmesis based on symmetry, shape, nipple-areola complex (NAC), scars, and radiation changes in 88% and 82% of patients at postoperative years 2 and 5, respectively.[17] This work highlights the durability of esthetics in oncoplastic reduction procedures.

The use of latissimus dorsi flaps in immediate oncoplastic procedures yields favorable esthetic

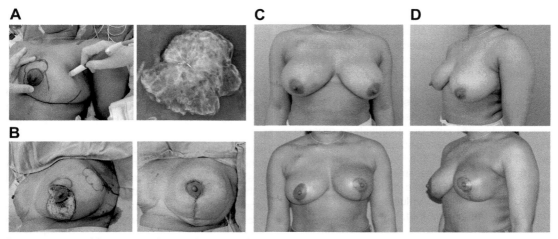

Fig. 1. A 45-year-old patient with an early-stage left upper outer breast cancer. (*A*) Resection was performed using a Savi Scout reflector (Merit Medical) to localize the tumor. The reflector was placed preoperatively, and the lumpectomy was performed using a handheld device which localizes it using nonradioactive radar waves. The 54-g lumpectomy specimen with reflector is confirmed intraoperatively with imaging. (*B*) An extended superomedial auto-augmentation technique was used to fill the defect and an additional 20 g of tissue was removed for shaping. A contralateral mastopexy was performed removing 90 g for symmetry. (*C*) Top row is before surgery. Bottom row is result is shown 1 year following left whole-breast external beam radiation therapy.

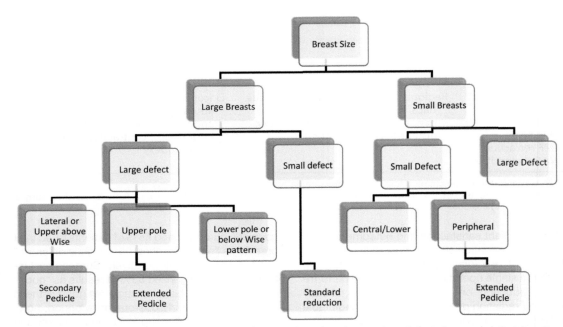

Fig. 2. Algorithm demonstrating oncoplastic techniques based on breast size, defect size, and defect location. *From* Losken A, Hart AM, Dutton JW, Broecker JS, Styblo TM, Carlson GW. The Expanded Use of Autoaugmentation Techniques in Oncoplastic Breast Surgery. *Plast Reconstr Surg.* 2018;141(1):10 to 19.

results according to patient-reported outcomes, clinical examinations, and panelist photographic assessment.[18,19] Hernanz and colleagues demonstrated good cosmetic outcomes by both patients and panelists, in which 81% of patients reported "excellent" outcomes and 19% reported "good" outcomes compared with a 44% "good" and a 56% "satisfactory" categorization by panelist assessment.[18] Although this study is limited in sample size (*n* = 16), it addresses revision rates for cosmesis. Out of 16 patients, 3 underwent revisions (1 for implant placement due to breast asymmetry and 2 for donor site scar revisions). Further research regarding the revision rate of oncoplastic procedures motivated by cosmetic as opposed to oncologic factors is warranted.

Veiga and colleagues prospectively compared patients who underwent oncoplastic breast surgery with traditional BCT without reconstruction via photographic assessment by a four-membered panel.[20] Esthetic elements evaluated included the following: volume, shape, breast location, inframammary fold, and scar. Superior scores were awarded to patients that underwent oncoplastic procedures. Of note, "volume" and "shape" were the two elements that received the lowest ratings in patients that underwent standard BCT without OPS. The esthetic result improved over time in the oncoplastic group, supporting the durability of OBS. In a comparison of OBS

with "latissimus dorsi mini flap" and skin-sparing mastectomy with immediate latissimus flap reconstruction, the oncoplastic cohort received significantly higher panel scores compared with the mastectomy cohort (3.8–2.9, respectively).[21] It is important to consider that much of the beauty of plastic and reconstructive surgery is subjective, and although it is difficult to demonstrate esthetic improvement objectively, it has been shown that patient satisfaction can be an adequate proxy.

Radiation Delivery in Breast Conservation

Part and parcel of BCT is the delivery of radiation, with the purpose of reducing the risk of local breast cancer recurrence which has been studied extensively.[22] The traditional method of radiation delivery is whole-breast radiation via external beam initiated 6 weeks after the operation, provided the patient is completely healed at that time. Radiation can be delivered via conventional or hypofractionated method. The delivery of a boost of radiation to the tumor bed (area of lumpectomy) has been shown to reduce recurrence risk.[23] Patients who receive a radiation boost have been shown to experience increased pain, induration, fibrosis, and edema.[24,25] Because there are variations in tissue rearrangement and architecture of the breast with OPS, the feasibility of delivering boost radiation has been debated. However, Gladwish and colleagues determined the ability to deliver boost radiation was not adversely affected comparing OPS with BCT.[26] Reliable placement of surgical clips to identify the resection bed is critical to accurately target boost radiation delivery.[27] Emerging technologies can help facilitate consistent identification of the resection cavity. Preliminary studies of three-dimensional bioabsorbable tissue markers placed at the time of surgery, including OPS, have shown promise with successful identification of the resection bed in preparation for boost radiation, in addition to low postoperative surgical site infection rates and preserved cosmetic outcomes.[28,29]

Accelerated partial breast irradiation (APBI) is a newer concept in comparison to whole-breast radiation. The risks of whole-breast radiation include damage to healthy breast tissue and toxicity to the heart and lungs. **Fig. 3** shows the progression of whole-breast radiation changes in a patient who underwent lumpectomy and oncoplastic reconstruction with reduction using inferior pedicle. Recurrence risk is highest at the site of the original tumor; therefore, delivery of radiation specifically to this area is the goal. ABPI can be delivered via brachytherapy, external beam radiotherapy, or intraoperative radiation therapy (IORT).[30] Few studies exist cataloging the effects of ABPI on the esthetic outcomes of OPS.

Brachytherapy for breast cancer treatment was introduced in the 1970s. It is performed under anesthesia by transcutaneous catheter insertion with subsequent radiation delivery through the catheters. Local tissue reactions at the catheter insertion sites are common, whereas this technique has been shown to be more protective of the thoracic organs. It is not done at many centers due to a steep learning curve and the invasive nature of the procedure.[31]

IORT is a single dose of radiation delivered at the time of surgery. The TARGIT-A trial showed no differences in oncologic outcomes between patients who received conventional whole-breast radiation and IORT.[32] Quality of life is improved and cost is reduced with the use of IORT as patients do not require repeat treatment visits. A study of 186 patients comparing whole-breast radiation to IORT in patients undergoing OPS showed a higher rate of fat necrosis and seroma with IORT, but no difference in cosmetic outcomes[33] (**Fig. 4**). Long-term breast fibrosis is not as common following IORT.

Recent research is focusing on identifying patients that would not benefit significantly from the receipt of radiation.[34] Although nomograms based on clinical and pathologic features were used to guide decision-making in the past, there are now

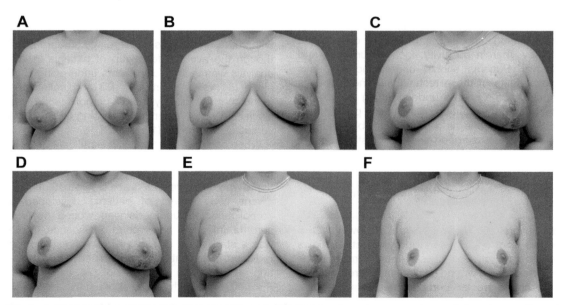

Fig. 3. A 37-year-old patient with macromastia and left invasive breast cancer who underwent neoadjuvant chemotherapy. (A) Before surgery. (B) After left lumpectomy with oncoplastic reduction using inferior pedicle and right symmetrizing reduction with inferior pedicle followed by completion of left whole-breast external beam radiation. Note hyperpigmentation of breast skin and loss of pigmentation of nipple-areolar complex. (C) Gradual recovery of left breast skin and nipple-areolar complex after radiation. (D) Continued recovery of left breast skin and nipple-areolar complex. (E) 1 year after surgery showing good symmetry and recovered pigmentation. (F) 2 years and 3 months after surgery showing stable result even with patient weight loss.

A 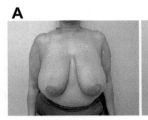 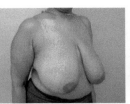   **B**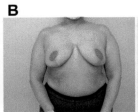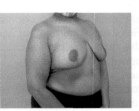

Fig. 4. A 59-year-old woman with right lower pole breast cancer who underwent a 75-g resection followed by IORT and a superomedial oncoplastic reduction with a total of 896 g resection. (*A*) Before surgery. She had a symmetrizing left reduction removing 920 g (*B*) Her result is shown at 1 year with good symmetry and minimal radiation fibrosis.

genomic molecular assays being used adjunctively to inform care. DCISionRT (PreludeDX, Laguna Hills, California) is a biomarker assay developed specifically for patients with ductal carcinoma in situ (DCIS), with the goal of de-escalating care and the need for radiation therapy in select patients.[35]

SAFETY OF ONCOPLASTIC SURGERY

OPS aims to optimize the final cosmetic appearance of the breast; however, breast esthetics are secondary in importance to oncologic efficacy and safety. Many oncoplastic techniques involve extensive rearrangement of local tissues, creation of additional incisions on the breast, or transposition of regional tissues into the tumor cavity. Legitimate concerns have been raised previously about how OPS techniques may affect overall risk of complications, subsequent delivery of adjuvant therapy, margin positivity, local recurrence, and survival. Patients should understand the risks and benefits of these techniques, and surgeons should have a shared understanding and agreement about the safety profile of these procedures. OPS is best done as a partnership between the ablative breast surgeon and the plastic surgeon, so that each can understand the goals and objectives of the other.

Surgical Complications Following Oncoplastic Breast Reconstruction

The overall complication rate following OPS ranges from 14% to 16% in systematic reviews and meta-analyses.[36,37] Common complications include delayed wound healing, fat necrosis, infection, nipple-areolar complex necrosis, seroma, and hematoma with individual incidence ranging from less than 1% to 4%.[36,38] Overall, the rate of complications requiring reoperation is likely around 3%.[37,39] In their NSQIP database analysis, Cil and colleagues identified multiple factors independently associated with a higher likelihood of developing a complication within 30 days of

surgery including obesity, smoking, American Academy of Anesthesiologists category 3 or 4, diabetes, bleeding disorder, chronic obstructive pulmonary disease, and a longer operative time.[40] The presence of bleeding disorder had the highest association with postoperative complications (odds ratio 1.8). Although smoking and nicotine use in reconstructive operations adds both morbidity and cost to a health care system, the cost-effectiveness of performing an ipsilateral oncoplastic operation at the time of cancer excision is significant as there is a high risk of complications of delayed OPS on a radiated breast.[41,42]

Oncoplastic techniques may have a comparable or slightly lower rate of complications compared with standard breast conservation therapy alone. A meta-analysis performed by Losken and colleagues demonstrated a rate of complications of 15.5% in patients undergoing OPS, compared with 25.9% in patients undergoing standard BCT, though the average follow-up of patients in this analysis was longer for patients undergoing BCT alone (64 vs 37 months).[37] Cil and colleagues found that the 30-day rate of complications was similar between patients undergoing OPS (1.7%) versus standard BCT(1.9%).[40]

When complications occur, a significant delay in initiation of adjuvant therapy may result. Kapadia and colleagues retrospectively reviewed 118 patients who underwent OPS at a single institution.[43] Twenty-two percent of patients developed a complication including delayed wound healing, seroma, infection, and wound dehiscence. There was a statistically significant delay in initiation of radiation in patients who developed a complication versus those who did not (74 vs 54 days, $P < .001$). Similarly, in a retrospective review of 150 patients undergoing OPS published by Hillberg and colleagues, initiation of adjuvant radiotherapy was delayed in 8.2% of patients due to a postoperative complication, though the overall complication rate was relatively high in this study (37.5%).[44] In a recent retrospective review published by Deigni and colleagues, 429 patients underwent OPS followed by either immediate contralateral symmetry procedure or symmetry procedure performed in a delayed fashion.[45] There was no significant difference in overall complications between the two groups. Although complications resulted in a delay in adjuvant therapy in 4.2% of patients overall, complications attributable to the contralateral symmetry procedure accounted for a delay in only 0.7% of patients. OPS in one study did not delay the time to delivery of adjuvant chemotherapy (29 days) when compared with lumpectomy alone (29.5 days).[46]

Local Recurrence, Disease Free, and Overall Survival

Given that OPS has only become a mainstream treatment option in the last two decades, long-term data about recurrence and survival are somewhat lacking. Numerous studies have demonstrated the significant impact that the oncoplastic approach has on improving margin control.[47,48] Margin positivity following partial mastectomy is known to predict local recurrence; however, tumor biology is also an important predictor of oncologic outcome. Oncoplastic surgical techniques extend the indications for breast conservation, including patients with larger and more aggressive tumors. In a retrospective cohort study of 1800 patients with breast cancer who underwent either standard breast conservation or oncoplastic breast conservation, Niinikoski and colleagues addressed the recurrence question.[49] After a median follow-up of 75 months, there was no difference in local recurrence-free survival between the two groups. Patients in the oncoplastic group had significantly larger tumors which were more often palpable and multifocal; in addition, their breast cancers had significantly higher histologic grade, T-stage, and lymph node involvement. There was no difference in positive margin rate between groups in this study. In a systematic review performed in 2016, De la Cruz and colleagues analyzed 6011 oncoplastic reconstruction patients with a mean follow-up of 50.5 months. Among 871 patients with at least 5 years follow-up, the rates of overall survival, disease-free survival, local recurrence, and distant recurrence were 93.4%, 85.4%, 6%, and 11.9%, respectively.[36] The investigators noted that these rates seem to correlate favorably with recurrence and survival rates after standard breast conservation, suggesting that surgical technique is not the primary predictor of oncologic outcome. The authors recently compared recurrence in 97 lumpectomy patients and 95 oncoplastic reduction patients with an average of 8 years follow-up and found that despite more advanced disease in the oncoplastic group there was a similar overall recurrence rate.[50] The multimodal treatment of breast cancer is such that more aggressive local control (as in a mastectomy) is not shown to reduce local/regional recurrence and that equivalent local/recurrence is often noted in the oncoplastic groups despite often having more aggressive cancers in those patients.[51]

In general, it seems that OPS techniques result in a generous resection and improved margin control, however, this does not translate into a recurrence benefit compared with standard breast conservation. Tumor recurrence, however, is not increased by the immediate reconstruction of these defects. OPS may be offered to patients with a broader range of tumor size and pathology, and the esthetic benefits of this approach do not seem to compromise cancer recurrence and survival.

Higher risk patients and more advanced disease are now not contraindicated when considering the oncoplastic approach (**Fig. 5**). Most studies have shown similar recurrence rates when compared with lumpectomy alone despite wider margins in the oncoplastic groups and higher risk patients (larger tumors, more human epidermal growth factor recepter (HER)2+ and triple negative, fewer estrogen recepter/progesterone recepter [ER/PR]+) in the oncoplastic groups. More aggressive local control with OPS might broaden the indications for breast conserving surgery (BCS), but the systemic and hormonal treatments have contributed to the recurrence safety in the oncoplastic approach. Although the true benefit on recurrence is difficult to demonstrate, there have been no studies showing it to be unsafe. The oncoplastic approach has allowed for more advanced disease to be treated with BCT. It has also found to be safe compared with mastectomy in tumors larger than 2 cm with similar overall survival rates (87.3 vs 87.1% at 10 years).[52] Several studies have shown similar locoregional recurrence and oncologic outcomes in large T2 tumors, locally advanced tumors, and DCIS when treated with oncoplastic breast conservation.[52–55] OPS has extended the indications even further with the technique being performed on patients with multifocal/multicentric tumors, extensive DCIS, or tumors greater than 5 cm with acceptable outcomes in a series of 39 patients.[56]

PATIENT SATISFACTION FOLLOWING ONCOPLASTIC SURGERY

The recent interest in patient-reported outcomes has generated some interesting data on patient satisfaction following OPS. Patient satisfaction

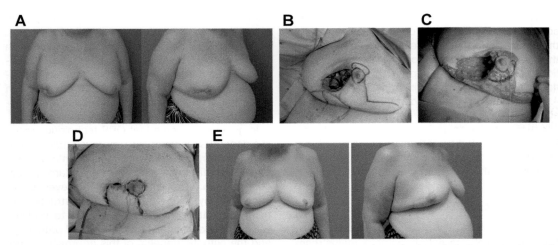

Fig. 5. A 56-year-old woman who underwent neoadjuvant chemotherapy for right ductal carcinoma in situ with comedonecrosis along with excisional biopsy. (*A*) Before surgery. (*B*) She underwent a 243-g quadrantectomy removing skin and breast tissue above the Wise pattern markings. (*C*) A superior pedicle was used for the nipple-areolar complex. (*D*) Skin was preserved from the lower pole of the breast to replace the resected skin. The symmetrizing left reduction removed 394 g of tissue. (*E*) Her result is shown 2 years following right whole-breast external beam radiation therapy with good symmetry.

following oncoplastic reconstruction has been shown to exceed satisfaction following standard breast conservation therapy, mastectomy alone, and mastectomy with reconstruction.[57–61] Rose and colleagues published the results of a survey study comparing patient-reported outcomes after OPS (107 patients) or standard breast conservation (657 patients).[57] Subjects were administered the Breast-Q validated questionnaire an average of 60.8 months from the time of surgery. The investigators found that despite having on average more advanced cancers, patients in the oncoplastic group had significantly higher self-reported psychosocial well-being. A comprehensive literature review of patient-reported outcome measures including Breast-Q was performed by Char and colleagues and found that OPS in general had the highest patient satisfaction scores among breast reconstructive choices.[61] Forty-three articles were included in this study looking at all forms of autologous tissue and implant-based reconstruction.

High levels of patient satisfaction have been reported after volume displacement techniques as well as volume replacement techniques.[58,62–64] In their survey of 624 patients undergoing a variety of different oncoplastic procedures, Rezai and colleagues demonstrated that there was no significant correlation between the method of oncologic reconstruction and the patient perception of the esthetic result.[65] Oncoplastic reconstruction with a reduction mammoplasty approach may have a particularly large impact

on patient-reported quality of life after surgery. Losken and colleagues performed a retrospective review of 353 patients undergoing oncoplastic breast reconstruction with a breast reduction technique.[12] The average reduction weight of patients in this study was 545 g. The investigators used the Breast-Q validated questionnaire to show that, compared with preoperative baseline, women undergoing oncoplastic reduction had increased self-confidence, feelings of attractiveness, emotional health, and satisfaction with sex life over 1 year postoperatively.

There is some evidence that suggests that oncologic status may affect patient-reported outcomes more than surgical technique. In their study of 120 patients undergoing oncoplastic breast reconstruction with volume displacement techniques, Gardfjell and colleagues showed that lower patient satisfaction seemed to correlate with need for axillary dissection and neoadjuvant chemotherapy.[62] In their comparison of 379 patients undergoing OPS or breast conservation alone, Ojala and colleagues showed that larger tumor diameter, multifocality, and oncoplastic reconstruction were predictive of poor patient-reported esthetic result; however, in this study, patients undergoing oncoplastic reconstruction were more likely to have larger, multifocal tumors with lymph node involvement.[66]

Patients undergoing oncoplastic reconstruction have high levels of satisfaction with their appearance, mental well-being, and overall perception of health, comparing favorably to other surgical breast cancer treatment modalities. This effect is somewhat expected and may be secondary to the attention to breast esthetics and symmetry that are the focus of oncoplastic techniques.

SUMMARY

Oncoplastic breast reconstruction is now a globally accepted option for treatment of breast cancer. This approach has a favorable safety profile and equivalent oncologic efficacy compared with standard breast conservation but has the major advantage of improved esthetic outcomes. Modern approaches include refinements in technique and a renewed focus on esthetics and outcomes including patient satisfaction and well-being. As more data are available demonstrating the safety of this approach, it is also being used on higher risk patients also with favorable outcomes.

CLINICS CARE POINTS

- In counseling patients about oncoplastic reconstruction in comparison with lumpectomy in the setting of breast-conserving therapy, plastic surgeons can inform patients that satisfaction with oncoplastic reconstruction is high and the risk of complications is low.
- When performing reconstruction of a lumpectomy defect, keep the principles of mastopexy, reduction, and auto-augmentation in mind to determine the best course of action.
- To avoid complications relating to radiation, it is advised to perform oncoplastic reconstruction before the receipt of radiation for breast-conserving therapy.
- To assess candidacy for oncoplastic reconstruction, plastic surgeons should consult with the breast surgical oncologist and radiation oncologist to formulate a multidisciplinary plan.

DISCLOSURE

Dr A Losken is a consultant for RTI surgical and has no relevant disclosures.

REFERENCES

1. Kelsall JE, McCulley SJ, Brock L, et al. Comparing oncoplastic breast conserving surgery with mastectomy and immediate breast reconstruction: case-matched patient reported outcomes. J Plast Reconstr Aesthet Surg 2017;70(10):1377–85.
2. Audretsch WP, Rezai M, Kolotas C, et al. Tumor-specific immediate reconstruction in breast cancer patients. Semin Plast Surg 1998;11(1):71–100.
3. Jonczyk MM, Jean J, Graham R, et al. Surgical trends in breast cancer: a rise in novel operative treatment options over a 12 year analysis. Breast Cancer Res Treat 2019;173(2):267–74.
4. Hernanz F, González-Noriega M, Sánchez S, et al. Oncoplastic breast conserving surgery with tailored needle-guided excision. Gland Surg 2017;6(6):698–705.
5. Macmillan RD, McCulley SJ. Oncoplastic breast surgery: what, when and for whom? Curr Breast Cancer Rep 2016;8:112–7.
6. Chatterjee A, Gass J, Patel K, et al. A consensus Definition and classification system of oncoplastic surgery developed by the American society of breast surgeons. Ann Surg Oncol 2019;26(11):3436–44.
7. Radtke C. Standards in oncoplastic breast reconstruction. Breast Care Basel Switz 2019;14(5):269–70.
8. Weber WP, Haug M, Kurzeder C, et al. Oncoplastic Breast Consortium consensus conference on nipple-sparing mastectomy. Breast Cancer Res Treat 2018;172(3):523–37.
9. Clough KB, Kaufman GJ, Nos C, et al. Improving breast cancer surgery: a classification and quadrant per quadrant atlas for oncoplastic surgery. Ann Surg Oncol 2010;17(5):1375–91.
10. Losken A, Brown CA. How to optimize aesthetics for the partial mastectomy patient. Aesthet Surg J 2020;40(Suppl 2):S55–65.
11. Kelemen P, Pukancsik D, Újhelyi M, et al. Comparison of clinicopathologic, cosmetic and quality of life outcomes in 700 oncoplastic and conventional breast-conserving surgery cases: a single-centre retrospective study. Eur J Surg Oncol 2019;45(2):118–24.
12. Losken A, Hart AM, Broecker JS, et al. Oncoplastic breast reduction technique and outcomes: an evolution over 20 years. Plast Reconstr Surg 2017;139(4):824e–33e.
13. Losken A, Hart AM, Dutton JW, et al. The expanded use of autoaugmentation techniques in oncoplastic breast surgery. Plast Reconstr Surg 2018;141(1):10–9.
14. Haloua MH, Krekel NMA, Winters HAH, et al. A systematic review of oncoplastic breast-conserving surgery: current weaknesses and future prospects. Ann Surg 2013;257(4):609–20.
15. Papanikolaou IG, Dimitrakakis C, Zagouri F, et al. Paving the way for changing perceptions in breast surgery: a systematic literature review focused on oncological and aesthetic outcomes of oncoplastic surgery for breast cancer. Breast Cancer Tokyo Jpn 2019;26(4):416–27.
16. Chan SWW, Cheung PSY, Chueng PSY, et al. Cosmetic outcome and percentage of breast

volume excision in oncoplastic breast conserving surgery. World J Surg 2010;34(7):1447–52.

17. Clough KB, Lewis JS, Couturaud B, et al. Oncoplastic techniques allow extensive resections for breast-conserving therapy of breast carcinomas. Ann Surg 2003;237(1):26–34.

18. Hernanz F, Regaño S, Redondo-Figuero C, et al. Oncoplastic breast-conserving surgery: analysis of quadrantectomy and immediate reconstruction with latissimus dorsi flap. World J Surg 2007;31(10): 1934–40.

19. Woerdeman LAE, Hage JJ, Thio EA, et al. Breast-conserving therapy in patients with a relatively large (T2 or T3) breast cancer: long-term local control and cosmetic outcome of a feasibility study. Plast Reconstr Surg 2004;113(6):1607–16.

20. Veiga DF, Veiga-Filho J, Ribeiro LM, et al. Evaluations of aesthetic outcomes of oncoplastic surgery by surgeons of different gender and specialty: a prospective controlled study. Breast Edinb Scotl 2011;20(5):407–12.

21. Gendy RK, Able JA, Rainsbury RM. Impact of skin-sparing mastectomy with immediate reconstruction and breast-sparing reconstruction with miniflaps on the outcomes of oncoplastic breast surgery. Br J Surg 2003;90(4):433–9.

22. Darby S, McGale P, Correa C, et al, Early Breast Cancer Trialists' Collaborative Group (EBCTCG). Effect of radiotherapy after breast-conserving surgery on 10-year recurrence and 15-year breast cancer death: meta-analysis of individual patient data for 10,801 women in 17 randomised trials. Lancet Lond Engl 2011;378(9804):1707–16.

23. Beddok A, Kirova Y, Laki F, et al. The place of the boost in the breast cancer treatment: state of art. Radiother Oncol J Eur Soc Ther Radiol Oncol 2022;170:55–63.

24. Chua BH, Link EK, Kunkler IH, et al. Radiation doses and fractionation schedules in non-low-risk ductal carcinoma in situ in the breast (BIG 3-07/TROG 07.01): a randomised, factorial, multicentre, open-label, phase 3 study. Lancet Lond Engl 2022; 400(10350):431–40.

25. Kelemen G, Varga Z, Lázár G, et al. Cosmetic outcome 1-5 years after breast conservative surgery, irradiation and systemic therapy. Pathol Oncol Res POR 2012;18(2):421–7.

26. Gladwish A, Didiodato G, Conway J, et al. Implications of oncoplastic breast surgery on radiation boost delivery in localized breast cancer. Cureus 2021;13(11):e20003.

27. Furet E, Peurien D, Fournier-Bidoz N, et al. Plastic surgery for breast conservation therapy: how to define the volume of the tumor bed for the boost? Eur J Surg Oncol 2014;40(7):830–4.

28. Kaufman CS, Cross MJ, Barone JL, et al. A three-dimensional bioabsorbable tissue marker for volume replacement and radiation planning: a multicenter study of surgical and patient-reported outcomes for 818 patients with breast cancer. Ann Surg Oncol 2021;28(5):2529–42.

29. Yehia ZA, Yoon J, Sayan M, et al. Does the use of BioZorb® result in smaller breast seroma volume? Anticancer Res 2022;42(6):2961–5.

30. Laplana M, García-Marqueta M, Sánchez-Fernández JJ, et al. Effectiveness and safety of intraoperative radiotherapy (IORT) with low-energy X-rays (INTRABEAM®) for accelerated partial breast irradiation (APBI). Clin Transl Oncol Off Publ Fed Span Oncol Soc Natl Cancer Inst Mex 2022; 24(9):1732–43.

31. Cozzi S, Augugliaro M, Ciammella P, et al. The role of interstitial brachytherapy for breast cancer treatment: an overview of indications, applications, and technical notes. Cancers 2022;14(10):2564.

32. Small W, Refaat T, Feldman SM, et al. Risk-stratified intraoperative radiation therapy as a definitive adjuvant radiation therapy modality for women with early breast cancer. Pract Radiat Oncol 2022;12(4): 320–3.

33. Cracco S, Semprini G, Cattin F, et al. Impact of intraoperative radiotherapy on cosmetic outcome and complications after oncoplastic breast surgery. Breast J 2015;21(3):285–90.

34. Allen SG, Speers C, Jagsi R. Tailoring the omission of radiotherapy for early-stage breast cancer based on tumor biology. Semin Radiat Oncol 2022;32(3):198–206.

35. Knowlton CA, Jimenez RB, Moran MS. Risk assessment in the molecular era. Semin Radiat Oncol 2022; 32(3):189–97.

36. De La Cruz L, Blankenship SA, Chatterjee A, et al. Outcomes after oncoplastic breast-conserving surgery in breast cancer patients: a systematic literature review. Ann Surg Oncol 2016;23(10):3247–58.

37. Losken A, Dugal CS, Styblo TM, et al. A meta-analysis comparing breast conservation therapy alone to the oncoplastic technique. Ann Plast Surg 2014; 72(2):145–9.

38. Piper ML, Esserman LJ, Sbitany H, et al. Outcomes following oncoplastic reduction mammoplasty: a systematic review. Ann Plast Surg 2016;76(Suppl 3):S222–6.

39. Fitoussi AD, Berry MG, Famà F, et al. Oncoplastic breast surgery for cancer: analysis of 540 consecutive cases [outcomes article]. Plast Reconstr Surg 2010;125(2):454–62.

40. Cil TD, Cordeiro E. Complications of oncoplastic breast surgery involving soft tissue transfer versus breast-conserving surgery: an analysis of the NSQIP database. Ann Surg Oncol 2016;23(10):3266–71.

41. Bloom JA, Asban A, Tian T, et al. A cost-utility analysis comparing immediate oncoplastic surgery with delayed oncoplastic surgery in smoking breast cancer patients. Ann Surg Oncol 2021;28(5):2579–88.

42. Bloom JA, Rashad R, Chatterjee A. The impact on mortality and societal costs from smoking cessation in aesthetic plastic surgery in the United States. Aesthet Surg J 2019;39(4):439–44.

43. Kapadia SM, Reitz A, Hart A, et al. Time to radiation after oncoplastic reduction. Ann Plast Surg 2019; 82(1):15–8.

44. Hillberg NS, Meesters-Caberg MAJ, Beugels J, et al. Delay of adjuvant radiotherapy due to postoperative complications after oncoplastic breast conserving surgery. Breast Edinb Scotl 2018;39:110–6.

45. Deigni OA, Baumann DP, Adamson KA, et al. Immediate contralateral mastopexy/breast reduction for symmetry can Be performed safely in oncoplastic breast-conserving surgery. Plast Reconstr Surg 2020;145(5):1134–42.

46. Khan J, Kahn J, Barrett S, et al. Oncoplastic breast conservation does not lead to a delay in the commencement of adjuvant chemotherapy in breast cancer patients. Eur J Surg Oncol J Eur Soc Surg Oncol Br Assoc Surg Oncol 2013;39(8):887–91.

47. Fitzal F, Bolliger M, Dunkler D, et al. Retrospective, multicenter analysis comparing conventional with oncoplastic breast conserving surgery: oncological and surgical outcomes in women with high-risk breast cancer from the OPBC-01/iTOP2 study. Ann Surg Oncol 2022;29(2):1061–70.

48. Barellini L, Marcasciano M, Lo Torto F, et al. Intraoperative ultrasound and oncoplastic combined approach: an additional tool for the oncoplastic surgeon to obtain tumor-free margins in breast conservative surgery-A 2-year single-center prospective study. Clin Breast Cancer 2020;20(3):e290–4.

49. Niinikoski L, Leidenius MHK, Vaara P, et al. Resection margins and local recurrences in breast cancer: comparison between conventional and oncoplastic breast conserving surgery. Eur J Surg Oncol J Eur Soc Surg Oncol Br Assoc Surg Oncol 2019;45(6): 976–82.

50. Losken A, Smearman EL, Hart AM, et al. The impact oncoplastic reduction has on long-term recurrence in breast conservation therapy. Plast Reconstr Surg 2022;149(5):867e–75e.

51. Pearce BCS, Fiddes RN, Paramanathan N, et al. Extreme oncoplastic conservation is a safe new alternative to mastectomy. Eur J Surg Oncol J Eur Soc Surg Oncol Br Assoc Surg Oncol 2020;46(1): 71–6.

52. De Lorenzi F, Loschi P, Bagnardi V, et al. Oncoplastic breast-conserving surgery for tumors larger than 2 centimeters: is it oncologically safe? A matched-cohort analysis. Ann Surg Oncol 2016;23(6):1852–9.

53. Chauhan A, Sharma MM. Evaluation of surgical outcomes following oncoplastic breast surgery in early breast cancer and comparison with conventional breast conservation surgery. Med J Armed Forces India 2016;72(1):12–8.

54. Song HM, Styblo TM, Carlson GW, et al. The use of oncoplastic reduction techniques to reconstruct partial mastectomy defects in women with ductal carcinoma in situ. Breast J 2010;16(2):141–6.

55. Broecker JS, Hart AM, Styblo TM, et al. Neoadjuvant therapy combined with oncoplastic reduction for high-stage breast cancer patients. Ann Plast Surg 2017;78(6S Suppl 5):S258–62.

56. Koppiker CB, Noor AU, Dixit S, et al. Extreme oncoplastic surgery for multifocal/multicentric and locally advanced breast cancer. Int J Breast Cancer 2019; 2019:4262589.

57. Rose M, Svensson H, Handler J, et al. Patient-reported outcome after oncoplastic breast surgery compared with conventional breast-conserving surgery in breast cancer. Breast Cancer Res Treat 2020;180(1):247–56.

58. Bazzarelli A, Baker L, Petrcich W, et al. Patient satisfaction following level II oncoplastic breast surgery: a comparison with mastectomy utililizing the breast-Q questionnaire will be published in surgical oncology. Surg Oncol 2020;35:556–9.

59. Chand ND, Browne V, Paramanathan N, et al. Patient-reported outcomes are better after oncoplastic breast conservation than after mastectomy and autologous reconstruction. Plast Reconstr Surg Glob Open 2017;5(7):e1419.

60. Hart AM, Pinell-White X, Egro FM, et al. The psychosexual impact of partial and total breast reconstruction: a prospective one-year longitudinal study. Ann Plast Surg 2015;75(3):281–6.

61. Char S, Bloom JA, Erlichman Z, et al. A comprehensive literature review of patient-reported outcome measures (PROMs) among common breast reconstruction options: what types of breast reconstruction score well? Breast J 2021;27(4):322–9.

62. Gardfjell A, Dahlbäck C, Åhsberg K. Patient satisfaction after unilateral oncoplastic volume displacement surgery for breast cancer, evaluated with the BREAST-Q™. World J Surg Oncol 2019;17(1):96.

63. Kim KD, Kim Z, Kuk JC, et al. Long-term results of oncoplastic breast surgery with latissimus dorsi flap reconstruction: a pilot study of the objective cosmetic results and patient reported outcome. Ann Surg Treat Res 2016;90(3):117–23.

64. van Paridon MW, Kamali P, Paul MA, et al. Oncoplastic breast surgery: achieving oncological and aesthetic outcomes. J Surg Oncol 2017;116(2): 195–202.

65. Rezai M, Kraemer S, Kimmig R, et al. Breast conservative surgery and local recurrence. Breast Edinb Scotl 2015;24(Suppl 2):S100–7.

66. Ojala K, Meretoja TJ, Leidenius MHK. Aesthetic and functional outcome after breast conserving surgery - comparison between conventional and oncoplastic resection. Eur J Surg Oncol J Eur Soc Surg Oncol Br Assoc Surg Oncol 2017;43(4):658–64.

Modern Approaches to Implant-Based Breast Reconstruction

Ara A. Salibian, MD[a], Nolan S. Karp, MD[b],*

KEYWORDS

- Breast reconstruction • Nipple-sparing mastectomy • Cohesive implant • Acellular dermal matrix

KEY POINTS

- Successful implant-based breast reconstruction requires a team approach between the breast surgeon and plastic surgeon.
- Patient selection, mastectomy flap quality, and surgical technique are critical in nipple-sparing mastectomy.
- Modern highly cohesive implants have esthetic benefits in breast reconstruction though preoperative discussion of all implant-related risks is paramount.
- Support materials including acellular dermal matrix have both risks and benefits in breast reconstruction and their use should be individualized.

INTRODUCTION

Implant-based reconstruction remains the most common form of breast reconstruction today.[1] Although many of the basic principles of implant-based reconstruction have not changed, several core components of these procedures have evolved toward what can be considered the "modern" approach. This approach is focused on a team-based paradigm,[2] in which the breast and plastic surgeons work together with the patient throughout all phases of care to optimize both oncologic and reconstructive outcomes.

Specific advances in this field include the evolution of mastectomy techniques, which allow for preservation of the skin envelope and nipple, when indicated to optimize esthetic results without compromising oncologic safety through nipple-sparing mastectomy (NSM).[3,4] The implant technology improved to offer more cohesive and form-stable implants[5] that are particularly beneficial in the reconstructive setting. On the other hand, the association of textured implants with breast implant-associated anaplastic large cell lymphoma (BIA-ALCL)[6,7] changed considerations with implant selection and resulted in the introduction of smooth, tabbed tissue expanders. The use of support materials such as acellular dermal matrix (ADM) helped minimize complications such as capsular contracture[8] and introduced new techniques such as immediate implant[9] and prepectoral reconstruction.[10] Moreover, evidence-based reporting in breast reconstruction has been incorporated within a greater, critical focus on patient-reported outcomes[11] and shared decision-making.[12,13]

The modern approach to implant-breast reconstruction encompasses the evolution in all of these techniques and considerations. In this article, the authors focus specifically on modern mastectomy considerations and how they impact implant-based breast reconstruction, current prosthesis choices and their impact on outcomes, and our current understanding of support materials in implant-based breast reconstruction.

a Division of Plastic and Reconstructive Surgery, University of California, Davis, 2335 Stockton Blvd., NAOB 6th floor, Sacramento, CA 95817, USA; b Hansjörg Wyss Department of Plastic Surgery, New York University Langone Health, 305 East 47th Street, Suite 1A, New York, NY 10017, USA
* Corresponding author.
E-mail address: nolan.karp@nyulangone.org

Clin Plastic Surg 50 (2023) 223–234
https://doi.org/10.1016/j.cps.2022.09.003

MODERN APPROACH TO MASTECTOMY
Mastectomy Flap Quality

The success of implant-based breast reconstruction is tied to the preceding mastectomy. The ablative and reconstructive surgeries, however, should not be considered as sequential events, but instead as interdependent components of the same procedure. The transition to this approach is dictated by the teamwork between the breast surgeon and the plastic surgeon, with proactive communication throughout the preoperative, intraoperative, and postoperative treatment of patients.[2]

A thorough understanding of the lamellar structure of the breast and its fascial system[14] is paramount in interpreting mastectomy flap quality. The corpus mammae are held within an irregular pseudocapsule from the surrounding adipose tissue. A distinct superficial layer of the superficial fascia, also referred to as the anterior lamina fascia, separates a thinner layer of subcutaneous fat from deeper, lobular anterior lamellar fat.[15] These fascial layers, along with the thickness of the subcutaneous tissue, can be visualized on preoperative breast MRI (**Fig. 1**) as well as ultrasound. Preoperative imaging can serve as a useful guide for both the breast and plastic surgeons to estimate the thickness of mastectomy flaps and their implications for implant-based reconstructive choices.

The thickness of the subcutaneous layer of the breast varies significantly among different patients, with an increased body mass index (BMI) correlating with a thicker layer of subcutaneous tissue.[16] Therefore, thick flaps do not necessarily equal well-perfused flaps and vice versa. Instead, the relative thickness of the preoperative subcutaneous layer of the breast to the thickness of the mastectomy flap plays a more important role in predicting perfusion, with ratios less than around 70% associated with ischemic complications of the skin envelope.[17]

The thickness of the subcutaneous layer also varies significantly within each breast, with breast tissue reaching the dermis at the vertical Cooper's ligaments. In this regard, surgical dissection along the appropriate anatomic planes is significantly more important than the absolute thickness of a flap with regard to perfusion. Overall flap thickness can have important implications for esthetic results, especially in prepectoral reconstruction where implant edges and rippling are more visible in thin patients. Aside from relative flap thickness, several other factors are important in assessment of mastectomy flap quality and can be used to predict potential ischemic complications of the skin envelope (**Box 1**).[18] Clinical assessment of incision edge bleeding, preservation of subcutaneous tissue, and the extent of visible dermis and cautery burns are all important variables. Adjunctive imaging modalities such as indocyanine green angiography can be useful tools for perfusion assessment.[19]

Nipple-Sparing Mastectomy

Mastectomy flap quality is particularly important in NSM as perfusion becomes an even more critical factor given the preservation of the entire skin envelope and nipple-areola complex (NAC). NSM has demonstrated equivalent oncologic outcomes[3] and superior esthetic and patient-reported outcomes[4] compared with its traditional mastectomy counterpart. Criteria for oncologic indications for NSM based on tumor-to-nipple distance continue to evolve. Although a 2-cm cutoff was traditionally used, more recent studies have demonstrated similar rates of pathologic nipple involvement[20] and locoregional recurrence[21] with tumor-to-nipple distances (TNDs) less than or equal to 1 cm, whereas other studies have found an increased locoregional recurrence rate below 1 cm.[22] Long-term recurrence rates with different cutoffs and consideration of other tumor characteristics are still needed.

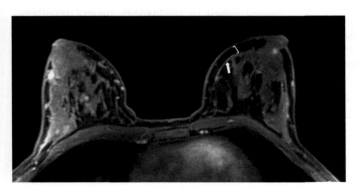

Fig. 1. Preoperative breast MRI can be useful in understanding the fascial layers of the breast and subcutaneous tissue thickness. The white arrow denotes the level of the breast pseudocapsule and the white brackets the thickness of the adipose tissue superficial to the mastectomy plane.

Box 1
Important factors in evaluating mastectomy flap quality

Preservation of subcutaneous tissue on underside of mastectomy flap

Extent of visible dermis

Bleeding at incision edges[a]

Relative mastectomy flap thickness[b]

Extent of electrocautery burns

Visible skin mottling

Adjunctive imaging modalities[a]

[a]Interpretation difficult if epinephrine-containing infiltration utilized.[b]Ratio of preoperative subcutaneous tissue thickness to postmastectomy flap thickness.

Incision planning is a critical component of NSM given its significant implications for esthetic results, perfusion of the skin envelope, and access for oncologic extirpation. Although multiple choices exist, certain trends have become readily apparent with the abundance of literature on this topic. A recent meta-analysis of 9975 NSMs confirmed the increased risk of nipple necrosis with periareolar incisions.[23] Similarly, inverted-T or wise-pattern incisions have also been associated with ischemic complications of the skin envelope[24,25] likely because of more significant disruption of the subdermal plexus and creation of a T-point. The inframammary fold (IMF) incision has become the most widely used NSM incision[23] given its esthetic location and low risk of ischemic skin envelope complications (Fig. 2).[25–27]

Patient selection, and therefore proper assessment of risk factors for complications, also plays an important role in NSM outcomes. Well-known risk factors for postoperative complications include elevated BMI,[26] tobacco use,[28] radiation,[26] and diabetes.[29] Other variables include mastectomy indication, as therapeutic NSMs have also been found to have a higher complication rate than prophylactic NSM[30] as well as reconstructive modality with immediate implant and autologous reconstruction associated with increased complication rates compared with two-stage tissue expander reconstruction.[31] Different risk calculators for complications after mastectomy and reconstruction are available[32,33] and can be particularly useful for preoperative patient counseling.

Increasing breast size as correlated by greater mastectomy weights[34] and ptosis[35] have also been found to be predictors of postoperative complications. NSM has been demonstrated to be safe after breast reduction and mastopexy.[36] Furthermore, staged breast reduction before NSM, originally described by Spear and colleagues,[37] has been found to decrease rates of major mastectomy flap necrosis in these patients (Fig. 3).[38] Immediate reconstruction and concomitant mastopexy has also been described in implant-based reconstruction. Several techniques can be used including the button-hole mastopexy[39,40] and wise and skin reduction patterns[41–44] with the NAC either pedicled on the dermal plexus or transposed as a free graft. Excellent mastectomy flap quality is paramount in these cases to maintain already-compromised perfusion to the NAC that is now being transposed.

MODERN IMPLANT CHOICES

The breast implant technology has undergone a significant evolution since its introduction. Today's line of breast implants are characterized by improved gel-fill ratios, better implant shell design, and increased gel-crosslinking aimed to decrease complications such as rippling, malposition, and gel bleed while improving form stability of implants and subsequently breast esthetics.[45] Several implant characteristics are variable within, and among different manufacturers, including implant cohesivity, texturing, shape, size, and projection.

Implant cohesivity is related to the degree of gel cross-linking and has important implications for shape, form, fill, firmness, and feel.[46] More cohesive implants will have greater form stability and upper pole projection but can feel firmer to patients which may be undesirable.[47] Modern highly cohesive, form-stable implants have been particularly useful in prepectoral breast reconstruction to minimize rippling and improve upper pole fill (Fig. 4),[48] both of which can be more challenging in thinner patients without the additional coverage provided by the pectoralis major. The degree of implant cohesivity should be individualized to each patient and mastectomy defect, importantly discussing all options and involving patients in the selection preoperatively.

The introduction of form-stable implants has also allowed for the development of anatomic, shaped implants that are suggested to provide a more natural appearance. Studies, however, have demonstrated similar postoperative patient satisfaction and quality-of-life metrics between round and shaped implants after breast reconstruction.[49,50] In addition, the association of macrotextured implants with BIA-ALCL[6] has had significant implications for implant choices, favoring the use of smooth, round implants, especially in the breast cancer population. Recent US Food

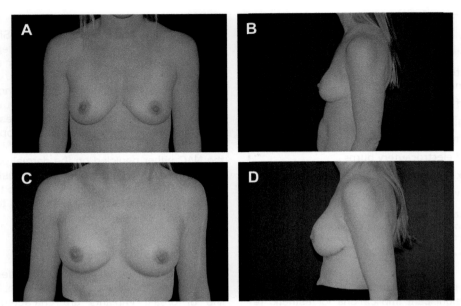

Fig. 2. Nipple-sparing mastectomy with implant-based reconstruction using inframammary fold incisions. Preoperative (A,B) and postoperative (C,D) photos of a 40-year-old woman with staged breast reconstruction with tissue expanders replaced with smooth round moderate profile 265-mL gel implants.

and Drug Administration (FDA) safety requirements for breast implants were also implemented which include a required patient decision checklist and a "black box" warning on all breast implants describing increasing lifetime risks of complications as well as associations with BIA-ALCL and symptoms of breast implant illness.[51] These changes further reinforce the importance of preoperative patient counseling and education for informed, shared decision-making.

SUPPORT MATERIALS IN IMPLANT RECONSTRUCTION
Acellular Dermal Matrix

The introduction of ADM for use in breast reconstruction by Breuing and colleagues ushered in a rapid adoption of ADM-assisted techniques in implant-based reconstructive procedures. "Dual-plane", or partial submuscular reconstruction, remains a widely used technique,[1] in which the ADM is typically used for inferolateral prosthesis coverage after being sutured to the cut edge of the pectoralis major muscle superiorly, and the IMF and anteriorly axillary line inferolaterally (Fig. 5).

In comparison to traditional total submuscular coverage, dual-plane ADM techniques have less morbidity as well as the ability to perform immediate implant reconstructions.[9] Esthetic results have also been suggested to be superior to total submuscular coverage[52,53] given improved control and

expansion of the lower pole (Fig. 6). Although several studies have cited faster tissue expander filling with dual-plane reconstruction,[54,55] these data, in addition to pain outcomes, are conflicting.[56]

The additional benefits of ADM use have also been described including decreasing periprosthetic fibrosis[57-59] and a subsequent association with lower rates of capsular contracture,[8] in addition to a potential protective effect against rippling[60] and radiation fibrosis.[61,62] With the "resurgence" of prepectoral reconstruction, ADM use has further been advocated as a means of defining the breast pocket, supporting the implant, and decreasing the inflammatory processes leading to capsular contracture.[10]

However, the complication profile of ADM cannot be ignored.[63] Certain initial concerns of significantly increased major complication rates with ADM[64] were improved with modifications to ADM processing from aseptic to sterile manufacturing that decreased rates of infection.[65] However, more recent meta-analyses still suggest an increased risk of certain complications with ADM-assisted reconstructions, particularly infection and seroma.[66,67] The significant cost of ADM use must also be considered,[63,68] especially when multiple sheets are needed as with certain prepectoral techniques.

Synthetic Mesh

The use of synthetic mesh in breast reconstruction has stemmed from an effort to decrease cost

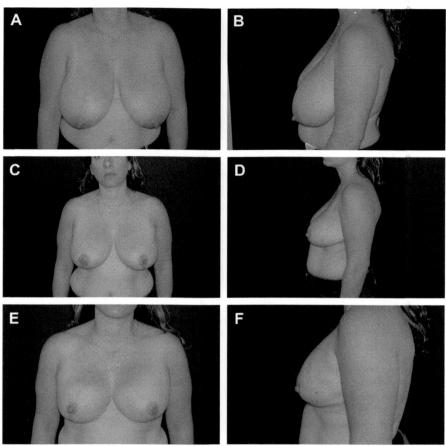

Fig. 3. Nipple-sparing mastectomy with breast reduction before implant-based breast reconstruction. A 38-year-old woman presented for breast reduction (*A, B*). Breast reduction with 380 gm removed on the right and 410 gm removed on the left (*C,D*). The patient subsequently underwent dual-plane NSM and immediate implant reconstruction using smooth high-profile silicone implants (*E,F*).

associated with biologic support materials. Retrospective series using polyglactin 910 in a dual-plane technique have demonstrated low complication rates[69,70] as well as a cost-benefit compared with ADM-assisted reconstruction.[71] Other types of synthetic mesh such as titanium-coated polypropylene have also been extensively studied[72] and demonstrated to have improved complication profiles to ADM in prospective trials.[73]

Synthetic mesh can also be used in conjunction with ADM to decrease cost. This is particularly useful in prepectoral immediate implant reconstruction that can require multiple sheets of ADM. Techniques include laying of ADM within synthetic mesh along the inferolateral border[74] or splitting ADM and synthetic mesh along the inferior and superior aspects of the implant, respectively (**Fig. 7**).[75] These studies have importantly demonstrated the short-term safety profile of synthetic

mesh as well as decreased material costs.[75] Long-term data on capsular contracture will be needed to determine the true utility of synthetic mesh in implant-based reconstruction.

Implant-Based Reconstruction Without Mesh

Since the introduction of biologic and synthetic meshes and the utilization of the prepectoral plane in breast reconstruction, reports of implant placement without support materials have also been described (**Fig. 8**). A recent 10-year series of 250 two-stage prepectoral reconstruction after NSM demonstrated a low short-term complication rate and a 4.0% rate of grade III/IV capsular contracture at an average of 55.5 months of follow-up.[76] The introduction of tabbed tissue expanders and the concept of mastectomy pocket tailoring has further brought into question the need for ADM solely as means of implant support. Recent

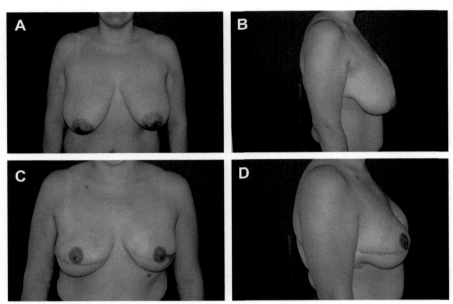

Fig. 4. Breast reconstruction with highly cohesive formal stable implants. Preoperative (*A, B*) and postoperative (*C, D*) photos of a 40-year-old woman with bilateral skin-sparing mastectomy (SSM)and prepectoral immediate implant reconstruction with ADM and vicryl mesh using highly cohesive gel implants: 605 mL. She subsequently had three-dimensional nipple-areola tattoos.

comparative studies in two-stage pectoral reconstruction with and without ADM have demonstrated comparable short-term complication rates[77],[78] as well as similar esthetic results and patient satisfaction with decreased cost.[78]

Immediate implant reconstruction without mesh support has also been described,[79] though much less frequently, likely due to concerns of implant support and control. The use of adipodermal flaps in wise-pattern skin reduction patterns has been suggested as a means of addressing these issues to offload the weight of the implant and define the pocket.[41],[42] Excellent perfusion of the mastectomy flaps with adequate tissue thickness is

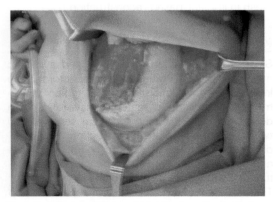

Fig. 5. Intraoperative photograph of dual-plane breast reconstruction with acellular dermal matrix sutured to pectoralis major border.

paramount in such cases, however, to avoid potentially significant complications. A 2021 systematic review of prepectoral reconstruction suggested similar rates of complications between mesh and no-mesh reconstructions, though data were inconclusive given the lack of comparative studies.[80]

Modern Approach to Support Materials

The use of support materials in breast reconstruction has changed significantly over the last 15 years. An initial surge in the use of these materials since their introduction may now be followed by a trend toward more selective usage. This can be attributed to increasing published data on outcomes and complications as well as newer prosthetic devices such as tabbed expanders. Furthermore, in March of 2019, the US FDA Medical Devices Advisory Committee reinforced that surgical mesh, including human-derived ADM, in breast reconstruction was considered nonhomologous use and not cleared or approved by the FDA with a need for further clinical evaluation.[81] This has prompted the use of ADM and synthetic mesh in breast reconstruction to fall under further scrutiny.

The modern approach to support materials in implant-based reconstruction requires an individualized protocol for each patient and mastectomy defect. Multiple variables are taken into account including patient desires, NAC preservation,

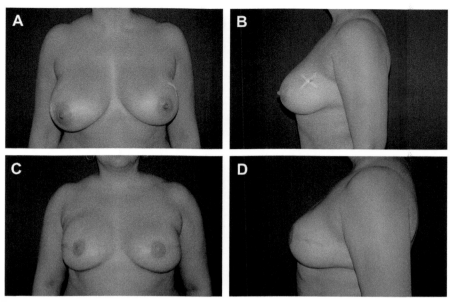

Fig. 6. Implant-based breast reconstruction with dual-plane technique. Preoperative (*A*, *B*) and postoperative (*C*, *D*) photos of a 42-year-old woman with staged dual-plane skin-sparing mastectomy with smooth round gel implants: 700 cc on the right and 750 cc on the left.

current and desired breast size, and intraoperative mastectomy flap thickness and quality. A spectrum of techniques can then be used based on the particular scenario including (1) total submuscular reconstruction, (2) dual-plane reconstruction with ADM, or (3) prepectoral reconstruction with anterior ADM coverage, combined ADM and synthetic mesh, or no support material.

Total submuscular reconstruction confers the most vascularized prosthesis protection in cases of mastectomy flap viability concern, though some may prefer to delay reconstruction all together if submuscular techniques are not preferred by the surgeon or patient. Dual-plane reconstruction allows for immediate implant placement in thinner patients that may otherwise

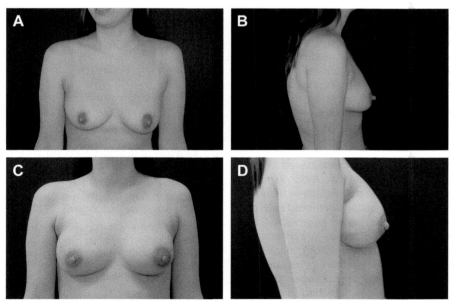

Fig. 7. Immediate implant breast reconstruction in the prepectoral plane with split mesh technique. Preoperative (*A*, *B*) and postoperative (*C*, *D*) photos of a 35 year old with right breast cancer and BRCA1 gene mutation who had NSM with prepectoral DTI using ADM and vicryl mesh and highly cohesive 325 mL implants.

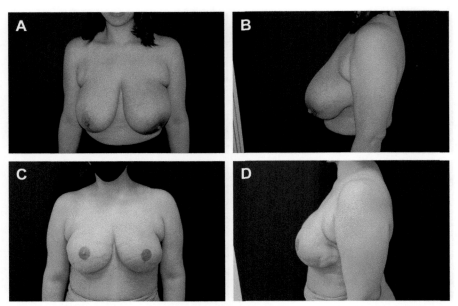

Fig. 8. Two-staged prepectoral breast reconstruction without ADM. Preoperative (*A, B*) and postoperative (*C, D*), photos of a 46 year old with left breast DCIS. The patient underwent skin-sparing mastectomies immediate tissue expander placement in the prepectoral plane without ADM. She subsequently underwent implant exchange to highly cohesive 750 smooth round gel implants. She had nipple reconstruction and tattoos.

have undesirable esthetic sequelae of prepectoral implants. The use of support material in prepectoral reconstruction often falls to surgeon preference, particularly with the advent of tabbed tissue expanders,[77] though most reports of prepectoral immediate implant placement use some form of biologic or synthetic mesh for immediate support.[82–85] Eventually, long-term capsular contracture data on prepectoral reconstruction with and without support will be needed. In the end, the ability to comfortably use any of these techniques and appropriately counsel patients on the risks and benefits of each option will afford the plastic surgeon the greatest ability to individualize results and optimize outcomes.

SUMMARY

The modern approach to implant-based breast reconstruction is a synthesis of evolution in surgical techniques, advancement in material technologies and focus on the patient-centered delivery of care through a team-oriented approach. Successful reconstructive outcomes are intimately tied to mastectomy quality in both skin- and nipple-sparing cases which requires close collaboration with the oncologic surgeon. Current implant models offer a wide selection of choices to optimize esthetic outcomes but continue to have inherent risks that must be thoroughly discussed with patients preoperatively. The use of

support materials in breast reconstruction, such as ADM, is evolving as modern tabbed expanders may not require the same degree of prosthesis support, though further research is necessary to refine indications. Optimizing outcomes requires knowledge of all current techniques and the flexibility to adapt surgical plans to individualize care for each patient undergoing implant-based breast reconstruction.

CLINICS CARE POINTS

- Successful implant-based reconstruction requires close collaboration between the plastic surgeon and breast surgeon with regard to mastectomy and reconstruction planning.
- Relative mastectomy flap thickness and mastectomy flap quality are critical factors in reconstructive outcomes.
- Inframammary fold incisions have the lowest complication rates in nipple-sparing mastectomy and immediate implant-based reconstruction.
- Highly cohesive implants may be particularly beneficial in prepectoral reconstruction to minimize rippling and improve upper pole fill at a tradeoff for increased implant firmness

- Acellular dermal matrix-assisted breast reconstruction has demonstrated low rates of capsular contracture but has also been associated with higher rates of infection and seroma. Further research is needed to refine indications and selective use may be warranted.

DISCLOSURE

Dr Karp owns shares in Surgical Innovations Associates.

REFERENCES

1. ASPS National Clearinghouse of Plastic Surgery Procedural Statistics. Plastic surgery statistics report. 2020. Available at: https://www.plasticsurgery.org/documents/News/Statistics/2020/plastic-surgery-statistics-full-report-2020.pdf. Accessed February 20, 2022.
2. Storm-Dickerson T, Sigalove N. Prepectoral breast reconstruction: the breast surgeon's perspective. Plast Reconstr Surg 2017;140(6S Prepectoral Breast Reconstruction):43S–8S.
3. Adam H, Bygdeson M, de Boniface J. The oncological safety of nipple-sparing mastectomy - a Swedish matched cohort study. Eur J Surg Oncol 2014; 40(10):1209–15.
4. Rossi C, Mingozzi M, Curcio A, et al. Nipple areola complex sparing mastectomy. Gland Surg 2015; 4(6):528–40.
5. Calobrace MB, Capizzi PJ. The biology and evolution of cohesive gel and shaped implants. Plast Reconstr Surg 2014;134(1 Suppl):6S–11S.
6. Clemens MW, Brody GS, Mahabir RC, et al. How to diagnose and treat breast implant-associated anaplastic large cell lymphoma. Plast Reconstr Surg 2018;141(4):586e–99e.
7. Rastogi P, Riordan E, Moon D, et al. Theories of etiopathogenesis of breast implant-associated anaplastic large cell lymphoma. Plast Reconstr Surg 2019;143(3S A Review of Breast Implant-Associated Anaplastic Large Cell Lymphoma): 23S–9S.
8. Salzberg CA, Ashikari AY, Koch RM, et al. An 8-year experience of direct-to-implant immediate breast reconstruction using human acellular dermal matrix (AlloDerm). Plast Reconstr Surg 2011;127(2): 514–24.
9. Choi M, Frey JD, Alperovich M, et al. Breast in a day": examining single-stage immediate, permanent implant reconstruction in nipple-sparing mastectomy. Plast Reconstr Surg 2016;138(2):184e–91e.
10. Sbitany H. Important considerations for performing prepectoral breast reconstruction. Plast Reconstr Surg 2017;140(6S Prepectoral Breast Reconstruction):7S–13S.
11. Pfob A, Mehrara BJ, Nelson JA, et al. Towards patient-centered decision-making in breast cancer surgery: machine learning to predict individual patient-reported outcomes at 1-year follow-up. Ann Surg 2021. https://doi.org/10.1097/SLA.0000000000004862. Online ahead of print.
12. Momoh AO, Griffith KA, Hawley ST, et al. Patterns and correlates of knowledge, communication, and receipt of breast reconstruction in a modern population-based cohort of patients with breast cancer. Plast Reconstr Surg 2019;144(2):303–13.
13. Lee CN, Ubel PA, Deal AM, et al. How informed is the decision about breast reconstruction after mastectomy?: a prospective, cross-sectional study. Ann Surg 2016;264(6):1103–9.
14. Duncan AM, Al Youha S, Joukhadar N, et al. Anatomy of the breast fascial system: a systematic review of the literature. Plast Reconstr Surg 2022; 149(1):28–40.
15. Rehnke RD, Groening RM, Van Buskirk ER, et al. Anatomy of the superficial fascia system of the breast: a comprehensive theory of breast fascial anatomy. Plast Reconstr Surg 2018;142(5): 1135–44.
16. Frey JD, Salibian AA, Choi M, et al. Optimizing outcomes in nipple-sparing mastectomy: mastectomy flap thickness is not one size fits all. Plast Reconstr Surg Glob Open 2019;7(1):e2103.
17. Frey JD, Salibian AA, Choi M, et al. Mastectomy flap thickness and complications in nipple-sparing mastectomy: objective evaluation using magnetic resonance imaging. Plast Reconstr Surg Glob Open 2017;5(8):e1439.
18. Frey JD, Salibian AA, Bekisz JM, et al. What is in a number? Evaluating a risk assessment tool in immediate breast reconstruction. Plast Reconstr Surg Glob Open 2019;7(12):e2585.
19. Diep GK, Hui JY, Marmor S, et al. Postmastectomy reconstruction outcomes after intraoperative evaluation with indocyanine green angiography versus clinical assessment. Ann Surg Oncol 2016;23(12): 4080–5.
20. Dent BL, Miller JA, Eden DJ, et al. Tumor-to-Nipple distance as a predictor of nipple involvement: expanding the inclusion criteria for nipple-sparing mastectomy. Plast Reconstr Surg 2017;140(1): 1e–8e.
21. Wu ZY, Kim HJ, Lee J, et al. Recurrence outcomes after nipple-sparing mastectomy and immediate breast reconstruction in patients with pure ductal carcinoma in situ. Ann Surg Oncol 2020;27(5): 1627–35.
22. Frey JD, Salibian AA, Lee J, et al. Oncologic trends, outcomes, and risk factors for locoregional recurrence: an analysis of tumor-to-nipple distance

and critical factors in therapeutic nipple-sparing mastectomy. Plast Reconstr Surg 2019;143(6): 1575–85.

23. Daar DA, Abdou SA, Rosario L, et al. Is there a preferred incision location for nipple-sparing mastectomy? A systematic review and meta-analysis. Plast Reconstr Surg 2019;143(5):906e–19e.

24. Munhoz AM, Aldrighi CM, Montag E, et al. Clinical outcomes following nipple-areola-sparing mastectomy with immediate implant-based breast reconstruction: a 12-year experience with an analysis of patient and breast-related factors for complications. Breast Cancer Res Treat 2013;140(3):545–55.

25. Frey JD, Salibian AA, Levine JP, et al. Incision choices in nipple-sparing mastectomy: a comparative analysis of outcomes and evolution of a clinical algorithm. Plast Reconstr Surg 2018;142(6): 826e–35e.

26. Colwell AS, Tessler O, Lin AM, et al. Breast reconstruction following nipple-sparing mastectomy: predictors of complications, reconstruction outcomes, and 5-year trends. Plast Reconstr Surg 2014; 133(3):496–506.

27. Donovan CA, Harit AP, Chung A, et al. Oncological and surgical outcomes after nipple-sparing mastectomy: do incisions matter? Ann Surg Oncol 2016; 23(10):3226–31.

28. McCarthy CM, Mehrara BJ, Riedel E, et al. Predicting complications following expander/implant breast reconstruction: an outcomes analysis based on preoperative clinical risk. Plast Reconstr Surg 2008; 121(6):1886–92.

29. Matsen CB, Mehrara B, Eaton A, et al. Skin flap necrosis after mastectomy with reconstruction: a prospective study. Ann Surg Oncol 2016;23(1):257–64.

30. Frey JD, Salibian AA, Karp NS, et al. Comparing therapeutic versus prophylactic nipple-sparing mastectomy: does indication inform oncologic and reconstructive outcomes? Plast Reconstr Surg 2018;142(2):306–15.

31. Frey JD, Choi M, Salibian AA, et al. Comparison of outcomes with tissue expander, immediate implant, and autologous breast reconstruction in greater than 1000 nipple-sparing mastectomies. Plast Reconstr Surg 2017;139(6):1300–10.

32. Frey JD, Salibian AA, Choi M, et al. Putting together the pieces: development and validation of a risk-assessment model for nipple-sparing mastectomy. Plast Reconstr Surg 2020;145(2):273e–83e.

33. Naoum GE, Ho AY, Shui A, et al. Risk of developing breast reconstruction complications: a machine-learning nomogram for individualized risk estimation with and without postmastectomy radiation therapy. Plast Reconstr Surg 2022;149(1):1e–12e.

34. Frey JD, Salibian AA, Karp NS, et al. The impact of mastectomy weight on reconstructive trends and outcomes in nipple-sparing mastectomy:

progressively greater complications with larger breast size. Plast Reconstr Surg 2018;141(6): 795e–804e.

35. De Vita R, Zoccali G, Buccheri EM, et al. Outcome evaluation after 2023 nipple-sparing mastectomies: our experience. Plast Reconstr Surg 2017;139(2): 335e–47e.

36. Alperovich M, Tanna N, Samra F, et al. Nipple-sparing mastectomy in patients with a history of reduction mammaplasty or mastopexy: how safe is it? Plast Reconstr Surg 2013;131(5):962–7.

37. Spear SL, Rottman SJ, Seiboth LA, et al. Breast reconstruction using a staged nipple-sparing mastectomy following mastopexy or reduction. Plast Reconstr Surg 2012;129(3):572–81.

38. Salibian AA, Frey JD, Karp NS, et al. Does staged breast reduction before nipple-sparing mastectomy decrease complications? A matched cohort study between staged and nonstaged techniques. Plast Reconstr Surg 2019;144(5):1023–32.

39. Salibian AH, Harness JK, Mowlds DS. Primary buttonhole mastopexy and nipple-sparing mastectomy: a preliminary report. Ann Plast Surg 2016; 77(4):388–95.

40. Movassaghi K, Stewart CN. The "smile mastopexy": a novel technique to aesthetically address the excess skin envelope in large, ptotic breasts while preserving nipple areolar complex during prosthetic breast reconstruction. Aesthet Surg J 2022;42(6): NP393–403.

41. Safran T, Al-Halabi B, Viezel-Mathieu A, et al. Skin-reducing mastectomy with immediate prepectoral reconstruction: surgical, aesthetic, and patient-reported outcomes with and without dermal matrices. Plast Reconstr Surg 2021;147(5):1046–57.

42. Mosharrafa AM, Mosharrafa TM, Zannis VJ. Direct-to-Implant breast reconstruction with simultaneous nipple-sparing mastopexy utilizing an inferiorly based adipodermal flap: our experience with prepectoral and subpectoral techniques. Plast Reconstr Surg 2020;145(5):1125–33.

43. Manrique OJ, Banuelos J, Abu-Ghname A, et al. Surgical outcomes of prepectoral versus subpectoral implant-based breast reconstruction in young women. Plast Reconstr Surg Glob Open 2019;7(3):e2119.

44. Aliotta RE, Scomacao I, Duraes EFR, et al. Pushing the envelope: skin-only mastopexy in single-stage nipple-sparing mastectomy with direct-to-implant breast reconstruction. Plast Reconstr Surg 2021; 147(1):38–45.

45. Chang EI, Hammond DC. Clinical results on innovation in breast implant design. Plast Reconstr Surg 2018;142(4S The Science of Breast Implants): 31S–8S.

46. Salibian AA, Karp NS. Cohesive implants in revisionary breast reconstruction: strategies for optimizing aesthetic outcomes. Ann Breast Surg 2020;4.

47. Ram E, Lavee J, Freimark D, et al. Improved long-term outcomes after heart transplantation utilizing donors with a traumatic mode of brain death. J Cardiothorac Surg 2019;14(1):138.

48. Sbitany H, Lee KR. Optimizing outcomes in 2-stage prepectoral breast reconstruction utilizing round form-stable implants. Plast Reconstr Surg 2019; 144(1S Utilizing a Spectrum of Cohesive Implants in Aesthetic and Reconstructive Breast Surgery): 43S–50S.

49. Khavanin N, Clemens MW, Pusic AL, et al. Shaped versus round implants in breast reconstruction: a multi-institutional comparison of surgical and patient-reported outcomes. Plast Reconstr Surg 2017;139(5):1063–70.

50. Macadam SA, Ho AL, Lennox PA, et al. Patient-reported satisfaction and health-related quality of life following breast reconstruction: a comparison of shaped cohesive gel and round cohesive gel implant recipients. Plast Reconstr Surg 2013;131(3):431–41.

51. U.S. Food and Drug Administration. Breast implants. 2021. Available at: https://www.fda.gov/medical-devices/implants-and-prosthetics/breast-implants. Accessed March 12, 2022.

52. Vardanian AJ, Clayton JL, Roostaeian J, et al. Comparison of implant-based immediate breast reconstruction with and without acellular dermal matrix. Plast Reconstr Surg 2011;128(5):403e–10e.

53. DeLong MR, Tandon VJ, Farajzadeh M, et al. Systematic review of the impact of acellular dermal matrix on aesthetics and patient satisfaction in tissue expander-to-implant breast reconstructions. Plast Reconstr Surg 2019;144(6):967e–74e.

54. Sbitany H, Sandeen SN, Amalfi AN, et al. Acellular dermis-assisted prosthetic breast reconstruction versus complete submuscular coverage: a head-to-head comparison of outcomes. Plast Reconstr Surg 2009;124(6):1735–40.

55. Sbitany H, Serletti JM. Acellular dermis-assisted prosthetic breast reconstruction: a systematic and critical review of efficacy and associated morbidity. Plast Reconstr Surg 2011;128(6):1162–9.

56. McCarthy CM, Lee CN, Halvorson EG, et al. The use of acellular dermal matrices in two-stage expander/ implant reconstruction: a multicenter, blinded, randomized controlled trial. Plast Reconstr Surg 2012; 130(5 Suppl 2):57S–66S.

57. Stump A, Holton LH 3rd, Connor J, et al. The use of acellular dermal matrix to prevent capsule formation around implants in a primate model. Plast Reconstr Surg 2009;124(1):82–91.

58. Basu CB, Leong M, Hicks MJ. Acellular cadaveric dermis decreases the inflammatory response in capsule formation in reconstructive breast surgery. Plast Reconstr Surg 2010;126(6):1842–7.

59. Tevlin R, Borrelli MR, Irizarry D, et al. Acellular dermal matrix reduces myofibroblast presence in the breast capsule. Plast Reconstr Surg Glob Open 2019;7(5):e2213.

60. Nahabedian MY, Glasberg SB, Maxwell GP. Introduction to "prepectoral breast reconstruction. Plast Reconstr Surg 2017;140(6S Prepectoral Breast Reconstruction):4S–5S.

61. Komorowska-Timek E, Oberg KC, Timek TA, et al. The effect of AlloDerm envelopes on periprosthetic capsule formation with and without radiation. Plast Reconstr Surg 2009;123(3):807–16.

62. Sbitany H, Wang F, Peled AW, et al. Immediate implant-based breast reconstruction following total skin-sparing mastectomy: defining the risk of preoperative and postoperative radiation therapy for surgical outcomes. Plast Reconstr Surg 2014;134(3): 396–404.

63. Ivey JS, Abdollahi H, Herrera FA, et al. Total muscle coverage versus AlloDerm human dermal matrix for implant-based breast reconstruction. Plast Reconstr Surg 2019;143(1):1–6.

64. Weichman KE, Wilson SC, Weinstein AL, et al. The use of acellular dermal matrix in immediate two-stage tissue expander breast reconstruction. Plast Reconstr Surg 2012;129(5):1049–58.

65. Weichman KE, Wilson SC, Saadeh PB, et al. Sterile "ready-to-use" AlloDerm decreases postoperative infectious complications in patients undergoing immediate implant-based breast reconstruction with acellular dermal matrix. Plast Reconstr Surg 2013; 132(4):725–36.

66. Zhao X, Wu X, Dong J, et al. A meta-analysis of postoperative complications of tissue expander/implant breast reconstruction using acellular dermal matrix. Aesthet Plast Surg 2015;39(6):892–901.

67. Lee KT, Mun GH. Updated evidence of acellular dermal matrix use for implant-based breast reconstruction: a meta-analysis. Ann Surg Oncol 2016; 23(2):600–10.

68. de Blacam C, Momoh AO, Colakoglu S, et al. Cost analysis of implant-based breast reconstruction with acellular dermal matrix. Ann Plast Surg 2012; 69(5):516–20.

69. Haynes DF, Kreithen JC. Vicryl mesh in expander/ implant breast reconstruction: long-term follow-up in 38 patients. Plast Reconstr Surg 2014;134(5): 892–9.

70. Meyer Ganz O, Tobalem M, Perneger T, et al. Risks and benefits of using an absorbable mesh in one-stage immediate breast reconstruction: a comparative study. Plast Reconstr Surg 2015;135(3): 498e–507e.

71. Tessler O, Reish RG, Maman DY, et al. Beyond biologics: absorbable mesh as a low-cost, low-complication sling for implant-based breast reconstruction. Plast Reconstr Surg 2014;133(2):90e–9e.

72. Dieterich M, Paepke S, Zwiefel K, et al. Implant-based breast reconstruction using a titanium-

coated polypropylene mesh (TiLOOP Bra): a multi-center study of 231 cases. Plast Reconstr Surg 2013;132(1):8e–19e.

73. Gschwantler-Kaulich D, Schrenk P, Bjelic-Radisic V, et al. Mesh versus acellular dermal matrix in immediate implant-based breast reconstruction - a prospective randomized trial. Eur J Surg Oncol 2016; 42(5):665–71.

74. Gfrerer L, Liao EC. Technique refinement in prepectoral implant breast reconstruction with vicryl mesh pocket and acellular dermal matrix support. Plast Reconstr Surg Glob Open 2018;6(4):e1749.

75. Karp NS, Salibian AA. Splitting the difference: using synthetic and biologic mesh to decrease cost in prepectoral immediate implant breast reconstruction. Plast Reconstr Surg 2021;147(3):580–4.

76. Salibian AH, Harness JK, Mowlds DS. Staged suprapectoral expander/implant reconstruction without acellular dermal matrix following nipple-sparing mastectomy. Plast Reconstr Surg 2017;139(1):30–9.

77. Salibian AA, Bekisz JM, Kussie HC, et al. Do we need support in prepectoral breast reconstruction? Comparing outcomes with and without ADM. Plast Reconstr Surg Glob Open 2021;9(8):e3745.

78. Manrique OJ, Huang TC, Martinez-Jorge J, et al. Prepectoral two-stage implant-based breast reconstruction with and without acellular dermal matrix: do we see a difference? Plast Reconstr Surg 2020; 145(2):263e–72e.

79. Viezel-Mathieu A, Alnaif N, Aljerian A, et al. Acellular dermal matrix-sparing direct-to-implant prepectoral breast reconstruction: a comparative study including cost analysis. Ann Plast Surg 2020;84(2): 139–43.

80. DeLong MR, Tandon VJ, Bertrand AA, et al. Review of outcomes in prepectoral prosthetic breast reconstruction with and without surgical mesh assistance. Plast Reconstr Surg 2021;147(2):305–15.

81. Committee USFaDAGaPSDPotMDA. Available at: https://www.fda.gov/media/122962/download. Accessed February 20, 2022.

82. Jafferbhoy S, Chandarana M, Houlihan M, et al. Early multicentre experience of pre-pectoral implant based immediate breast reconstruction using Braxon((R)). Gland Surg 2017;6(6):682–8.

83. Jones G, Yoo A, King V, et al. Prepectoral immediate direct-to-implant breast reconstruction with anterior AlloDerm coverage. Plast Reconstr Surg 2017; 140(6S):31S–8S. Prepectoral Breast Reconstruction).

84. Reitsamer R, Peintinger F. Prepectoral implant placement and complete coverage with porcine acellular dermal matrix: a new technique for direct-to-implant breast reconstruction after nipple-sparing mastectomy. J Plast Reconstr Aesthet Surg 2015;68(2):162–7.

85. Becker H, Lind JG 2nd, Hopkins EG. Immediate implant-based prepectoral breast reconstruction using a vertical incision. Plast Reconstr Surg Glob Open 2015;3(6):e412.

Prepectoral Breast Reconstruction

Francis D. Graziano, MD, Jocelyn Lu, MD, Hani Sbitany, MD*

KEYWORDS

- Prepectoral breast reconstruction • Breast reconstruction • Acellular dermal matrix
- Implant-based reconstruction

KEY POINTS

- Prepectoral breast reconstruction has become a popular method of postmastectomy breast reconstruction due to its numerous benefits in properly selected patients.
- Prepectoral reconstruction, as compared with retropectoral position, provides the benefit of leaving the pectoralis major muscle in its anatomic position, resulting in decreased acute and chronic pain, avoidance of animation deformity, and improved upper extremity strength.
- Careful patient selection and intraoperative mastectomy flap evaluation are critical to obtaining optimal results in prepectoral breast reconstruction.
- Acellular dermal matrices allow for control of the breast envelope and implant position, resulting in high levels of patient satisfaction and esthetic outcomes.

INTRODUCTION

Implant-based reconstruction continues to be the most commonly performed procedure for postmastectomy breast reconstruction in the United States, with over 103,000 cases performed in 2020.[1,2] Traditional methods of submuscular or partial submuscular/partial acellular dermal matrix (ADM) (dual-plane) are still commonly used.[3] Although the submuscular implant reconstruction technique offers the benefit of reliable vascularized coverage, it disrupts the native anatomy of the chest wall. This is due to the elevation and often disinsertion of the pectoralis major muscle during implant pocket creation. Prepectoral breast reconstruction involves placement of the breast implant or tissue expander above the pectoralis and serratus muscles, thus leaving the chest wall muscles in their original positions.[4] The reported benefits of the prepectoral breast reconstruction technique include decreased acute and chronic postoperative pain, avoidance of animation deformity, precise control of the implant pocket, and high levels of patient satisfaction.[5,6] Also, prepectoral reconstruction technique avoids enveloping the implant in the pectoralis muscle, which can become fibrotic and tight, especially in the setting of postmastectomy radiation.[7] The fibrotic pectoralis muscle can cause translational force on the implant leading to malposition and capsular contracture.[7] As the prosthesis is placed closer to the skin with less vascularized soft tissue coverage, it is critical for the surgeon to assess preoperative and perioperative factors to ensure optimal outcomes. Through proper patient selection and ideal surgical technique, prepectoral breast reconstruction can be performed with high esthetic and patient satisfaction while also minimizing patient morbidity.

PREOPERATIVE CONSIDERATIONS
Patient Selection

As with any operation, patient selection is critical for optimal results. A full assessment of the patient's past medical and surgical history should be performed with particular attention to conditions that can affect wound healing and

Division of Plastic and Reconstructive Surgery, Department of Surgery, Icahn School of Medicine at Mount Sinai, New York, NY, USA
* Corresponding author. 425 West 59th Street, 7th Floor, New York, NY 10019.
E-mail address: Hani.Sbitany@mountsinai.org

Clin Plastic Surg 50 (2023) 235–242
https://doi.org/10.1016/j.cps.2022.09.004
0094-1298/23/© 2022 Elsevier Inc. All rights reserved.

mastectomy vascular supply. Conditions that can impair mastectomy flap perfusion include peripheral vascular disease, diabetes, preoperative radiation, smoking, and obesity. Conditions that may cause delayed wound healing include immunosuppression, steroid use, and connective tissue disorders (ie, Ehlers-Danlos). Poorly controlled diabetes (hemoglobin A1c > 7.0), obesity (body mass index [BMI] greater than 35), and active/recent smoking are considered contraindications to prepectoral breast reconstruction and are associated with an increased risk of mastectomy flap necrosis and implant infection or extrusion.[8]

Although prepectoral breast reconstruction is typically used in the immediate setting after mastectomy, prepectoral technique can also be considered in a delayed fashion. Most commonly, this is seen in the group of patients who underwent a prior mastectomy and submuscular implant reconstruction, and now present with complaints of chronic pain, capsular contracture, and/or animation deformity. In these patients, the implant can be converted from subpectoral to prepectoral position, often with the aid of ADM for implant support. These patients largely have immediate relief of animation deformity and improved pain.[6] Lastly, patients who underwent no reconstruction at the time of mastectomy can be candidates for prepectoral reconstruction. In this group of patients, the mastectomy flaps have undergone the delay phenomena, and therefore raising these mastectomy flaps with placement of prepectoral tissue expander or implant can be performed relatively reliably.

Radiation status
Another important consideration is the radiation status of the patient. Patients who underwent preoperative radiation therapy have an increased risk of dehiscence and wound healing complications due to impaired microcirculation.[9] In our opinion, these patients typically benefit from autologous rather than prepectoral implant-based reconstruction. However, in contrast, patients who are planning to receive postmastectomy radiation therapy (PMRT) can be considered for prepectoral breast reconstruction. Although rates of complications are increased in patients who undergo PMRT after prepectoral reconstruction, they are similar to complication rates in patients undergoing submuscular implant reconstruction with PMRT.[10,11] In fact, some authors have suggested that prepectoral breast reconstruction in the setting of PMRT significantly decreases the rate of capsular contracture and implant migration when compared with submuscular reconstruction.[12,13] As such, prepectoral

breast reconstruction can be considered in this subset of patients who require PMRT, as prepectoral reconstruction allows for potentially more predictable esthetic outcomes following radiation.

Oncologic considerations
In addition to assessing patient-specific comorbidities, oncologic considerations should be analyzed preoperatively. From a tumor-specific standpoint, patients with tumors that invade the chest wall fascia or come within 0.5 cm of the chest wall are contraindicated for prepectoral breast reconstruction.[14] Given the location of the tumor, these patients have a higher chance of chest wall recurrence.[15] If prepectoral reconstruction was to be performed in patients with chest wall tumors, recurrence would be difficult to detect due to the overlying breast implant. Therefore, patients with chest wall tumors or tumors within 0.5 cm of the chest wall should be considered for submuscular reconstruction. Submuscular implant-based reconstruction allows for the chest wall to be more easily palpated by self-exam or on clinical exam.

Additional oncologic considerations include inflammatory breast cancer, patients with stage IV breast cancer, or patients with the aggressive axillary disease. These disease processes are relative contraindications to prepectoral breast reconstruction given their needs for aggressive adjuvant therapy.[16] Lastly, although not a contraindication to prepectoral breast reconstruction, superficial tumors can lead to varying amounts of skin resection, which can lead to distortion of the mastectomy skin envelope and subsequent abnormal implant positioning. Planned skin pattern resection and resultant esthetic outcomes should be discussed with the patient preoperatively to set expectations.

Infection control
Special attention should be given to preventing postoperative infections in prepectoral breast reconstruction. Without vascularized muscle coverage over the implant, postoperative infection can threaten implant loss. Patients should have nasal swabs for Methicillin-resistant *Staphylococcus aureus* (MRSA), and if positive, topical mupirocin is recommended for decolonization.[17] All patients, regardless of MRSA status, are recommended to perform Hibilcens showers the night before surgery. On the day of surgery, intravenous Ancef (or Clindamycin for patients with allergies) should be injected within 60 minutes of incision to decrease the rate of surgical site infections.

INTRAOPERATIVE TECHNIQUES
Intraoperative Mastectomy Flap Assessment

It is critical to examine the soft tissue of the mastectomy skin following completion of the mastectomy before proceeding with prepectoral reconstruction. Mastectomy flaps must be assessed for adequate perfusion and viability. This process starts with a clinical examination of the mastectomy, assessing for dermal bleeding at the mastectomy flap margin and the presence of subcutaneous tissue along the underside of the mastectomy flap. Presence of subcutaneous tissue on the mastectomy flap indicates the preservation of the subdermal plexus, and is more likely to be well perfused. Areas with exposed dermis on the underside require caution and careful clinical consideration, depending on the area. If near the mastectomy flap margin then the authors opt to excise these portions. However, if areas of exposed dermis are not easily amenable to excision, then the authors typically prefer to delay the reconstruction to allow for the mastectomy flaps to revascularize and recover. Delayed prepectoral breast reconstruction can then take place typically at a minimum of 3 weeks after the mastectomy. Another option in the setting of exposed dermis on the underside of the skin flap is subpectoral reconstruction if this is deemed safe and aligns with the patient's goals.

Although thicker mastectomy flaps can often signify improved vascularity, thin flaps do not necessarily mean a poorly perfused flap. Patients with thinner body habitus and lower BMI often have a thinner layer of subcutaneous tissue before the breast capsule.[18] Therefore, in this patient population, thin mastectomy flaps are expected and often have adequate perfusion.

In cases where patients have thin but viable mastectomy flaps, the senior author suggests performing two-stage breast reconstruction with tissue expanders. In these cases, tissue expanders are placed with minimal to no fill, therefore decreasing the amount of tension and stretch on the skin. This can result in less venous congestion relative to aggressive tissue expander fill or large direct to implant placement.[19]

In addition, perfusion assessment devices can provide useful information regarding mastectomy skin flap perfusion.[20–22] Most commonly used perfusion devices often use indocyanine green angiography and allow for real-time assessment of mastectomy flap perfusion. These devices allow for the assessment of nonviable areas which allows for direct excision at the time of immediate reconstruction.[23] The perfusion data can also be used to inform the decision to proceed with either prepectoral or subpectoral reconstruction. These devices can be useful adjuncts to clinical examination.

Acellular Dermal Matrices Use

Proper utilization of ADMs for implant support and breast pocket control has become an essential aspect of successful prepectoral breast reconstruction.[24] Advocates for using ADM in prepectoral reconstruction cite higher rates of implant exposure and capsular contracture in cases where implants are placed subcutaneously without ADM support.[25] The advent of ADM use has made prepectoral breast reconstruction safer with a decreased inflammatory response to implant placement, thus improving esthetic results.[26] Prior studies have shown that prepectoral breast reconstruction with ADM is equally safe as subpectoral reconstruction.[27,28]

Various ADM products exist on the market with different qualities including meshing and thickness. The senior author of this study prefers thin ADM for prepectoral reconstruction due to improved engraftment with the mastectomy skin flaps. Studies have found that the use of thicker ADMs can lead to higher rates of seroma, longer need for drains, and decreased rates of engraftment.[29,30] For this reason, we recommend using ADM sheets with a maximal thickness of 2 mm, or thinner, for soft tissue support in prepectoral reconstruction.

ADM allows for precise control of the boundaries of the reconstruction and therefore it is critical to identify anatomic borders of the breast. Although it is the breast surgeon's primary objective to provide oncologic safety, it can be common for the breast surgeon to remove soft tissue beyond the borders of the breast. In these cases, it is important to use preoperative markings along with manual palpation to identify the original inframammary fold (IMF), medial, lateral, and superior borders of the breast. After borders of the breast have been identified, then ADM can be used to re-establish these borders of the reconstructed breast.

ADM is used to cover the entire anterior surface and varying amounts of the posterior surface based on the surgeon's preferred technique.[31–33] The senior author recommends using a two-layer cuff technique at the inferior aspect of the implant to bolster the recreated IMF (**Fig. 1**). This technique is performed by placing the most inferior portion of the ADM posterior to the inferior aspect of the implant and suturing the ADM to the chest wall. Then as the ADM transitions from the posterior to the anterior aspect of the implant, the most

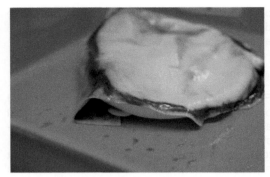

Fig. 1. Senior author's preferred method of ADM inset for anterior implant coverage, showing the two-layer cuff technique at the inferior aspect of the implant.

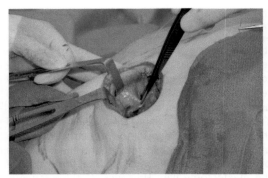

Fig. 3. After the implant is placed in the ADM pocket, the two-layer cuff is created by placing the most inferior portion of the ADM posterior to the inferior aspect of the implant and suturing the ADM to the chest wall. Roughly a 2 to 3 cm cuff of ADM is placed posterior to the implant.

inferior portion of the sling is sutured to the chest wall. This double cuff at the IMF helps ensure long-term support at the IMF and decreases the risk of implant descent.[8] In the case of nipple-sparing mastectomy through an inframammary approach, the superior and lateral/medial aspects of the ADM are inset in place, followed by implant placement and two-layer cuff creation (Figs. 2–6). In the case of skin-sparing mastectomy, the two-layer cuff is created first, then the lateral, medial, and superior borders of the ADM are fixated in place after implant placement. In both ADM inset techniques, the whole anterior aspect of the implant is covered with ADM. ADM inset allows for precise control of the reconstructed breast pocket and can result in long-term esthetic results (Fig. 7A and B).

Larger amounts of ADM are used in prepectoral reconstruction when compared with dual-plane reconstruction. This is of particular importance as ADM has been found to have higher rates of

seroma postoperatively.[34,35] Consideration must be given to proper drain management to prevent seromas and allow for incorporation of ADM with surrounding soft tissues. The senior recommends leaving at least one drain in place for 2 to 3 weeks. In the case of larger breasts, two drains can be placed, one drain in the potential space between the mastectomy flap and the ADM and one drain in the breast pocket. It may be beneficial to use ADM with fenestrations to allow for fluid egress and prevention of seroma formation.[36]

Preventing and Addressing Postoperative Rippling

An issue that can arise postoperatively in implant-based reconstruction is the occurrence of rippling.[37] This can be an issue in prepectoral reconstruction, where the upper pole cannot be buffered underneath the pectoralis muscle. Placement of ADM itself can help provide additional soft tissue coverage and potentially prevent implant

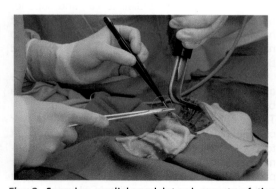

Fig. 2. Superior, medial, and lateral aspects of the ADM are inset first in the case of a nipple sparing mastectomy.

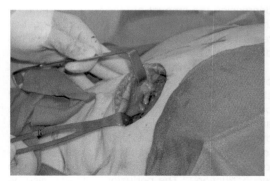

Fig. 4. Superior aspect of the cuff can be seen sutured to the chest wall.

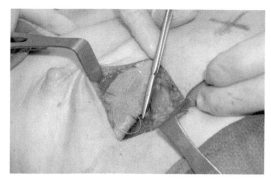

Fig. 5. Most inferior aspect of the ADM is then sutured in place.

rippling, especially in low BMI patients with thin mastectomy flaps.[38] The senior author has three main techniques to both address and prevent implant rippling. First, in the setting of two-stage breast reconstruction, it is advisable to underfill the tissue expander relative to the anticipated final implant size. In the senior author's practice, the final volume of the tissue expander is, on average, 150 to 200 cc less than the estimated implant volume. This technique is performed so that the permanent implant is placed in a tight breast envelope, therefore minimizing rippling in the final reconstruction.

Second, implant selection with regard to implant cohesivity and base width is critical for preventing implant rippling. The senior author's preference is to use a smooth, round, filled to capacity silicone implant with high cohesivity. High-capacity fill decreases the amount of rippling on the implant surface which translates to decrease visible rippling externally in the final reconstruction. It is also important to select an implant with a base width that closely matches the base width dimension of the ADM pocket. Implants that have base

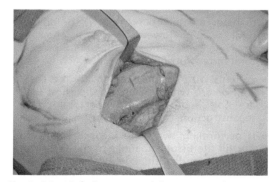

Fig. 6. Most inferior aspect of the ADM can been seen sutured to chest wall. At this point, the ADM is fully inset to the chest wall.

widths that are narrower than the ADM base width pocket are more susceptible to rippling. Choosing an implant with high cohesivity can also mitigate the potential for postoperative rippling.

Third and lastly, fat grafting can be used as an adjunctive procedure in prepectoral breast reconstruction. Fat grafting can help increase mastectomy flap thickness, especially in the upper pole, and subsequently decrease visible rippling.[39,40] This technique also has the benefit of improving upper pole contour, which may be an issue in prepectoral reconstruction. As the pectoralis muscle is not draping over the superior aspect of the implant, patients can develop an abrupt, unnatural transition from the chest wall to implant. Fat grafting to the area can improve this transition between the chest wall and implant while also reducing any rippling that may be present. In the senior author's experience, fat grafting can typically be performed at the time of tissue expander to implant exchange. These three techniques can be used to both prevent and address potential postoperative rippling in prepectoral reconstruction.

POSTOPERATIVE CONSIDERATIONS AND COMPLICATIONS
Postoperative Dressings

Postoperative dressings are typically based on surgeon preference. The senior author recommends reinforcing the skin closure with a watertight dressing, either surgical skin glue or steri-strips. This can be further reinforced with a nonadherent gauze bandage and semiocclusive dressing. Drain site dressings have been a topic of debate, with a recent study showing no decrease in infectious complications in immediate tissue expander reconstruction with use of Biopatch drain cover (Ethicon, Somerville, NJ).[41] Whether to use a drain dressing or not is a surgeon-dependent issue.

Infections

As with any implant-based reconstruction, surgical site infections require immediate attention. This is especially true in prepectoral breast reconstruction. With no pectoralis muscle, any breakdown of the skin can lead to ADM and implant exposure. Patients with suspected surgical site infections should be given oral antibiotics and followed closely as an outpatient. If a patient develops any systematic symptoms or has signs of a threatened implant exposure then the patient requires immediate surgical debridement, threatened skin excision, implant exchange, and intravenous antibiotics. It is critical to treat possible

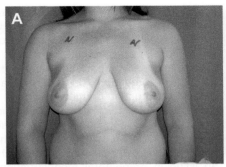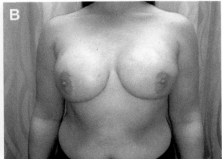

Fig. 7. (*A*) A 38-year-old woman presented with BRCA 1 positive status, and made a decision to undergo bilateral nipple-sparing mastectomies. She desired a large size postoperatively, and thus underwent bilateral prepectoral tissue expander placement. Mastectomies were done through an inframammary approach, and with a wedge excision of lower pole skin to alleviate her pseudoptosis in each breast. At the second stage, the expanders were exchanged for round cohesive silicone gel implants. (*B*) At 2 years postoperatively, she maintains a stable, soft breast reconstruction on each side.

implant infections early and aggressively due to the risk of biofilm formation. Biofilms are difficult to eradicate and often lead to persistent infections, even with long-term intravenous antibiotic use. Prior studies have shown infection rates for implant-based reconstruction to range between 10% and 15% after two-stage reconstruction and direct to implant; however, no differences in infection rate were seen between prepectoral and subpectoral reconstruction.[42,43]

SUMMARY

Prepectoral breast reconstruction has become a popular technique for postmastectomy breast reconstruction due to its numerous benefits. Prepectoral reconstruction provides the benefit of decreased acute and chronic pain, avoidance of animation deformity, improved upper extremity strength, high patient satisfaction, and esthetic outcomes. Preoperatively, patient selection is key to minimize the risk of postoperative complications and optimize outcomes. Oncologic factors should be considered preoperatively to assess if the patient is a candidate for prepectoral reconstruction. Intraoperatively, mastectomy flap perfusion and viability assessment with clinical examination and perfusion devices are critical for successful reconstructive outcomes. ADM is used to re-establish natural breast borders, provide long-term implant support and minimize capsular contracture. Fat grafting and proper implant selection can help minimize or prevent rippling. Reconstructive surgeons should critically assess preoperative patient characteristics and intraoperative surgical techniques to obtain optimal outcomes in prepectoral breast reconstruction.

CLINICS CARE POINTS

Pearls:

- Intraoperative mastectomy skin flap assessment is crucial for successful outcomes. Both clinical examination (assessing for dermal bleeding at skin edges, presence of subcutaneous tissue present on the underside of the mastectomy flap) and indocyanine green angiography perfusion devices can help determine the viability of the skin flaps.

- ADM provides an important adjunctive role in recreating the breast borders, allowing for precise control of the breast pocket while also providing long-term support of the implant. It is important to use drains and to leave them in place for 2 to 3 weeks to minimize the potential for seroma formation.

Pitfalls:

- Do not perform prepectoral breast reconstruction in patients with preoperative radiation therapy, recent/active smoking, uncontrolled diabetes (hemoglobin A1c > 7), or obesity (BMI > 35). However, patients who are receiving PMRT can be considered for prepectoral reconstruction.

- Patients with tumors that invade the chest wall or are within 5 mm of the chest wall are not candidates for prepectoral breast reconstruction.

- If performing two-stage reconstruction, do not fill the tissue expander to the same size as the intended final implant as this can lead to postoperative rippling. Instead aim to fill to 150 to 200 cc less than the planned permanent implant size.

FINANCIAL DISCLOSURE STATEMENT

Dr Sbitany is a consultant for Allergan, Inc. He received no compensation or support for this article. The remaining authors have no disclosures related to the content of this article.

REFERENCES

1. American Society of Plastic Surgeons. 2020 plastic surgery procedural statistics. https://www.plasticsurgery.org/documents/News/Statistics/2020/plastic-surgery-statistics-full-report-2020.pdf. [Accessed 27 July 2022].
2. Sbitany H, Amalfi AN, Langstein HN. Preferences in choosing between breast reconstruction options: a survey of female plastic surgeons. Plast Reconstr Surg 2009;124(6):1781-9.
3. Wang F, Peled AW, Garwood E, et al. Total skin-sparing mastectomy and immediate breast reconstruction: an evolution of technique and assessment of outcomes. Ann Surg Oncol 2014;21(10):3223-30.
4. Becker H, Lind JG 2nd, Hopkins EG. Immediate implant-based prepectoral breast reconstruction using a vertical incision. Plast Reconstr Surg Glob Open 2015;3(6):e412.
5. Sigalove S, Maxwell GP, Sigalove NM, et al. Prepectoral implant-based breast reconstruction: rationale, indications, and preliminary results. Plast Reconstr Surg 2017;139(2):287-94.
6. Sbitany H, Piper M, Lentz R. Prepectoral breast reconstruction: a safe alternative to submuscular prosthetic reconstruction following nipple-sparing mastectomy. Plast Reconstr Surg 2017;140(3):432-43.
7. Srinivasa DR, Holland M, Sbitany H. Optimizing perioperative strategies to maximize success with prepectoral breast reconstruction. Gland Surg 2019;8(1):19-26.
8. Sbitany H. Important considerations for performing prepectoral breast reconstruction. Plast Reconstr Surg 2017;140(6S Prepectoral Breast Reconstruction):7s-13s.
9. Bettinger LN, Waters LM, Reese SW, et al. Comparative study of prepectoral and subpectoral expander-based breast reconstruction and clavien IIIb score outcomes. Plast Reconstr Surg Glob Open 2017;5(7):e1433.
10. Graziano FD, Shay PL, Sanati-Mehrizy P, et al. Prepectoral implant reconstruction in the setting of post- mastectomy radiation. Gland Surg 2020;10(1):411-6.
11. Sbitany H, Gomez-Sanchez C, Piper M, et al. Prepectoral breast reconstruction in the setting of post-mastectomy radiation therapy: an assessment of clinical outcomes and benefits. Plast Reconstr Surg 2019;143(1):10-20.
12. Sigalove S. Prepectoral breast reconstruction and radiotherapy-a closer look. Gland Surg 2019;8(1):67-74.
13. Sinnott CJ, Persing SM, Pronovost M, et al. Impact of postmastectomy radiation therapy in prepectoral versus subpectoral implant-based breast reconstruction. Ann Surg Oncol 2018;25(10):2899-908.
14. Vidya R, Berna G, Sbitany H, et al. Prepectoral implant-based breast reconstruction: a joint consensus guide from UK, European and USA breast and plastic reconstructive surgeons. Ecancermedicalscience 2019;13:927.
15. Buchanan CL, Dorn PL, Fey J, et al. Locoregional recurrence after mastectomy: incidence and outcomes. J Am Coll Surg 2006;203(4):469-74.
16. Mohamed MM, Al-Raawi D, Sabet SF, et al. Inflammatory breast cancer: new factors contribute to disease etiology: a review. J Adv Res 2014;5(5):525-36.
17. Hart A, Desai K, Yoo J, et al. Incidence of methicillin-resistant staphylococcus aureus (MRSA) carrier status in patients undergoing post-mastectomy breast reconstruction. Aesthet Surg J 2017;37(1):35-43.
18. Robertson SA, Rusby JE, Cutress RI. Determinants of optimal mastectomy skin flap thickness. Br J Surg 2014;101(8):899-911.
19. Sbitany H, Wang F, Peled AW, et al. Tissue expander reconstruction after total skin-sparing mastectomy: defining the effects of coverage technique on nipple/areola preservation. Ann Plast Surg 2016;77(1):17-24.
20. Phillips BT, Lanier ST, Conkling N, et al. Intraoperative perfusion techniques can accurately predict mastectomy skin flap necrosis in breast reconstruction: results of a prospective trial. Plast Reconstr Surg 2012;129(5):778e-88e.
21. Mazdeyasna S, Huang C, Bonaroti AR, et al. Intraoperative optical and fluorescence imaging of blood flow distributions in mastectomy skin flaps for identifying ischemic tissues. Plast Reconstr Surg 2022;150(2):282-7.
22. Pruimboom T, Schols RM, Van Kuijk SM, et al. Indocyanine green angiography for preventing postoperative mastectomy skin flap necrosis in immediate breast reconstruction. Cochrane Database Syst Rev 2020;4(4):Cd013280.
23. Mattison GL, Lewis PG, Gupta SC, et al. SPY imaging use in postmastectomy breast reconstruction patients: preventative or overly conservative? Plast Reconstr Surg 2016;138(1):15e-21e.
24. Johnson AC, Colakoglu S, Siddikoglu D, et al. Impact of dermal matrix brand in implant-based breast reconstruction outcomes. Plast Reconstr Surg 2022;150(1):17-25.

25. Snyderman RK, Guthrie RH. Reconstruction of the female breast following radical mastectomy. Plast Reconstr Surg 1971;47(6):565–7.
26. Basu CB, Jeffers L. The role of acellular dermal matrices in capsular contracture: a review of the evidence. Plast Reconstr Surg 2012;130(5 Suppl 2):118s–24s.
27. Sbitany H, Sandeen SN, Amalfi AN, et al. Acellular dermis-assisted prosthetic breast reconstruction versus complete submuscular coverage: a head-to-head comparison of outcomes. Plast Reconstr Surg 2009;124(6):1735–40.
28. Colwell AS, Damjanovic B, Zahedi B, et al. Retrospective review of 331 consecutive immediate single-stage implant reconstructions with acellular dermal matrix: indications, complications, trends, and costs. Plast Reconstr Surg 2011;128(6):1170–8.
29. Rose JF, Zafar SN, Ellsworth Iv WA. Does acellular dermal matrix thickness affect complication rate in tissue expander based breast reconstruction? Plast Surg Int 2016;2016:2867097.
30. Hur J, Han HH. Outcome assessment according to the thickness and direction of the acellular dermal matrix after implant-based breast reconstruction. Biomed Res Int 2021;2021:8101009.
31. Gui G, Gui M, Gui A, et al. Physical characteristics of surgimend meshed biological ADM in immediate prepectoral implant breast reconstruction. Plast Reconstr Surg Glob Open 2022;10(6):e4369.
32. Tierney BP, De La Garza M, Jennings GR, et al. Clinical outcomes of acellular dermal matrix (simpliderm and alloderm ready-to-use) in immediate breast reconstruction. Cureus 2022;14(2):e22371.
33. Khan A, Tasoulis MK, Teoh V, et al. Pre-pectoral one-stage breast reconstruction with anterior biological acellular dermal matrix coverage. Gland Surg 2021;10(3):1002–9.
34. Ho G, Nguyen TJ, Shahabi A, et al. A systematic review and meta-analysis of complications associated with acellular dermal matrix-assisted breast reconstruction. Ann Plast Surg 2012;68(4):346–56.
35. Lee KT, Mun GH. A meta-analysis of studies comparing outcomes of diverse acellular dermal matrices for implant-based breast reconstruction. Ann Plast Surg 2017;79(1):115–23.
36. Maisel Lotan A, Ben Yehuda D, Allweis TM, et al. Comparative study of meshed and nonmeshed acellular dermal matrix in immediate breast reconstruction. Plast Reconstr Surg 2019;144(5):1045–53.
37. Safran T, Al-Badarin F, Al-Halabi B, et al. Aesthetic limitations in direct-to-implant prepectoral breast reconstruction. Plast Reconstr Surg 2022;150(1):22e–31e.
38. Nahabedian MY, Glasberg SB, Maxwell GP. Introduction to "prepectoral breast reconstruction". Plast Reconstr Surg 2017;140(6S Prepectoral Breast Reconstruction):4s–5s.
39. Spear SL, Coles CN, Leung BK, et al. The safety, effectiveness, and efficiency of autologous fat grafting in breast surgery. Plast Reconstr Surg Glob Open 2016;4(8):e827.
40. Goodreau AM, Driscoll CR, Nye A, et al. Revising prepectoral breast reconstruction. Plast Reconstr Surg 2022;149(3):579–84.
41. Weichman KE, Clavin NW, Miller HC, et al. Does the use of biopatch devices at drain sites reduce perioperative infectious complications in patients undergoing immediate tissue expander breast reconstruction? Plast Reconstr Surg 2015;135(1):9e–17e.
42. Baker BG, Irri R, MacCallum V, et al. A prospective comparison of short-term outcomes of subpectoral and prepectoral strattice-based immediate breast reconstruction. Plast Reconstr Surg 2018;141(5):1077–84.
43. Bennett KG, Qi J, Kim HM, et al. Comparison of 2-year complication rates among common techniques for postmastectomy breast reconstruction. JAMA Surg 2018;153(10):901–8.

Direct to Implant Reconstruction

Jordan M.S. Jacobs, MD[a], Charles Andrew Salzberg, MD[b],*

KEYWORDS

• Direct-to-implant • One-stage • Subpectoral • Prepectoral • Acellular dermal matrix

KEY POINTS

• Direct-to-implant reconstruction can be successfully performed in both the subpectoral and prepectoral tissue planes in patients with adequate skin envelope quality and quantity.
• Proper patient selection and implant sizing improve chances of successful outcomes.
• Implant coverage with acellular dermal matrix provides a biologic scaffold with good strength and long-term lower pole support.

INTRODUCTION

Breast cancer treatment remains, primarily, a surgical disease, and there has been an increase in the percentage of patients who choose mastectomy over breast conservation.[1] Implant-based breast reconstruction continues to be the most common restorative surgery after mastectomy. This type of reconstruction involves either a one-stage, direct-to-implant insertion or a staged approach with immediate tissue expander insertion followed by exchange to a permanent prosthesis at a secondary surgery. Improvements in surgical techniques as well as technological advances have made direct-to-implant insertion at the time of mastectomy a much more feasible option.

The concept of a one-stage, direct-to-implant reconstruction, was first introduced in 2001 by the senior author.[2] Since that time, it has gained wide acceptance and is now performed in approximately 20% of reconstructions.[3] In the nipple-sparing patient not requiring skin expansion, it offers a "one-step" reconstruction, thereby reducing the number of surgical procedures and shortening the time to completion of reconstruction (Fig. 1).

Complete coverage of the implant or tissue expander is generally accepted to reduce the incidence of exposure, bottoming out, and loss of control of the inframammary fold. The pectoralis major and serratus anterior muscle bellies are commonly used, which provide durable, vascularized tissue. They are easily accessible in the surgical field and have reliable anatomical borders with well-defined vascular supplies. Other options for soft tissue coverage of the implant lower pole include rectus abdominus fascia, external oblique fascia, and acellular dermal matrices (ADMs).[4–10] These biologic materials all have the benefit of low infection rates due to complete revascularization of the implant pocket. Synthetic mesh has also been used for partial and complete implant coverage and has shown good pocket control with reduced material costs.[11]

The success of direct to implant reconstruction has been greatly facilitated by the development of ADMs from either human or porcine origin. These biologic scaffolds provide an off-the-shelf dermal matrix with good strength and pliability. Removal of all cellular components with various processing techniques avoids the potential for inflammation and rejection.[12] The acellular scaffold becomes completely integrated into the overlying skin envelope through angiogenesis and revascularization. Although complete implant coverage with muscle and/or fascial flaps typically leads to a contracted lower pole shape, ADM or synthetic mesh allows creation of a malleable pocket with complete coverage of the underlying implant and good long-term lower pole

a Icahn School of Medicine, Mount Sinai Hospital, 1 Gustave Levy Place, New York, NY 10029, USA; b Cleveland Clinic Florida, 3555 10th Ct, Vero Beach, Fl 32960, USA
* Corresponding author.
E-mail address: asalzbergmd@yahoo.com

Clin Plastic Surg 50 (2023) 243–248
https://doi.org/10.1016/j.cps.2022.11.003

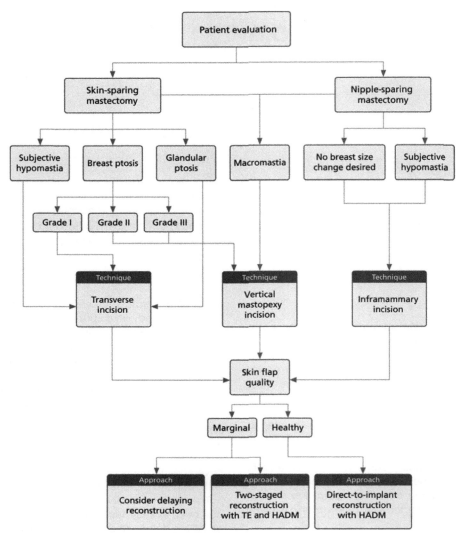

Fig. 1. Algorithm for direct to implant reconstruction. (*From* Salzberg CA, Ashikari AY, Koch RM, Chabner-Thompson E. An 8-year experience of direct-to-implant immediate breast reconstruction using human acellular dermal matrix (AlloDerm). Plast Reconstr Surg. 2011;127(2):514-524.)

support.[13,14] Its ability to stretch postoperatively and increase the lower pole length allows a more natural appearing reconstruction. In addition, refinements in dermal matrix processing as well as surgical techniques have resolved initial concerns of increased infection and seroma rates.[15–17]

Although direct-to-implant reconstruction was originally described using a subpectoral implant placement, it can also be safely and successfully performed in the prepectoral tissue plane.[18]

Increased size and thickness options of ADMs have led to an increase in the popularity of this technique.[19–21] With the pectoralis major muscle left undisturbed in its native position and complete coverage of the breast prosthesis provided mainly by ADM, patient recovery is quicker with less morbidity.[22–24] Typical patients for this technique are younger and more active, with the need to maintain maximum range of motion of the shoulder and upper extremity. The prepectoral reconstruction also avoids the potential for an animation deformity, which results from adhesion between the pectoralis major muscle and overlying skin envelope. The resultant contour animation deformities that patients experience while contracting their pectoralis major muscle can be distressing and is difficult to correct without complete separation of the muscle flap from the skin flap.

Perhaps, the most crucial variable to a successful outcome is adequate perfusion to the mastectomy skin flaps. Skin flap perfusion must be accurately assessed after the breast tissue has been removed before deciding to proceed with direct-to-implant reconstruction. The development of indocyanine green angiography has allowed more accurate assessments of skin viability and decreased the incidence of necrosis, which can have devastating implications such as exposure, infection, and need for secondary surgeries.[25,26]

Below, we describe our most updated approach to direct-to-implant reconstruction in both the subpectoral and prepectoral planes.

TECHNIQUE

As with any type of reconstruction, the pathway to a successful outcome is multifactorial. Proper patient selection begins with a comprehensive consultation and, for us, a three-dimensional imaging session. The risks and benefits of all reconstructive options are discussed and the patient goals are defined. Patients who undergo either skin-sparing or nipple-sparing mastectomies are typically good candidates for direct-to-implant insertion. However, all patients must understand that the final decision to proceed with immediate implant insertion is made intraoperatively once the perfusion and viability of the skin envelope has been determined.

The ideal candidate for direct-to-implant reconstruction is a woman with up to full C cup volume and Grade 1 to 2 ptosis. Larger breasts can be done with this technique in the hands of experienced surgeons.

SUBPECTORAL DIRECT TO IMPLANT

The preoperative markings include the sternal midline, inframammary fold, lateral mammary fold, and medial breast border. Nipple-preserving mastectomies are typically performed through an inframammary incision measuring 10 to 13 cm, depending on the breast size. An axillary counter-incision is made or sometimes access through the inframammary fold (IMF) is possible if axillary lymph node sampling is indicated. Incisions around the areolar border have been shown to compromise the circulation the nipple areolar complex (NAC).[27] Skin-sparing approaches are performed through a peri-areolar approach, usually with the scar orientation based on preoperative areolar dimensions.

Once the mastectomy has been completed, the skin pocket is irrigated copiously with warm saline to remove avascular fat particles because these are a potential nidus for infection and seroma

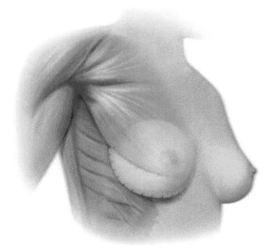

Fig. 2. Retropectoral construct in direct to implant reconstruction. (*From* Salzberg CA. Nonexpansive immediate breast reconstruction using human acellular tissue matrix graft (AlloDerm). Ann Plast Surg. 2006;57(1):1-5.)

formation. The lateral border of the pectoralis major muscle is then identified and raised with electrocautery and the loose areolar plane is developed up to the second rib superiorly, to the sternal fibers medially, and to the anterior axillary line laterally. The origins are then released off the chest wall up the 4 o'clock position on the right breast and the 8 o'clock position on the left breast. The ADM, which has been prepared in saline baths for 10 minutes is then placed dermis side up and brought up to the breast pocket. Starting medially and proceeding laterally, a 3-0 Vicryl suture is then used to secure the superior edge of the ADM to the released inferior edge of the pectoralis muscle in a simple running fashion. The lateral and medial borders of the ADM are then fixated down to the chest wall, starting a new suture medially and again using a 3-0 Vicryl suture in simple running fashion (**Fig. 2**). A sterile sizer may be inserted temporarily if desired to help determine a "hand in glove" fit to the reconstruction.

Intraoperative skin flap perfusion analysis is performed at this time with the implant/sizer in place. We typically perform postimage processing and use relative perfusion data points for areas that show marginal perfusion. As long as the skin flap viability is adequate, the appropriate-sized implant is placed under the pectoralis major/ADM pocket through the inframammary fold opening. Once the implant position is confirmed, the ADM is fixated down to the inferior chest wall at the level of desired IMF using the 2 sutures previously started. Mastectomy skin flap redraping is

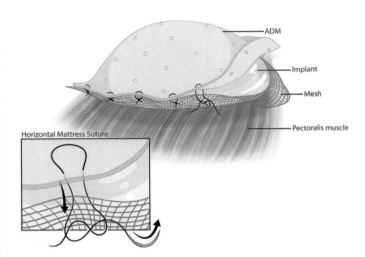

Fig. 3. "Empanada" prepectoral construct in direct to implant reconstruction. Printed with permission from © Mount Sinai Health System.

essential to place the NAC in the perfect position and may be sutured to the underlying dermis or muscle using a fine, absorbable suture. Placement of 2 drains on each side and layered skin closure completes the reconstruction.

PREPECTORAL DIRECT TO IMPLANT

The prepectoral direct-to-implant technique involves complete coverage of the breast prosthesis with ADM. We typically perform this reconstruction using a large (16 × 20 cm), thick piece of ADM, or 2 smaller pieces sutured together. There are 2 main techniques we use: fixation of the ADM to the anterior and lateral chest walls followed by implant placement through an inframammary fold access, or ex vivo construction of an implant/ADM/mesh construct, the so-called "empanada" technique[17] (Fig. 3).

Both techniques provide a natural breast shape with a shorter recovery period but typically require a secondary procedure to correct postoperative rippling and/or step-off deformities.

COMPLICATIONS

Complications of direct-to-implant reconstruction include skin breakdown/necrosis, seroma, hematoma, implant exposure, implant malposition, capsular contracture, infection, and implant loss. The most predictable risk factors include smoking, obesity, nonnipple-sparing mastectomy, and implant size greater than 600 mL, and the overall incidence of complications is 8% to 10%.[28,29] Previous radiation therapy as well as postoperative radiation are both associated with higher complication rates. Capsular contracture rates have remained low in both the nonirradiated and irradiated breasts and the incidence has been

shown to be inversely related the implant size.[14] Maintaining strict inclusion criteria and making decisions based on critical intraoperative skin perfusion analysis will significantly reduce the incidence of complications.

Revision rates of direct-to-implant reconstruction are 3% to 5% in the first year. The most common reasons for revision include implant size change, implant malposition, and rippling or other contour deformities. The use of 3D imaging preoperatively has allowed more precise sizing and a greater ability to meet patient size goals. The revision rates for contour deformities are higher in prepectoral reconstruction due to almost universal rippling of the upper pole.

DISCUSSION

Direct-to-implant reconstruction has been safely performed by the senior author for the past 20 years. Although initially described in a subpectoral plane, it can be safely performed in the prepectoral plane as well. The subpectoral plane offers upper pole muscular and lower pole ADM coverage with less rippling and a more natural appearance in one-stage. However, the recovery is typically longer than that of the prepectoral technique and there is potential for animation deformities as well as upper limb weakness and range of motion limitations.

The prepectoral direct-to-implant reconstruction is an excellent option for the young, fit, and active patients who want a quicker recovery with less potential for prolonged activity restrictions. However, the prepectoral reconstructive patients need to be prepared for the likelihood of secondary fat grafting to correct rippling and contour deformities. We typically perform this secondary procedure 3 months after the initial reconstruction in the patient not requiring adjuvant chemotherapy and/or radiation therapy. In the patients requiring adjuvant treatment, secondary reconstruction is typically delayed until this has been completed.

Direct-to-implant reconstruction has been safely performed in both patients with previous radiation therapy or the need for adjuvant radiation after mastectomy.[14] Although there is an increase in the incidence of capsular contracture in the setting of radiation therapy, this risk also exists with immediate tissue expander insertion, and must be considered if performing these procedures.

The use of prepectoral breast reconstruction and the use of synthetic mesh both have the downside of not knowing the long-term consequences. It is certainly possible that the advantage we have seen in the past of decreased capsular contracture and long-term excellent fold creation with the use of ADM may be obviated by using synthetic materials.

As with most surgeries, proper patient selection and setting expectations is paramount to the success of direct-to-implant reconstruction.

SUMMARY

Implant-based breast reconstruction remains the most commonly performed type of restorative surgery after mastectomy for breast cancer. Direct-to-implant reconstruction provides a one-stage, final implant insertion, thereby bypassing the need for serial tissue expansion. With proper patient selection, successful preservation of the breast skin envelope, and accurate implant size and placement, direct-to-implant reconstruction has a very high rate of success and patient satisfaction.

CLINICS CARE POINTS

- Direct-to-implant reconstruction involves a one-stage restorative procedure with good long-term safety and results.
- Although classically described in the subpectoral plane, direct-to-implant reconstruction can be performed in the prepectoral plane with complete ADM coverage.
- Preoperative patient selection, accurate intraoperative decision-making with skin flap angiography, and proper postoperative management are keys to successful outcomes.
- Advances in breast implant technology have improved the postoperative results in direct-to-implant reconstruction.

DISCLOSURE

There are no financial relationships to disclose for either author.

REFERENCES

1. Kummerow KL, Du L, Penson DF, et al. Nationwide trends in mastectomy for early-stage breast cancer. JAMA Surg 2015 Jan;150(1):9–16.
2. Salzberg CA. Nonexpansive immediate breast reconstruction using human acellular tissue matrix graft (AlloDerm). Ann Plast Surg 2006;57:1–5.
3. https://www.plasticsurgery.org/documents/News/ Statistics/2018/reconstructive-breast-procedures-age-2018.pdf (Accessed June 2022).
4. Little JW III, Golembe EV, Fisher JB. The "living bra" in immediate and delayed reconstruction of the breast follow- ing mastectomy for malignant and nonmalignant disease. Plast Reconstr Surg 1981; 68:392–403.
5. Isken T, Onyedi M, Izmirli H, et al. Abdominal fascial flaps for providing total implant coverage in one-stage breast reconstruction: an autologous solution. Aesthetic Plast Surg 2009;33:853–8.
6. Breuing KH, Warren SM. Immediate bilateral breast recon- struction with implants and inferolateral Allo-Derm slings. Ann Plast Surg 2005;55:232–9.
7. Gamboa-Bobadilla GM. Implant breast reconstruction using acellular dermal matrix. Ann Plast Surg 2006;56:22–5.
8. Breuing KH, Colwell AS. Inferolateral AlloDerm hammock for implant coverage in breast reconstruction. Ann Plast Surg 2007;59:250–5.
9. Zienowicz RJ, Karacaoglu E. Implant-based breast reconstruction with allograft. Plast Reconstr Surg 2007;120:373–81.
10. Topol BM, Dalton EF, Ponn T, et al. Immediate single-stage breast reconstruction using implants and human acellular dermal tissue matrix with adjustment of the lower pole of the breast to reduce unwanted lift. Ann Plast Surg 2008;61:494–9.
11. Faulkner HR, Shikowitz-Behr L, McLeod M, et al. The use of absorbable mesh in implant-based breast reconstruction: a 7-year review. Plast Reconstr Surg 2020;146(6):731e–6e.
12. Livesey S., Atkinson Y., Call T., et al. An acellular dermal transplant processed from human allograft skin retains normal extracellular matrix components and ultrastructural characteristics. Poster presented at the American Association of Tissue Banks Conference, August 20–24, 1994.
13. Salzberg CA, Ashikari AY, Koch RM, et al. An 8-year experience of direct-to-implant immediate breast reconstruction using human acellular dermal matrix (AlloDerm). Plast Reconstr Surg 2011;127(2): 514–24.

14. Salzberg CA, Ashikari AY, Berry C, et al. Acellular Dermal matrix-assisted direct-to-implant breast reconstruction and capsular contracture: a 13-year experience. Plast Reconstr Surg 2016;138(2): 329–37.

15. Sbitany H, Sandeen SN, Amalfi AN, et al. Acellular dermis-assisted prosthetic breast recon- struction versus complete submuscular coverage: a head-to- head comparison of outcomes. Plast Reconstr Surg 2009;124:1735–40.

16. Nahabedian MY. AlloDerm performance in the setting of prosthetic breast surgery, infection, and irradiation. Plast Reconstr Surg 2009;124:1743–53.

17. Preminger BA, McCarthy CM, Hu QY, et al. The influence of AlloDerm on expander dynamics and complications in the setting of immediate tissue expander/im- plant reconstruction: a matched-cohort study. Ann Plast Surg 2008;60:510–3.

18. Sayegh F, Zoghbi Y, Jacobs J, et al. The "empanada" construct: prepectoral technique refinement utilizing a composite acellular dermal matrix mesh wrap. Plast Reconstr Surg 2021;147(6):1082–3.

19. Ter Louw RP, Nahabedian MY. Prepectoral breast reconstruction. Plast Reconstr Surg 2017;140(5S Advances in Breast Reconstruction):51S–9S.

20. Safran T, Al-Halabi B, Viezel-Mathieu A, et al. Direct-to-implant prepectoral breast reconstruction: patient-reported outcomes. Plast Reconstr Surg 2021;148(6):882e–90e.

21. Antony AK, Robinson EC. An algorithmic approach to prepectoral direct-to-implant breast reconstruction: version 2.0. Plast Reconstr Surg 2019 May; 143(5):1311–9.

22. Sbitany H. Important considerations for performing prepectoral breast reconstruction. Plast Reconstr Surg 2017;140(6S Prepectoral Breast Reconstruction):7S–13S.

23. Bonomi S, Sala L, Cortinovis U. Prepectoral breast reconstruction. Plast Reconstr Surg 2018 Aug; 142(2):232e–3e.

24. Urquia LN, Hart AM, Liu DZ, et al. Surgical outcomes in prepectoral breast reconstruction. Plast Reconstr Surg Glob Open 2020;8(4):e2744.

25. Chattha A, Bucknor A, Chen AD, et al. Indocyanine green angiography use in breast reconstruction: a national analysis of outcomes and cost in 110,320 patients. Plast Reconstr Surg 2018;141(4):825–32.

26. Lauritzen E, Damsgaard TE. Use of Indocyanine green angiography decreases the risk of complications in autologous- and implant-based breast reconstruction: a systematic review and meta-analysis. J Plast Reconstr Aesthet Surg 2021;74(8):1703–17.

27. Daar DA, Abdou SA, Rosario L, et al. Is there a preferred incision location for nipple-sparing mastectomy? A systematic review and meta-analysis. Plast Reconstr Surg 2019;143(5):906e–19e.

28. Hunsicker LM, Ashikaria AY, Berry C, et al. Short-term complications associated with acellular dermal matriz-assisted direct-to-implant breast reconstruction. Ann Plast Surg 2017;78(1):35–40.

29. Colwell AS, Damjanovic B, Zahedi B, et al. Retrospective review of 331 consecutive immediate single-stage implant reconstructions with acellular dermal matrix: indications, comlications, trends, and costs. Plast Reconstr Surg 2011;128(6):1170–8.

A Spectrum of Disease
Breast Implant-Associated Anaplastic Large Cell Lymphoma, Atypicals, and Other Implant Associations

Megan E. Fracol, MD[a], Megan M. Rodriguez, BS[a,b], Mark W. Clemens, MD, MBA[a,*]

KEYWORDS

- Breast implant-associated anaplastic large cell lymphoma • Textured breast implants
- Breast reconstruction • Breast augmentation • Inflammatory malignancies

KEY POINTS

- Breast implant-associated anaplastic large cell lymphoma (BIA-ALCL) is an uncommon and still emerging malignancy caused by textured surface breast implants.
- Effective October 1, 2022, the 2023 edition of the International Classification of Diseases, Tenth Revision, Clinical Modification (ICD-10-CM) now describes BIA-ALCL by diagnosis code C84.7A BIA-ALCL as anaplastic large cell lymphoma, ALK-negative breast when combined with additional code Z98.82 to identify breast implant status.
- BIA-ALCL is a sequela of exposure to a textured device and no confirmed pure smooth implant cases have ever been reported to date.
- World Health Organization criteria for BIA-ALCL include (1) large anaplastic cell morphology, (2) confluent CD30 immunohistochemistry staining, (3) a single T cell clone on flow cytometry, (4) arising in continuity with a breast implant.
- Surgical management includes device explantation, total capsulectomy, resection of associated capsular masses with negative margins, excisional biopsies of lymphadenopathy, with immediate or delayed reconstruction based on patient preference.

INTRODUCTION

Breast implant-associated anaplastic large cell lymphoma (BIA-ALCL) is an uncommon and still emerging malignancy caused by textured surface breast implants. BIA-ALCL was described in 1997 case report.[1] BIA-ALCL was the first described implant-associated malignancy, although several more inflammatory-mediated tumors arising around implants (B-cell lymphomas [BCL] and squamous cell carcinoma [SCC]) have subsequently been described over the past decade.[2,3] BIA-ALCL is the result of a chronic monoclonal T-cell stimulation, and is a purely T-cell lymphoma.[4] Rising physician awareness and public attention of this disease entity has contributed to an increasing number of case reports and series over the past two decades. The purpose of this article is to review the history of the disease, epidemiology, diagnostic work-up, treatment strategies, prognosis, and future directions in this field.

[a] Department of Plastic Surgery, MD Anderson Cancer Center, University of Texas, 1400 Pressler Street, Houston, TX 77030, USA; [b] University of Texas, Houston School of Medicine, Houston, TX, USA
* Corresponding author. Department of Plastic Surgery, The University of Texas, MD Anderson Cancer Center, 1400 Pressler Street, Unit 1488 Houston, TX 77030.
E-mail address: MWClemens@mdanderson.org
Twitter: @clemensmd (M.W.C.)

Clin Plastic Surg 50 (2023) 249–257
https://doi.org/10.1016/j.cps.2022.12.001
0094-1298/23/© 2022 Elsevier Inc. All rights reserved.

History and Current Incidence

The first textured surface implants were introduced to the US market over 50 years ago in 1968.[5] Surface texturization was developed in an effort to prevent parallel alignment of collagen fibers in the capsule, thereby disrupting organized scar formation and theoretically preventing capsular contracture. Textured surface implants gained popularity as a way to combat capsular contracture in the late 1980s and were briefly the most popular type of breast implant in the late 1990s but fell out of favor in the early 2000s and supplanted by smooth surface implants in the United States.[6] Textured implants have been by far the most common implant used in Europe, Oceania, Asia, and South America, exceeding 95% of these markets.[7] However, practice patterns have shifted considerably around the world following the US FDA Class I device recall of Allergan Biocell implants in 2019 which precipitated a worldwide Biocell ban as well as regulatory actions against textured implants in numerous countries.

The first case of BIA-ALCL was reported in 1997.[1] The patient was a 41-year-old woman who presented with a history of Biocell textured saline breast implants that had been in place for 5 years when a mass presented in the right breast. She was treated with chemotherapy and radiation, however, was lost to follow up shortly thereafter.[8] Reports of BIA-ALCL remained relatively infrequent until January 2011 with the release of an United States food and drug administration (FDA) safety communication warning about "the possible association" of ALCL and breast implants.[9] Greater public awareness led to the establishment of the PROFILE registry (www.thepsf.org/PROFILE) to prospectively track US cases.[10] The World Health Organization classified BIA-ALCL as a novel T-cell lymphoma in 2016, which also contributed to greater awareness.[11] To date, BIA-ALCL has only been reported either in patients with textured devices (either implants or tissue expanders), with a history of textured implants, or with an unknown history.[12] There have been no cases reported in patients who have a confirmed history of smooth implants only.

Not all surface texture is the same. Various classification schemes exist to describe surface texturization, but they all largely rely on total surface area and/or depth of peaks and valleys to describe the extent of texturization.[13–15] The degree of texturization depends on how the implant surface is processed. Processing techniques to roughen the surface include polyurethane foam coating (Highest surface area texturization), salt loss (High surface area texturization: Biocell, Allergan Aesthetics, An Abbvie Corporation, Irvine, CA), and negative imprinting (Moderate surface area texturization: Siltex, Mentor; A Johnson & Johnson Company, New Brunswick, NJ).[16,17] Polyurethane was discontinued in the United States in 1992 due to concerns about the release of the carcinogenic compound 2,4-toluene diamine as the implant surface degrades over time. The US FDA recall of Allergan Biocell implants occurred in 2019[18] due to a disproportionate risk of BIA-ALCL as approximately 91% of known BIA-ALCL cases involved a Biocell implant when clinical history was known.[19]

The risk of BIA-ALCL seems to be proportionate to the degree of surface texturization.[20] This risk is highest in women with the Allergan Biocell implants at 1:2200.[21] The highest risk estimate quoted to date came out of Memorial Sloan Kettering Cancer Center, where one case was seen out of every 355 patients which has been updated since publication by Dr Cordeiro to 1:100.[22] When counseling patients on their risk of developing BIA-ALCL from an implant, it is important to keep in mind that this estimate depends on the type of implant being used. For women undergoing placement of smooth breast implants, the risk is essentially that of ALCL in the general population, approximately one in four million.[23]

Diagnosis

Patients with a history of textured breast implants (or unknown surface texture history) with a late onset seroma (>1 year from implant placement), asymmetric swelling, or implant-associated mass should undergo testing to rule out BIA-ALCL. Evaluation begins with an ultrasound to assess for a peri-prosthetic fluid collection or mass. The lymph nodes can also be examined at this time for involvement. A small seroma (<5–10 cc) can be normal, but symptomatic fluid collections should be sampled with fine needle aspiration and cytology. Typically, a minimum of 50 cc of fluid is required for adequate analysis. Previous repeated aspirations may have a dilutional effect and therefore require even larger quantity of sample to obtain a definitive diagnosis. Cytology includes both H&E stains to evaluate cell morphology as well as immunohistochemical stains for cell surface markers. H&E will show abnormally large (3-4x normal) lymphocytes with horseshoe or kidney-shaped nuclei.[19] ALCL is a T-cell lymphoma, and as such the cell surface will stain positive for various T-cell markers. As it is a monoclonal proliferation, there should be an abundance and near confluence of CD30+ T cells. Note that approximately 1% to 2% of normal circulating lymphocytes normally express CD30; therefore,

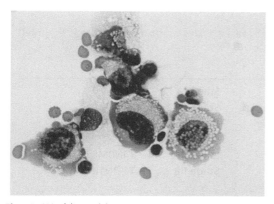

Fig. 1. World Health Organization criteria for BIA-ALCL includes large anaplastic cell morphology arising in continuity with a breast implant.

scant positivity of normal cells is a benign and common finding.[24] ALK-negativity is another hallmark of ALCL and therefore is not useful as a screening test as anaplastic lymphoma kinase (ALK) will always be negative even in the presence of BIA-ALCL. ALK is useful once a diagnosis has been established to differentiate BIA-ALCL from the much more aggressive ALK- systemic ALCL. Pathology evaluation of capsule specimens should be performed with CD30 immunohistochemistry regional sampling in 12 distinct regions to ensure proper screening of the tissue for tumor invasion.[25] For suspicious lesions, additional stains may be warranted to rule out less common implant-associated malignancies, such as BCLs (CD138, PAX5, CD20, human herpesvirus-8, Epstein Barr virus [EBV]) and SCC with cytokeratin stains.[26] Note that routine pathology of a breast implant capsule should always be sent for evaluation of breast cancer which is significantly more common than any of the former malignancies. World Health Organization criteria for BIA-ALCL include (1) large anaplastic cell morphology, (2) confluent CD30 immunohistochemistry staining, (3) a single T-cell clone on flow cytometry, and (4) arising in continuity with a breast implant (Fig. 1). Increasingly, surgeons are encountering patients with pathology specimens meeting one or two criteria, but not achieving the diagnosis of BIA-ALCL. These lesions are collectively referred to as atypical and represent diagnostic challenges. It is currently not possible to define the clinical significance or malignant potential of an atypical lesion and whether these represent a precursor lesion, in situ form, or simply an abundance of inflammation. If ultrasound is inadequate, then MRI can be performed as an adjunctive imaging procedure. An updated mammogram (within 12 months) should be obtained to evaluate for

breast cancer, although it should be noted that mammograms have poor sensitivity for lymphoma. If there are any solid masses identified on imaging, then core needle biopsy should be performed, with the stains as described above.

Although genetic sequencing is not routinely used in the workup of this tumor, it is notable that recent research has shown the JAK-STAT3 pathway to be constitutively activated in a majority of cases.[27] In addition, genetic sequencing may have prognostic value as the presence of p53 has been theorized as a marker for more aggressive disease and portends a worse prognosis. Underlying genetic alterations may represent a target for therapy in the future.

Staging

Non-Hodgkin lymphoma is most commonly staged as a liquid tumor by the Ann Arbor staging system. However, staging of BIA-ALCL is performed according to the MD Anderson Cancer Center solid tumor "tumor node metastasis (TNM)" classification[28] (Table 1). Tumor extent, or "T", is based on the degree of infiltration into, or beyond, the capsule. T1 tumors are confined to an effusion on the luminal side of the capsule. T2 tumors demonstrate early capsule infiltration. T3 tumors demonstrate cell aggregates or sheets infiltrating the capsule. T4 tumors demonstrate lymphoma infiltrates beyond the capsule. Lymph node involvement is broken down into "N0" or none, "N1" or one regional lymph node, and "N2" or multiple regional lymph nodes. Last, metastasis is simply broken down into whether distant spread is present or absent. Stage I disease is all confined to the breast capsule. Stage II disease shows infiltrates beyond the capsule but without lymph node involvement OR infiltrates confined to the capsule with only one regional lymph node involved. Stage III disease demonstrates regional lymph node involvement, and stage IV disease demonstrates distant metastasis. See Table 1 for the TNM staging system. This TNM staging system is now supported by the World Health Organization and the National Comprehensive Cancer Network (NCCN).

Management

Once a diagnosis of BIA-ALCL has been established, PET–CT scanning is indicated to determine if lymph node involvement or distant metastasis exists. Importantly, fresh inflammation may be indistinguishable from active malignancy on PET; therefore, imaging must be performed before any surgical intervention. Suspicious lymph nodes may undergo fine needle aspiration with cytology as described above; however, an excisional

Table 1
MD Anderson cancer center solid tumor TNM staging of breast implant-associated anaplastic large cell lymphoma

	TNM Classification		Staging	
T1	Limited to luminal side of capsule	Stage IA	T1N0M0
T2	Early capsule invasion	Stage IB	T2N0M0
T3	Sheets or aggregates of cells invading capsule	Stage IC	T3N0M0
T4	Lymphoma present beyond the capsule		
		Stage IIA	T4N0M0
N0	No lymph node involvement	Stage IIB	T1-3N1M0
N1	One regional lymph node involved		
N2	More than 1 regional lymph node involved	Stage III	T4N1M0 or anyTN2M0
M0	No distant metastasis	Stage IV	AnyTAnyNM1
M1	Distant metastasis present		

biopsy of lymph nodes may be required to achieve a reliable diagnosis as fine needle aspiration (FNA) can be frequently indeterminate.

The mainstay of treatment is complete surgical resection. This usually involves total en bloc capsulectomy with the removal of the implant[29] (Fig. 2A–C). The posterior capsule in a subpectoral implant may be particularly challenging to resect off of the rib cage; however, complete resection is essential to achieve cure and minimize disease recurrence. Targeted lymph node dissection of involved lymph nodes is performed at the time of explantation.

Adjuvant therapy is reserved for cases of positive margins, lymph node involvement, recurrent disease, or distant metastasis. Positive margins can occasionally be seen when the tumor involves the chest wall or in regional lymph node metastasis. Adjunct radiation (25–30g) is an option in these choices, although complete surgical excision is still the preferred treatment of choice as this has been shown to have superior disease-free survival compared with all other treatment modalities. Anthracycline-based chemotherapy with or without stem cell transplant has traditionally been used for systemic ALCL, and more recently NCCN guidelines have allowed for primary use of brentuximab vedotin as a monotherapy for patients with advanced BIA-ALCL. Brentuximab is a well-tolerated immunotherapy which has been described both as an adjunct and in the neoadjuvant setting to shrink chest wall tumors to optimize subsequent surgical management of disease. The most common side effect of brentuximab is peripheral neuropathies which may be temporary or permanent.

Management of the contralateral breast is recommended due to the risk of occult bilateral BIA-ALCL. It is reasonable to perform implant removal

with total capsulectomy on the non-affected side as well, since bilateral BIA-ALCL has been reported in 2% to 4% of cases.[21] Bilateral disease may or may not be apparent on pre-op PET–CT; thus, contralateral total capsulectomy in an asymptomatic breast is recommended for all patients.

Reconstruction

As BIA-ALCL is caused by textured implants, it is reasonable to offer an immediate reconstruction with smooth implants or autologous flaps in these patients.[30] Reconstruction may be performed either immediately or in a delayed setting. A study from MD Anderson Cancer Center treating 66 consecutive patients with BIA-ALCL noted that 18 patients (27%) underwent reconstruction after implant removal. Seven (39%) of these were immediate, whereas 11 (61%) were delayed based on invasive chest wall disease at time of diagnosis. The authors recommend delayed reconstruction in cases of advanced disease (stage IIA and beyond or disease beyond the capsule) so that adjuvant chemotherapy can be delivered before final reconstruction. In this series, most patients were reconstructed with smooth implants (n = 13, 72%), whereas two patients (11%) underwent immediate mastopexy alone, one patient (6%) underwent reconstruction with bilateral deep inferior epigastric artery perforator flap and one patient (6%) underwent serial fat grafting. Seventeen patients (94%) were highly satisfied with the reconstruction.

Prognosis

Overall, prognosis is very good for patients diagnosed with BIA-ALCL confined to the capsule, with complete remission rates of 93% and 5-year overall survival at 97.9%.[25] Complete remission rates go down to 72% when a tumor mass is

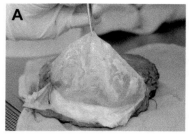 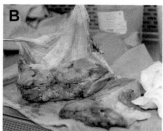 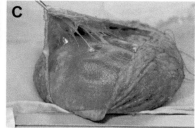

Fig. 2. BIA-ALCL en bloc resection specimens demonstrate a vigorous capsular response (A), viscous seroma reaction (B), and associated capsular tumors (C).

present and 5-year overall survival drops to 75% with lymph node involvement.[31] For this reason, chemotherapy and/or radiation are justified in these patients. Lymph node involvement likewise decreases remission rates and overall survival. Regardless, this is significantly better than 5-year progression free survival of peripheral ALK-negative ALCL, which has been reported at 36%.[32]

Case Reporting

Systematic collection of case reports has helped significantly to identify patterns in disease presentation, response to therapies, and optimization of NCCN treatment guidelines as the global standard of care for this disease. As such, the American Society of Plastic Surgery, the Plastic Surgery Foundation, and the FDA established the PROFILE registry in 2012.[10] This online registry prospectively tracks case reports of BIA-ALCL in the United States, and the FDA specifically recommends that all surgeons encountering such cases to report this clinical data to PROFILE.

Insurance Coverage

Insurance coverage of BIA-ALCL continues to be a challenge within the United States. One study looked at a cross-sectional analysis of US insurance companies and their coverage for BIA-ALCL.[33] This group found that only 30% of companies surveyed had a policy on BIA-ALCL coverage. Policies providing coverage for implant removal in the affected breast remains sporadic and is not guaranteed. Regarding the contralateral breast, only two-thirds of these companies covered removal for medically necessary implants (ie, originally placed for breast reconstruction) and only 43% of companies covered removal of the contralateral implant for cosmetic augmentations. Most companies (70%) covered implant reinsertion, but usually only in cases of breast reconstruction. Only 17% of companies covered implant reinsertion for cases of cosmetic augmentation. Many companies have clearly stated within their policies explicit denials of any cancer therapy of

BIA-ALCL if the patient has a prior history of cosmetic augmentation. Effective October 1, 2022, the 2023 edition of the ICD-10-CM now describes BIA-ALCL by diagnosis code C84.7A BIA-ALCL as anaplastic large cell lymphoma, ALK-negative breast when combined with additional code Z98.82 to identify breast implant status.

Management of Asymptomatic Patients with Textured Implants

Patients with a textured breast implant may have a relative indication for prophylactic removal based on the risks and benefits of the procedure.[41,42] Implant removal alone or combined with capsulectomy may or may not prevent the future development of BIA-ALCL. En bloc capsulectomy has associated morbidity which should be weighed along with patient preexisting comorbidities. The risk of developing BIA-ALCL in textured implant patients remains low, and BIA-ALCL generally has a good prognosis when diagnosed early and treated appropriately. Attempts should be made to inform textured implant patients of the risk of BIA-ALCL so that adequate implant surveillance screening can be performed and allow earlier diagnosis in cases that do develop.

Other Implant-Associated Malignancies

Beyond BIA-ALCL, there have also been reports of BCLs and SCCs arising from within breast implant capsules as well as other types of surgically implantable devices. These case reports are limited, and not nearly as numbered as those for BIA-ALCL, with approximately 20 cases of SCC and 30 cases of various BCLs (Table 2). In the largest series of BCLs arising around breast implants, we previously reported that all cases involved an active infection of EBV, a known driver of B-cell lymphotropism and oncoviral properties. Therefore, EBV is a likely key component to pathogenesis within implant-associated BCLs.[2] The FDA and American Society of Plastic Surgeons (ASPS) released a statement on September 8, 2022, to inform the public of these risks.[34,35] It is important

Table 2
Comparison between breast implant-associated anaplastic large cell lymphoma and implant associated B-cell lymphomas and squamous cell carcinoma

	BIA-ALCL	IA-BCL	IA-SCC
Number of case reports	> 1000	~30	~20
Predominant cell type	T cells	B cells	Squamous cells
Implant type	Textured surface, both saline and silicone	Both textured and smooth surface, both saline and silicone	Both textured and smooth surface, both saline and silicone
Length of device placement before presentation	Average 10 y	Variable, 10–20 y	Average 20 y
Typical presentation	Unilateral swelling, erythema, pain, periprosthetic effusion	Unilateral swelling, erythema, pain, periprosthetic effusion	Unilateral swelling, erythema, pain, more likely to present as a mass with extracapsular spread
Pathology	Sheets of abnormal T cells with horseshoe or kidney shaped nuclei, CD30+, ALK-	Sheets of abnormal B cells, CD20+, various other B-cell markers (depending on the type of B-cell lymphoma), EBV + frequently	Sheets of keratin producing cells, p63+, CK5/6+
Treatment	En bloc capsulectomy, implant removal, responds to bretuximab and anthracycline-based chemotherapy, radiation	En bloc capsulectomy, implant removal, responds to CHOP-based chemotherapy	En bloc capsulectomy with removal of any invading masses, less responsive to chemotherapy or radiation
Prognosis	Very good: complete remission achieved in 93% who present with limited disease	Unclear, may behave similar to BIA-ALCL	Poor: up to 43% mortality at 6 months

CHOP, cyclophosphamide, doxorubicin hydrochloride (hydroxydaunorubicin), vincristine sulfate (Oncovin), and prednisone is a chemotehrapy regimen

to note that characteristics of BIA-SCC differ significantly from BIA-ALCL. For one, BIA-SCC seems have a more aggressive phenotype, with approximately 50% mortality rate at short-term follow-up reported in known cases. Extracapsular spread is more common than contained disease at the time of diagnosis. Although all types of implants have been reported within the clinical history of these patients, it is still unclear whether a specific type of implant common to all implants serves as an oncologic driver similar to textured implants and BIA-ALCL. The average time that the devices have been in place before diagnosis is long term, over 20 years. This seems to suggest it could be similar in etiology to a Marjolin ulcer, whereby SCC arises through chronic inflammation in the capsule. Please refer to **Table 2** for additional comparisons between BIA-ALCL, BIA-BCL, and BIA-SCC.

Although pathogenesis is beyond the scope of this review article, it is important to note that surgeon technique has not been shown to effect the future development of BIA-ALCL.[36] Physicians must seek out reputable sources of research as there is an abundance of misinformation currently being circulated on BIA-ALCL.[37] BIA-ALCL patients do not have distinct microbiomes, and Ralstonia bacteria are no longer implicated in pathogenesis.[38] Current research focuses on a mechanism of perpetual exhaustive phagocytosis whereby macrophages digest silicone particulate, becoming overwhelmed and releasing inflammatory cytokines and allergic inflammation cascade. Lymphocytes are highly replicative with selection for JAK/STAT mutations. A key mediator of all these implants seems to be an immune suppressed and hypoxic interface between the implant and the surrounding tissue.[39,40]

SUMMARY

In conclusion, BIA-ALCL is an uncommon and still emerging malignancy that has only become readily recognized over the past decade. Much research is now available elucidating best practice for diagnosis and treatment to ensure optimal outcomes for BIA-ALCL patients. Case reports have risen with increasing recognition of this disease but the current COVID pandemic may have impeded or delayed recent reporting. BIA-ALCL usually presents with disease isolated to the implant capsule and generally has a good prognosis when treated appropriately. Complete surgical excision consists of en bloc capsulectomy with implant removal and removal of associated masses with negative margins. Diagnosis should be established; consultation with oncology as well as imaging must be performed before any surgical intervention. Future research will focus on better understanding of BIA-ALCL within the context of a larger spectrum of inflammatory mediated malignancies so that ultimately, we may progress from cure to prevention.

CLINICS CARE POINTS

- When breast implant -associated anaplastic large cell lymphoma (BIA-ALCL) is suspected, aspirate and test for disease before any surgical intervention.
- Suspicious fluid collections should be tested for CD30 immunohistochemistry to rule out disease.
- Pathology evaluation generally requires at least 50 mL of aspirant and may require higher volumes if the patient has had prior repeated aspirations.
- Confirmed diagnosis should receive metastatic workup with PET/CT and oncology consult before attempting explantation.
- Complete surgical treatment includes explantation, total capsulectomy, resection of associated masses with negative margins, and excision of involved lymph nodes.
- Reconstruction may be performed in the immediate or delayed setting.
- Disease surveillance includes imaging every 6 months for 2 years after surgical treatment.
- Breast implant informed consent should include the risk of BIA-ALCL, squamous cell carcinoma, and B-cell lymphoma.

DISCLOSURE

MD Anderson Cancer Center participates in FDA clinical trials for Abbvie Allergan, Mentor Corporation, and Establishment Labs. All authors report no financial conflicts of interest.

REFERENCES

1. Keech JA Jr, Creech BJ. Anaplastic T-cell lymphoma in proximity to a saline-filled breast implant. Plast Reconstr Surg 1997;100(2):554–5.
2. Medeiros LJ, Marques-Piubelli ML, Sangiorgio VFI, et al. Epstein-Barr-virus-positive large B-cell lymphoma associated with breast implants: an analysis of eight patients suggesting a possible pathogenetic relationship. Mod Pathol 2021;34(12):2154–67.
3. Whaley RD, Aldrees R, Dougherty RE, et al. Breast implant capsule-associated squamous cell carcinoma: report of 2 patients. Int J Surg Pathol 2022;30(8):900–7.
4. Marra A, Viale G, Pileri SA, et al. Breast implant-associated anaplastic large cell lymphoma: a comprehensive review. Cancer Treat Rev 2020;84(3):101963.
5. Ashley FL. Further studies on the natural-Y breast prosthesis. Plast Reconstr Surg 1972;49:414–9.
6. Clemens MW. Discussion: anaplastic large cell lymphoma in the plastic Surgery practice: has it influenced practice patterns? Plast Reconstr Surg 2016;138(5):819e–20e.
7. Jalalabadi F, Doval J, Andres F, et al. Breast implant utilization trends in USA versus Europe and the impact of BIA-ALCL publications. Plast Reconstr Surg Glob Open 2021;9(3):e3449.
8. Miranda RN, Medeiros LJ, Ferrufino-Schmidt MC, et al. Pioneers of breast implant-associated anaplastic large cell lymphoma: history from case report to global recognition. Plast Reconstr Surg 2019;143(3S A Review of Breast Implant-Associated Anaplastic Large Cell Lymphoma):7S–14S.
9. US Food & Drug Administration. Breast implant-associated anaplastic large cell lymphoma (BIA-ALCL). Available at: http://www.fda.gov/MedicalDevices/ProductsandMedicalProcedures/ImplantsandProsthetics/BreastImplants/ucm239995.htm. Accessed November 5th, 2022.
10. McCarthy CM, Loyo-Berríos N, Qureshi AA, et al. Patient registry and outcomes for breast implants and anaplastic large cell lymphoma etiology and epidemiology (PROFILE): initial report of findings, 2012-2018. Plast Reconstr Surg 2019;143(3S A Review of Breast Implant-Associated Anaplastic Large Cell Lymphoma):65S–73S.
11. Swerdlow SH, Campo E, Pileri SA, et al. The 2016 revision of the World Health Organization

classification of lymphoid neoplasms. Blood 2016; 127(20):2375–90.

12. Asaad M, Offodile A, Santanelli Di Pompeo F, et al. Management of symptomatic patients with textured implants. Plast Reconstr Surg 2021;147(5S): 58S–68S.

13. International Organization for Standardization. The ISO 14607:2018. Non-active surgical implants—mammary implants—particular requirements. Available at: https://www. iso.org/standard/63973.html. Accessed October 1, 2020.

14. Rebiere B, Petit E, Cot D. Instiut Europeen des Membranes. Definition d'une gamme de texturation pour les implants mammaires. Available at: www. iemm.univ-montp2.fr. Accessed October 1, 2020.

15. Atlan M, Nuti G, Wang H, et al. Breast implant surface texture impacts host tissue response. J Mech Behav Biomed Mater 2018;88:377–85.

16. Safety of polyurethane-covered breast implants. Expert panel on the safety of polyurethane-covered breast implants. Can Med Assoc J 1991;145: 1125–32.

17. Munhoz AM, Clemens MW, Nahabedian MY. Breast implant surfaces and their impact on current practices: where we are now, and where we are going? PRS Glob Open 2019;7(10th):e2466.

18. US Food and Drug Administration. The FDA requests Allergan voluntarily recall Natrelle BIOCELL textured breast implants and tissue expanders from the market to protect patients: FDA safety communication. US Food and Drug Administration. Available at: https://www.fda.gov/medical-devices/ safety-communications/fda-requests- allergan-voluntarily-recall-natrelle-biocell-textured-breast-implants-and-tissue. Accessed November 5, 2022.

19. FDA News Release. FDA takes action to protect patients from risk of certain textured breast implants; requests Allergan voluntarily recall certain breast implants and tissue expanders from market. 2019. Available at: https://www.fda.gov/news-events/ press-announcements/fda-takes-action-protect- patients-risk-certain-textured-breast-implants-irequests-allergan. Accessed November 5, 2022.

20. American Society of Plastic Surgeons. Breast implant-associated anaplastic large cell lymphoma (BIA-ALCL). Available at: https://www.plasticsurgery. org/patient-safety/breast-implant-safety/bia-alcl-summary. Accessed November 5, 2022.

21. Clemens MW, McGuire PA. Discussion: a prospective approach to inform and treat 1340 patients at risk for BIA-ALCL. Plast Reconstr Surg 2019;144(1):57–9.

22. Cordeiro PG, Ghione P, Ni A, et al. Risk of breast implant associated anaplastic large cell lymphoma (BIA-ALCL) in a cohort of 3546 women prospectively followed long term after reconstruction with textured breast implants. J Plast Reconstr Aesthet Surg 2020; 73:841–6.

23. de Jong D, Vasmel WL, de Boer JP, et al. Anaplastic large-cell lymphoma in women with breast implants. JAMA 2008 5;300(17):2030–5.

24. Clemens MW, Jacobsen ED, Horwitz SM. 2019 NCCN consensus guidelines on the diagnosis and treatment of breast implant-associated anaplastic large cell lymphoma (BIA-ALCL). Aesthet Surg J 2019;39(Suppl_1):S3–13.

25. Jaffe ES, Ashar BS, Clemens MW, et al. Best practices guideline for the pathologic diagnosis of breast implant-associated anaplastic large-cell lymphoma. J Clin Oncol 2020;38(10):1102–11.

26. Santanelli di Pompeo F, Clemens MW, Atlan M, et al. 2022 practice recommendation updates from the world consensus conference on BIA-ALCL. Aesthet Surg J 2022;42(11):1262–78.

27. Oishi N, Miranda RN, Feldman AL. Genetics of breast implant-associated anaplastic large cell lymphoma (BIA-ALCL). Aesthet Surg J 2019;39(Suppl_1):S14–20.

28. Clemens MW, Medeiros LJ, Butler CE, et al. Complete surgical excision is essential for the management of patients with breast implant-associated anaplastic large cell lymphoma. J Clin Oncol 2016; 34(2):160–8.

29. Tevis S, Hunt KH, Clemens MW. Stepwise en-bloc resection of breast implant associated ALCL with oncologic considerations. Aesthet Surg J Open Forum 2019;1(1):ojz005.

30. Lamaris GA, Butler CE, Clemens MW. Breast reconstruction following breast implant–associated anaplastic large cell lymphoma. Plast Reconstr Surg 2019;143(3S):51S–8S.

31. Ferrufino-Schmidt MC, Medeiros LJ, Liu H, et al. Clinicopathologic features and prognostic impact of lymph node involvement in patients with breast implant-associated anaplastic large cell lymphoma. Am J Surg Pathol 2018;42(3):293–305.

32. Miranda RN, Aladily TN, Prince HM, et al. Breast implant-associated anaplastic large-cell lymphoma: long-term follow-up of 60 patients. J Clin Oncol 2014;32(2):114–20.

33. Ha M, Ngaage LM, Zhu K, et al. Breast implant-associated anaplastic large cell lymphoma (BIA-ALCL): are you covered? Aesthet Surg J 2021; 41(12):NP1943–9.

34. American Society of Plastic Surgeons. ASPS statement on breast implant associated-squamous cell carcinoma (BIA-SCC). Available at: https://www. plasticsurgery.org/for-medical-professionals/ publications/psn-extra/news/asps-statement-on- breast-implant-associated-squamous-cell- carcinoma. Accessed November 5th, 2022.

35. U.S. Food and Drug Administration. Breast implants: reports of squamous cell carcinoma and various lymphomas in capsule around implants: FDA safety communication. Available at: https://www.fda.gov/

medical-devices/safety-communications/breast-implants-reports-squamous-cell-carcinoma-and-various-lymphomas-capsule-around-implants-fda. Accessed November 5th, 2022.

36. DeCoster RC, Lynch EB, Bonaroti AR, et al. Breast implant-associated anaplastic large cell lymphoma: defining future research priorities. Clin Plast Surg 2021;48(1):33–43.

37. Swanson E. Concerns regarding dishonesty in reporting a large study of patients treated with allergan Biocell breast implants. Ann Plast Surg 2022; 88(6):585–8.

38. Walker JN, Hanson BM, Pinkner CL, et al. Insights into the microbiome of breast implants and periprosthetic tissue in breast implant-associated anaplastic large cell lymphoma. Sci Rep 2019;9(1):10393.

39. Doloff JC, Veiseh O, de Mezerville R, et al. The surface topography of silicone breast implants mediates the foreign body response in mice, rabbits and humans. Nat Biomed Eng 2021;5(10):1115–30.

40. Oishi N, Hundal T, Phillips JL, et al. Molecular profiling reveals a hypoxia signature in breast implant-associated anaplastic large cell lymphoma. Haematologica 2021;106(6):1714–24.

41. Di Pompeo FS, Panagiotakos D, Firmani G, Sorotos M. BIA-ALCL epidemiological findings from a retrospective study of 248 cases extracted from relevant case reports and Series: a systematic review. Aesthet Surg J 2022;sjac312. https://doi.org/10.1093/asj/sjac312. Epub ahead of print. PMID: 36441968.

42. Clemens MW. Commentary on: BIA-ALCL epidemiological findings from a retrospective study of 248 cases extracted from relevant case reports and series: a systematic review. Aesthet Surg J 2023; sjad004. https://doi.org/10.1093/asj/sjad004. Epub ahead of print. PMID: 36624630.

Modern Approaches to Pedicled Latissimus Dorsi Flap Breast Reconstruction with Immediate Fat Transfer

Salma A. Abdou, MD, Karina Charipova, MD, David H. Song, MD, MBA*

KEYWORDS

- Autologous breast reconstruction • Latissimus dorsi pedicled flap • Fat grafting • Lipotransfer

KEY POINTS

- One of the main limitations of the latissimus dorsi pedicled flap for breast reconstruction is insufficient volume. This often requires supplementation with an implant, predisposing patients to risks inherent to introducing a prosthesis that includes implant exposure, capsular contracture, infection, and need for reoperation.
- The latissimus dorsi flap with immediate fat transfer (LIFT) offers a single-stage breast reconstruction with high-volume fat transfer to provide sufficient volume with the patient's own tissue.
- The LIFT procedure is a viable breast reconstruction option for patients who desire autologous breast reconstruction but are not candidates for free tissue transfer, as well as a salvage option for women in whom a prior reconstruction has failed or produced unsatisfactory outcomes.

INTRODUCTION

Several studies have shown that autologous breast reconstruction provides superior esthetic and patient-reported outcomes as compared with implant-based reconstruction.[1-3] Analysis of breast questionnaire (BREAST-Q) responses of over 2,000 women showed that at 2-year follow-up, women who underwent autologous reconstruction were more satisfied with their reconstructive outcome and had better psychosocial and sexual well-being than those who underwent implant-based reconstruction.[1] Furthermore, total 2-year health care costs associated with autologous reconstruction have also been shown to be lower than those of implant-based surgery despite the lower index cost of implant-based reconstruction.[3] Microsurgical abdominal-based free flaps are considered the gold standard for autologous breast reconstruction; however, not all patients are candidates (eg, patients with significant comorbidities that preclude them from prolonged anesthesia, history of abdominoplasty, or inadequate donor site volume). If this is the case in a patient who desires autologous breast reconstruction, the pedicled latissimus dorsi (LD) flap is commonly used as an alternative.

One of the main limitations of the LD pedicled flap for breast reconstruction is insufficient volume.[4] A variation of the LD flap, the extended LD flap, initially described by Hokin in 1983, sought to address this by incorporating lumbar fat extensions.[5] The extended LD flap has since evolved to include the parascapular and scapula "fat fascia."[5] Although they address the issue of insufficient volume, these technical modifications have had limited applications due to risk of increased donor site morbidity, which largely include increased seroma rates, wound dehiscence, and contour deformity.[5]

The use of an implant to supplement LD flap reconstruction is a popular breast reconstruction

Department of Plastic Surgery, MedStar Plastic and Reconstructive Surgery, Washington, DC, USA
* Corresponding author. 3800 Reservoir Road Northwest, PHC Building First Floor, Washington, DC 20007.
E-mail address: David.H.Song@medstar.net

Clin Plastic Surg 50 (2023) 259–265
https://doi.org/10.1016/j.cps.2022.10.004
0094-1298/23/Published by Elsevier Inc.

plasticsurgery.theclinics.com

modality, but brings with it additional risk factors, including infection, extrusion, capsular contracture, and need for exchange in the future.[6,7] In a study of late results of LD flap with implant reconstruction at 10-year follow-up, 50% of patients required late reoperation for revision or removal of the implant with a total failure rate of 10%, reflecting those patients who required definitive implant removal.[6] Within the same study, formal measurements of breast position, patient questionnaires, and photographic assessments indicated that symmetry and overall esthetic outcomes of LD flap and implant reconstruction trended toward poor, suggesting that even those patients for whom surgery is successful are dissatisfied and frequently seek further revision with fat grafting to improve volume and contour.[6,8,9] Fat grafting as a method of augmenting volume in patients with prior LD flap reconstruction has been shown to significantly improve patient satisfaction (ie, 20% satisfied and 80% very satisfied) with minimal complications (eg, minor local infection, fat necrosis).[9]

Although the majority of the existing literature has focused on the use of lipotransfer as a secondary revision procedure following both autologous and implant-based reconstruction, fat grafting as the primary modality for volume enhancement of the LD flap at the time of reconstruction (LD and immediate fat transfer, ie, latissimus dorsi flap with immediate fat transfer [LIFT]) has been recently introduced as a viable option to address the volume limitations of the LD flap.[8,9] This approach not only mitigates many of the historical issues seen with the use of a prosthesis, but also allows for a single-stage reconstruction using all the patient's own tissue, making it a highly valuable technique in the plastic surgeon's armamentarium for breast reconstruction. Importantly, the LIFT procedure can also be offered to patients as a salvage option after either failed microsurgical or implant-based reconstructive efforts.

PATIENT SELECTION AND PREOPERATIVE COUNSELING

Several factors and patient characteristics must be considered during the initial discussion of and evaluation for autologous breast reconstruction including oncologic treatment plan, medical comorbidities, current breast volume/contour, body habitus, reconstructive goals, and patient preference. The abdomen is frequently the preferred donor site in microsurgical autologous reconstruction. Several abdominal-based free flaps for breast reconstruction have been described, which differ in the amount of abdominal muscle incorporated, for example, muscle-sparing transverse rectus abdominis flap (MS-TRAM), and deep inferior epigastric perforator (DIEP) flap. However, eligible patients must have sufficient abdominal fat to create the desired breast size. Furthermore, patients with a history of abdominal surgery that may have damaged or sacrificed source vessels, angiosomes, and perforators may not be eligible.[10,11] Patient comorbidities, including hypercoagulable state and tobacco use, must be considered before surgery and patients must be advised accordingly. A candid conversation should be had with each patient and her support system regarding complications to set expectations early. Patients should be made aware that certain comorbidities, such as hypercoagulable state, diabetes mellitus, and obesity inherently predispose them to increased risk of specific complications (eg, microvascular failure, delayed wound healing, infection). When discussing various options for autologous reconstruction, flap- and donor site-specific complications should also be noted given, for instance, the known associations between abdominal flaps and hernia risk (0% to 10%) and LD flaps and seroma formation (5% to 25%).[10]

When the patient desires autologous breast reconstruction, we offer the LIFT procedure in addition to the gold standard option of microsurgical reconstruction. The LIFT is preferred for patients who cannot safely receive prolonged anesthesia, have hypercoagulable disorders, or have a history of previous abdominal surgery, which makes their inferior epigastric system unreliable (**Box 1**). We do offer it as a fully autologous alternative with faster recovery, less anesthesia time, and no flap monitoring.[10,11] There exists a

---

Box 1
Indications for a latissimus flap with immediate fat transfer (LIFT)

Indications for LIFT

- Patient desires autologous reconstruction
- Patient is a poor microvascular reconstruction candidate due to comorbidities (active smoking, hypercoagulable state, and obesity)
- Patient cannot undergo prolonged anesthesia
- Patient does not have alternative donor sites due to lack of adequate volume or previous surgery (eg, abdominal liposuction)
- Patient desires reduced recovery time and hospital length of stay

single study comparing the LIFT to abdominally based microsurgical breast reconstruction.[12] Patients who undergo the LIFT procedure for breast reconstruction have significantly shorter operative times and significantly shorter lengths of hospital stay than microsurgical breast reconstruction.

SURGICAL TECHNIQUE
Preoperative Markings

The LD flap is marked over the thoracolumbar fat pad with the patient upright in the preoperative area, considering patient preferences regarding the esthetic position of donor-site scars. Care is taken to orient the skin paddle along the natural creases of the back while allowing a gentle arch of rotation at the time of flap inset. The pinch test confirms no undue tension with closure of the donor site. Fat harvest sites vary depending on patient body habitus but commonly include the abdomen, thighs, and flanks. Fat harvest sites are similarly marked in the preoperative area. The orientation of the skin paddle is carefully reassessed in the operating room as adjustments may be indicated based on need for soft tissue coverage, especially in instances of concurrent mastectomy.

Fat Harvest

Fat is harvested and processed according to the manufacturer's instructions. We use a mixture of 50 mL of lidocaine 1% with epinephrine 1:100,000 diluted into 1 L of normal saline for tumescence and hemostasis. The fat is aspirated with a 3-mm liposuction cannula directly into a REVOLVE fat processing system (LifeCell, Co., Bridgewater, NJ). The fat is rinsed and processed according to manufacturer's instructions and then divided into 10-mL aliquots for the final transfer.

Immediate Fat Transfer

The LD flap is harvested in the lateral decubitus position. Although some authors describe performing both flap and fat harvest simultaneously, using a two-team approach to decrease operative time, this may not always be possible. Importantly, the LD flap is not immediately released from its bony attachments at the spinous processes. Performing the fat grafting with the LD in situ serves the important purpose of providing stabilization to increase efficiency of the lipotransfer. This allows for a high-volume fat transfer; nearly a twofold increase in the volume of fat that can be safely transferred.

There are four primary locations for injecting the harvested fat: the LD skin paddle, the LD muscle,

the mastectomy skin flaps, and the chest wall muscles (ie, pectoralis muscle, serratus muscle). Within the LD muscle and subcutaneous tissue, the fat is preferentially distributed in the portion that will ultimately form the lower breast pole upon final inset. Fat injection is done in a retrograde and fanlike fashion to allow for even distribution and smooth contour. Fat grafting directly into the LD muscle is safe given the absence of a large venous plexus. Furthermore, animal and clinical studies have shown that muscle is an appropriate recipient for lipotransfer owing to its robust blood supply.

Care is taken to avoid injection surrounding the vascular pedicle and the skin paddle is monitored closely for any signs of congestion. When the flap has been sufficiently augmented, the LD muscle is dis-originated from its bony attachments, denervated, and tunneled through the lateral thoracic tunnel to the anterior chest where it is inset to create the breast. Fat grafting before disinserting the flap is an important modification championed by the senior author to increase efficiency of the lipotransfer. In our experience, this technique results in an average of 66% fat take at 3 months follow-up. The most frequent complications following the LIFT procedure include donor-site seroma and delayed wound healing.

Postoperative Care

As patients undergoing LIFT do not require flap monitoring, patients have the option of leaving the same day or choosing to stay overnight in the hospital. In the senior author's practice, most patients who chose postoperative admission are discharged home within 24 to 48 h, making the LIFT a potentially more cost-effective option of reconstruction when compared with free tissue transfer. As all patients leave with at least one drain, follow-up is scheduled within one week of surgery to monitor incisional healing and drain outputs. Given the intrinsic increased risk of donor site seroma associated with the LD flap, the LIFT procedure is associated with longer time to drain removal compared with abdominally based flaps. Seromas are a known complication following the LD flap. There are reports on use of quilting sutures to decrease dead space, thus reducing drain output. However, the literature on this topic is largely composed of small case series. Furthermore, in the senior author's experience, use of quilting sutures may increase risk of hematoma without significantly reducing risk of seroma. We have not found that all patients who undergo LIFT require physical therapy, but all patients are monitored for ipsilateral upper extremity weakness or limited range of motion throughout follow-up and have the option of referral to outpatient therapy if they choose.

DISCUSSION

In 2009, the American Society of Plastic Surgeons reversed the moratorium on fat grafting. Since then, this technique has been widely used by plastic surgeons for both reconstructive and esthetic purposes. With regard to breast reconstruction, fat grafting is useful for revision to improve contour and symmetry after both autologous and implant baes reconstruction. High-volume fat grafting at the time of LD flap reconstruction has made the LIFT an attractive option for autologous breast reconstruction in patients who may not be candidates for microsurgical breast reconstruction. The senior author's technical modifications, which include performing lipotransfer before disorigination and denervation of the flap increases the speed and efficiency of fat grafting.[4]

Zhu and colleagues[13] provided an algorithm for the recommended recipient sites in fat grafted, volume-enhanced LD flap based on timing (immediate versus delayed) and indication (breast cancer versus prophylactic mastectomy) of reconstruction. In cases of immediate reconstruction after breast cancer removal, the chest wall muscles are not grafted to avoid dissemination of any residual tumor tissues. Furthermore, fat is not injected into the mastectomy skin flaps

following mastectomy for breast cancer to avoid vascular compromise of the skin flaps.[13] In instances of immediate breast reconstruction following prophylactic mastectomy, residual fat may be further injected into the mastectomy flaps or chest wall for additional volume. Despite early concerns that fat transfer following breast cancer treatment may play a role in promoting tumorigenesis and angiogenesis, this has not been corroborated with clinical data.[14]

Compared with the 10-case series presented by Zhu and colleagues[13] in which the mean volume of fat grafting was 176 mL per breast, the senior author has shown that a nearly twofold increase in fat volume can be safely transferred in cases of immediate reconstruction without risk of flap loss. This increased graft take may indeed result from injection directly into a well-vascularized recipient site (ie, the LD muscle) as well as meticulous technique to ensure that fat is spread evenly within and across all injection sites.

The senior author's experience showcases that using the aforementioned techniques, especially maximization of volume enhancement using fat grafting, the LIFT procedure is now considered interchangeable with the DIEP flap in patients who have both options available to them.[12] As noted, patients with elevated body mass index and those who prefer to avoid prolonged hospitalization may be more inclined to pursue LIFT over abdominally based microsurgical reconstruction. In fact, the senior author's practice highlights that patients with prior history of unilateral DIEP

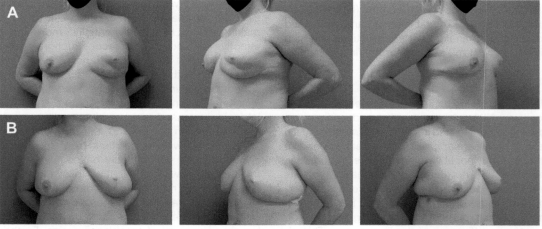

Fig. 1. A 46-year-old woman who presents 4 years following right nipple-sparing mastectomy and left skin-sparing mastectomy. The patient is unhappy with her implant-based reconstruction, mainly scar retraction and nipple asymmetry, and desires autologous breast reconstruction (*A*). The patient underwent latissimus dorsi flap reconstruction with immediate fat grafted from her abdomen. Photos above are 4 weeks postoperatively (*B*).*From* Allen R, Chen C, LoTiempo M. Deep Inferior Epigastric Artery Perforator Flap for Breast Reconstruction. In: Levine K, Vasile J, Chen C Allen R Sr, eds. Perforator Flaps for Breast Reconstruction. Edition 1, 2016, Thieme.

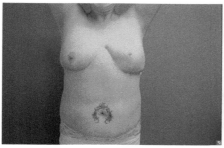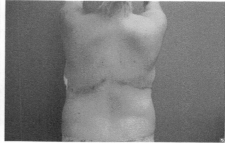

Fig. 2. Denervation of the flap ensures no animation deformities (*left*). Marking the skin paddle in preop with the patient standing up ensures scars are camouflaged in natural skin creases of the back.

flap can undergo subsequent contralateral LIFT with comparable results. This significantly supplements the armamentarium of non-microsurgeons to offer fully autologous options for breast reconstruction and in doing so, greatly increases accessibility for patients.

CASE DEMONSTRATION
Case 1

A 46-year-old woman with a history of breast cancer gene 2 (BRCA 2) mutation underwent right prophylactic mastectomy followed by implant-based reconstruction. Four years later, she presented to the senior author's practice to discuss options for breast revision due to dissatisfaction with her reconstruction. Her major concerns stemmed from multiple deformities, including scar retraction most notable at the inferior pole of the left breast, as well as nipple asymmetry. She underwent bilateral implant removal with anterior capsulectomy and bilateral LIFT with fat grafting from her abdomen (**Fig. 1**). Denervation of the flap ensures no animation deformities (**Fig. 2**).

Case 2

A 54-year-old woman with a history of left invasive ductal carcinoma with associated ductal carcinoma in situ underwent left lumpectomy and axillary dissection. Approximately 27 years later, patient was diagnosed with a new metaplastic carcinoma of the left breast and presented to the senior author's practice to discuss autologous options for immediate reconstruction. She underwent bilateral skin-sparing mastectomy with left sentinel lymph node biopsy and immediate bilateral LIFT with fat grafting from her abdomen (**Fig. 3**). Of note, patient was very active preoperatively and was able to return to return to her baseline level of activity including an intensive

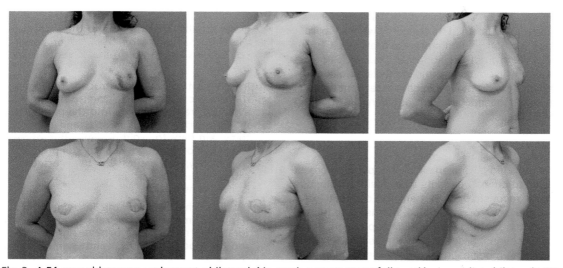

Fig. 3. A 54-year-old woman underwent a bilateral skin-sparing mastectomy followed by immediate bilateral LIFT with fat grafting from her abdomen.

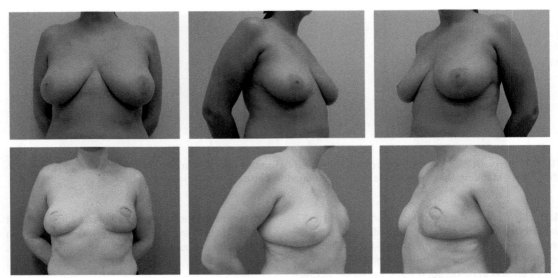

Fig. 4. A 46-year-old woman with left node-positive multicentric breast cancer and Factor V Leiden mutation underwent a bilateral skin-sparing mastectomy followed by bilateral LIFT for breast reconstruction.

weight-lifting regimen less than 2 months after breast reconstruction.

Case 3

A 46-year-old woman with a history of Factor V Leiden mutation complicated by provoked saddle pulmonary embolus on Xarelto presented to the senior author's practice to discuss reconstructive options in the setting of newly diagnosed left node-positive multicentric breast cancer. Patient primarily expressed interest in autologous options as she desired to avoid prosthetic devices and the need for replacement procedures. Patient was recommended for LIFT due to her extensive history of hypercoagulable state. She underwent bilateral skin-sparing mastectomy with left axillary node dissection and immediate bilateral LIFT with fat grafting from her abdomen (**Fig. 4**). She was treated with Lovenox in the immediate postoperative period and more recently underwent bilateral nipple reconstruction with additional fat grafting to left breast.

SUMMARY

The pedicled LIFT is an excellent option for breast reconstruction in patients who desire autologous breast reconstruction but are not candidates for microsurgical reconstruction. Furthermore, use of fat grafting to augment the LD flap mitigates the complications associated with use of implant. Technical modifications such as performing lipotransfer before disinsertion of the muscle allow for safe, efficient, and high-volume fat grafting.

As compared with the gold standard abdominally based microsurgical breast reconstruction, LD flap with immediate transfer offers patients shorter operative times and recovery.

CLINICS CARE POINTS

- Harvesting an extended latissimus dorsi flap and injecting fat in situ before release of the muscle from the spinous processes maximizes the surgeon's control while injecting fat into the flap.

- Preferentially injecting fat into the aspect of the flap that will form the inferior breast pole allows for a more natural contour to the flap.

- In immediate breast reconstruction following therapeutic mastectomy, care is taken to avoid fat transfer directly into the pectoralis major muscle, serratus muscle, and mastectomy skin flaps to avoid dissemination of residual tumor cells and vascular compromise, respectively; these sites can be injected in cases of prophylactic mastectomy and delayed reconstruction.

- Patients who undergo the latissimus dorsi flap with immediate fat transfer procedure for breast reconstruction have significantly shorter operative times and significantly shorter length of hospital stay than microsurgical breast reconstruction

DISCLOSURE

Dr D.H. Song receives royalties from Elsevier for Plastic Surgery, 3rd and 4th Editions, and Biomet Microfixation for Sternalock. The remaining authors have no financial disclosures, commercial associations, or any other conditions posing a conflict of interest to report.

REFERENCES

1. Santosa K, Qi J, Kim H, et al. Long-term patient-reported outcomes in postmastectomy breast reconstruction. JAMA Surg 2018;153(10):891–9.
2. Toyserkani N, Jorgensen M, Tabatabaeifar S, et al. Autologous versus Autologous versus implant-based breast reconstruction: a systematic review and meta-analysis of Breast-Q patient-reported outcomes-nbased bre. J Plast Reconstr Aesthet Surg 2020;73(2):278–85.
3. Lemaine V, Schilz S, Van Houten H, et al. Autologous breast reconstruction versus implant-based reconstruction: how do long-term costs and health care use compare? Plast Reconstr Surg 2020;145(2): 303–11.
4. Economides JM, Song DH. Latissimus dorsi and immediate fat transfer (LIFT) for complete autologous breast reconstruction. Plast Reconstr Surg Glob Open 2018;6(1):1–6.
5. Chang D, Youssef A, Cha S, et al. Autologous breast reconstruction with the extended latissimus dorsi flap. Plast Reconstr Surg 2002;110(3):751–9.
6. Tarantino I, Banic A, Fischer T. Evaluation of late results in breast reconstruction by latissimus dorsi flap and prosthesis implantation. Plast Reconstr Surg 2006;117(5):1387–94.
7. Chang DW, Barnea Y, Robb GL. Effects of an autologous flap combined with an implant for breast reconstruction: an evaluation of 1000 consecutive reconstructions of previously irradiated breasts. Plast Reconstr Surg 2008;122(2):356–62.
8. Thekkinkattil DK, Salhab M, McManus PL. Feasibility of autologous fat transfer for replacement of implant volume in complicated implant-assisted latissimus dorsi flap breast reconstruction. Ann Plast Surg 2015;74(4):397–402.
9. Sinna R, Delay E, Garson S, et al. Breast fat grafting (lipomodelling) after extended latissimus dorsi flap breast reconstruction: a preliminary report of 200 consecutive cases. J Plast Reconstr Aesthet Surg 2010;63(11):1769–77.
10. Nahabedian MY, Patel K. Autologous flap breast reconstruction: surgical algorithm and patient selection. J Surg Oncol 2016;113(8):865–74.
11. Rozen W, Garcia-Tutor E, Alonso-Burgos A, et al. The effect of anterior abdominal wall scars on the vascular anatomy of the abdominal wall: a cadaveric and clinical study with clinical implications. Clin Anat 2009;22(7):815–22.
12. Black CK, Zolper EG, Economides JM, et al. Comparison of the pedicled latissimus dorsi flap with immediate fat transfer versus abdominally based free tissue transfer for breast reconstruction. Plast Reconstr Surg 2020;146(2):137e–46e.
13. Zhu L, Mohan AT, Vijayasekaran A, et al. Maximizing the volume of latissimus dorsi flap in autologous breast reconstruction with simultaneous multisite fat grafting. Aesthet Surg J 2016;36(2):169–78.
14. Petit JY, Lohsiriwat V, Clough KB, et al. The oncologic outcome and immediate surgical complications of lipofilling in breast cancer patients: a multicenter study-milan-paris-lyon experience of 646 lipofilling procedures. Plast Surg Complet Clin Masters PRS- Breast Reconstr 2015;14–9. https://doi.org/10.1097/PRS.0b013e31821e713c.

Modern Approaches to Abdominal-Based Breast Reconstruction

Michael Borrero, MD, Hugo St. Hilaire, MD, Robert Allen, MD*

KEYWORDS

• Deep inferior epigastric perforator • DIEP • SIEA • DCIA • Autologous breast reconstruction

KEY POINTS

- Abdominal-based reconstruction remains at the forefront of autologous breast reconstruction.
- Preoperative imaging and proper patient selection reduces complexity and expedites surgery.
- Muscle-sparing flaps including the deep inferior epigastric perforator (DIEP) and superficial inferior epigastric artery (SIEA) have increasingly high success rates and less abdominal wall morbidity.
- The deep circumflex iliac artery flap provides either additional abdominal soft tissue to augment the DIEP/SIEA flaps or its own flap when these flaps are unavailable.
- Surgeons should be familiar with delay phenomenon and its role in abdominal-based flaps.

INTRODUCTION

Breast reconstruction has evolved over the last few decades but one thing is for certain: the lower abdomen remains the preferred donor site for autologous breast reconstruction (ABR). Tissue volume is often robust and emulates healthy breast tissue. Perforator-based flaps have decreased abdominal wall morbidity. The patient is left with a single, low transverse scar as the only evidence of their surgery. Innovation has favored the field over the last 3 decades, including extended abdominal flaps, stacked flaps, delay procedures, neurotization, and perforator exchange techniques. Modern approaches to abdominal-based breast reconstruction need to be delineated to ensure excellent patient outcomes and professional success.

Today, it is estimated that about 1 in 8 US women will develope invasive breast cancer, and this year alone, it is estimated that there will be 287,850 and 51,400 new cases of invasive and noninvasive (in situ) breast cancer, respectively.[1] Although implant-based reconstruction has surpassed autologous in the past, a recent study has shown that ABRs are increasing.[2]

The history of abdominal-based breast reconstruction dates to the early 1980s. It is during this time that Dr Carl Hartrampf pioneered the transverse rectus abdominus myocutaneous flap, colloquially known as the transverse rectus abdominis myocutaneous (TRAM) flap.[3] To his credit, and that of his team, the 1982 article detailing the TRAM flap procedure gained notoriety and sparked innovation within the realm of breast reconstruction. Moreover, although the TRAM flap remains a viable and successful reconstruction option to-date, the drawbacks soon became apparent, notably in the form of abdominal wall morbidity—hernias and bulging.

It was not long after that the senior author, Dr Allen, developed a solution—the deep inferior epigastric perforator (DIEP) flap. This was introduced in 1992 after thorough investigation of abdominal wall perforator anatomy. This was a major step in muscle-sparing breast reconstruction, and its innovation stimulated microsurgical advances. The benefits were apparent—equivocal success rates, inconspicuous scar, and complete avoidance of muscle harvest.

As the paradigm shifted toward muscle-sparing techniques, the superficial inferior epigastric flap

LSU Department of Surgery, 1542 Tulane Avenue, New Orleans, LA 70112, USA
* Corresponding author.
E-mail address: boballen@diepflap.com

Clin Plastic Surg 50 (2023) 267–279
https://doi.org/10.1016/j.cps.2022.10.007
0094-1298/23/© 2022 Elsevier Inc. All rights reserved.

also came to the forefront. The origin of this flap was well established for soft tissue reconstruction of the head and neck. The first published article regarding its use by Antia and Buch was in 1971.[4] Anatomic studies were published thereafter.[5] The flap was first used for free tissue transfer in breast reconstruction by the senior author in 1989.[6] This flap shares the same soft tissue components of the DIEP flap; however, the primary benefit is that it does not require abdominal fascial incision. Unfortunately, due the unreliable presence and caliber of the artery, a significant number of patients are not candidates for the flap, and those that undergo reconstruction with the SIEA flap are at an increased risk for arterial compromise and partial or total flap loss.[7] With that being said, the SIEA is the least invasive abdominal-based flap for breast reconstruction, and advances in imaging as well at using the delay phenomenon have increased SIEA utility and success.

To add to the abdominal-based flaps, the deep circumflex iliac artery (DCIA) flap has gained attention. This was initially described in 1979 by Taylor and colleagues[8] as the dominant supply for the groin flap. This pedicle perfuses the abdominal wall lateral and superior to the anterior superior iliac spine (ASIS), notably the flanks or "love handle." This area is often rich with soft tissue and underutilized.[9] It is also not reliably perfused by the DIEP or SIEA alone. It has the potential to provide ample soft tissue when the abdominal wall is inaccessible or does not provide enough volume for reconstruction.

PATIENT SELECTION AND CONSIDERATIONS

Recent trends have shown that ABR seems to be increasing. Indications for using abdominal-based flaps for breast reconstruction often include patient preference, severe soft tissue damage secondary to radiation therapy, and even failed implant reconstruction. Contraindications are few but include previous abdominoplasty or any procedure that has disrupted the inferior epigastric vascular supply to the abdominal wall. Considerations should always be made regarding the patient's known comorbidities. Nicotine products greatly influence flap outcomes, and therefore, all patients are counseled on smoking cessation for at least 1 month before and after surgery. This can be confirmed with a preoperative nicotinine test.

After determining that the patient is a surgical candidate for flap reconstruction, a thorough assessment of donor sites follows. There are multiple options but the priority flap is the DIEP flap. Assessing breast and donor volume concordance is critical. This depends on unilateral or bilateral reconstruction. If there is a significant discrepancy between the breast and abdominal donor sites, consideration for extended (eg, DCIA), stacked or hybrid flap reconstruction should be made and discussed with the patient. Fat grafting is often performed in the second stage. Stacked and extended abdominal flaps will be discussed briefly; however, they are beyond the purview of this article.

Of note, history of radiation therapy, or anticipation thereof, affects the decision-making process. Most commonly, in anticipation for adjuvant radiation therapy, flap reconstruction is delayed until the therapy is completed. A temporary or "bridge" expander if often considered to maintain as much of the skin envelope as possible until time of reconstruction.

Anatomy

Deep inferior epigastric
Abdominal wall anatomy including both the deep and superficial inferior epigastric systems are well described and have been corroborated in numerous studies, many of which by the senior author. The abdominal zones of arterial perfusion were initially described by Hartrampf.[10]

The deep inferior epigastric artery originates off the terminal aspect of the external iliac artery deep to the inguinal ligament. The artery courses superomedially through the abdominal wall and enters the rectus abdominis muscle, mostly commonly at the mid-rectus.[11,12] The branching pattern is variable, with perforators often originating within 6 cm caudal to the umbilicus.[13] Most perforators are musculocutaneous. Rarely, septocutaneous perforator wrapping around the medial edge of the rectus muscle may be encountered. A pedicle length of 10 cm can be easily achieved, artery diameter being 3 to 3.5 mm at its origin[14] (**Fig. 1**).

Superficial inferior epigastric
The superficial inferior epigastric flap is based off the named vessel. This artery most commonly originates from the common femoral artery approximately 2 to 3 cm inferior to the inguinal ligament such as the deep inferior epigastric. The origin can be variable, and it may also share a common trunk with the superficial circumflex iliac. The artery runs superiorly and will pierce the superficial fascia before branching and irrigating the anterior abdominal wall. Arterial presence and diameter are variable. Traditionally, the SIEA was recognized as being present in less than 50% of patients, and of adequate caliber for microvascular transfer is only ~50% of these

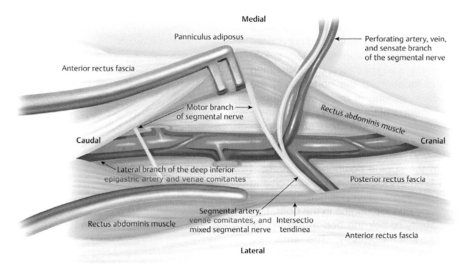

Medial

Panniculus adiposus

Perforating artery, vein, and sensate branch of the segmental nerve

Anterior rectus fascia

Motor branch of segmental nerve

Rectus abdominis muscle

Caudal   Cranial

Lateral branch of the deep inferior epigastric artery and venae comitantes

Posterior rectus fascia

Segmental artery, venae comitantes, and mixed segmental nerve

Rectus abdominis muscle

Intersectio tendinea

Anterior rectus fascia

Lateral

Fig. 1. Anatomy of abdominal wall, deep inferior epigastric pedicle, motor nerves perforating vessels (*From* Allen R, Chen C, LoTiempo M. Deep Inferior Epigastric Artery Perforator Flap for Breast Reconstruction. In: Levine K, Vasile J, Chen C Allen R Sr, eds. Perforator Flaps for Breast Reconstruction.)

patients.[5,15] Adequate caliber is typically defined as 1.5 mm in diameter or greater.

The superficial venous system is also important to recognize. The superficial inferior epigastric artery is often accompanied by venae comitantes. This is distinct from the superficial inferior epigastric vein, which drains the same soft tissues but courses separately and often medially away from the artery before draining into the common femoral vein.[15] SIEA pedicle length can be up to 8 cm and diameter ranges typically from 1.1 to 1.9 mm.

Deep circumflex iliac

The DCIA originates from the external iliac near the deep inferior epigastric artery. Similarly, there are 2 venae that accompany the artery. The artery travels laterally toward the ilium before piercing the transversalis fascia and giving off musculocutaneous perforators.[16] Immediately superior and lateral to the ASIS, the DCIA gives off and ascending branch, providing blood supply to the abdominal wall.[17] A lateral branch is also given off by the pedicle. This pedicle pierces the abdominal wall muscles to supply the overlying skin and subcutaneous tissues. Anatomic studies have shown that on average, there are less than 2 DCIA perforators and they are found 5 to 11 cm posterior to the ASIS and 1 to 35 mm superior to the iliac crest, establishing a zone of perfusion approximately 10 to 15 cm longitudinal by 20 to 30 cm transverse.[16,18]

Imaging

Preoperative imaging includes computed tomographic angiography (CTA), magnetic resonance

angiography (MRA), and duplex ultrasonography. Preoperative imaging is performed routinely at our institution in the form of CTA with thin cuts (1 mm or less) for evaluation of the perforators. Vascular 3-dimensional reconstruction may be beneficial in some cases but is usually unnecessary.

Imaging aids the surgeon in the perforator selection process, which expedites the surgery and decreases complexity. Perforator location is confirmed at the time of surgery with preoperative Doppler localization on the abdominal skin (Fig. 2).

Surgical techniques

Deep inferior epigastric perforator flap At the time of surgery, the patient's abdomen is marked preoperatively in the standing position similar to

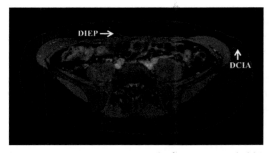

DIEP→

↑ DCIA

Fig. 2. Preoperative MRA with flap protocol (thin 1 mm cuts). Arrows denote right DIEA and left DCIA perforators. (*From* Allen RJ et al. The Stacked Hemiabdominal Extended Perforator Flap for Autologous Breast Reconstruction. Plast Reconstr Surg. 2018;142(6):1424-34.)

that of a traditional abdominoplasty. Landmarks include low transverse incision in the abdominal fold or 7 to8 cm above the introitus, and curvilinear extension to the anterior superior iliac spine. Based on abdominal wall volume, laxity, skin pinch assessment and location of the perforators, the superior incisional marking is made at or above the umbilicus. Preoperative imaging is routinely used to map perforators for selection, and the perforators are marked on the skin surface using a Doppler ultrasound probe before incision while the patient is in the supine position. The present or anticipated breast footprint is marked on the chest wall also in the standing position.

The patient is positioned supine in the operating room with capability to flex the bed at the hip for abdominal closure if necessary. The arms are tucked, if possible, otherwise they are draped sterilely with access to manipulate the arm boards intraoperatively, especially during microsurgical anastomosis.

A 2-team approach is preferred so that chest recipient vessels can be exposed simultaneously with flap elevation. This especially expedites the surgery in delayed reconstruction.

Flap elevation begins with the low transverse incision. The surgery is performed under loupe magnification. Careful dissection 6 to 8 cm lateral to the midline is performed to identify the superficial venous system. The superficial veins are routinely identified and dissected distally below the superficial fascia until an adequate length and caliber vessel is achieved, typically 6 cm and 2 mm, respectively.

After the superficial vein has been isolated and ligated, flap elevation proceeds, usually from lateral to medial. Dissection is carried down to the abdominal wall muscular fascia, at which time careful dissection proceeds with bipolar electrocautery and Westcott microsurgical scissors. Target perforator(s) are identified and dissected circumferentially. If multiple perforators are being selected, it is beneficial to identify all perforators before fascial incision so that the incision can be properly oriented.

Once the perforators have been selected, the anterior rectus fascia is opened sharply, being mindful that the perforator may run immediately under the fascia. The fascia is opened longitudinally, connecting multiple perforators, if necessary, with gentle curve laterally in anticipation of the trajectory of the inferior epigastric pedicle. Most perforators are musculocutaneous, and their muscular courses are variable. The rectus muscle is split parallel to their axis of orientation (Fig. 3). Circumferential dissection of the pedicle is performed, and side branches are ligated.

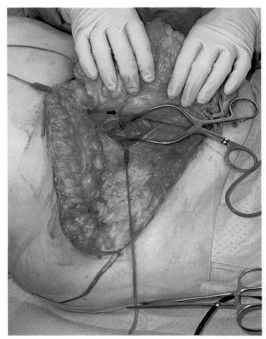

Fig. 3. Elevation of right hemiabdomen DIEP flap after intramuscular perforator dissection.

Preservation of motor nerve branches is critical to reduce abdominal wall morbidity.

The deep inferior epigastric vessels are dissected distally toward the origin until an adequate length and caliber is achieved. Typically, there are 2 veins. The remaining flap is elevated off the abdominal wall, and the midline incision is completed. At this time, the flap is completely perfused by the pedicle. The pedicle is ligated after the recipient vessels have been exposed and prepared. This limits ischemia time of the flap. Each vessel should be ligated separately. Often, the veins are marked with a surgical pen to establish orientation and prevent kinking or twisting after transfer to the recipient site. The flap is weighed, transferred to the chest, and secured in place.

Superficial inferior epigastric artery flap

The beauty of the SIEA flap is the ease of dissection. The same principles of flap elevation apply, except there is no fascial incision or muscular dissection. The flap is elevated in a similar manner, beginning with the inferior incision. The superficial vein and inferior epigastric artery are identified, and careful microsurgical dissection is performed craniocaudal until adequate length and caliber of the vessels have been achieved. The preferred length is 6 to 8 cm and a diameter greater than 1.5 mm. After circumferential dissection of the vessels has been performed, the flap is elevated off the abdominal wall, ligating all perforators from the deep system. The flap is harvested, weighed, transferred, and inset in the same manner as previously discussed.

Deep circumflex iliac artery flap

The DCIA flap is often combined with the DIEP and SIEA flaps, what is colloquially known as a "stacked flap." The term "stacked" describes the use of multiple flaps, either conjoined, placed side-to-side, or on top of each other. The combination of flaps creates additional volume for reconstruction. Stacked flaps will be described in detail in a separate article; however, it is important to note their role in abdominal-based breast reconstruction.

DCIA flap markings differ if the flap is isolated or combined with the DIEP or SIEA.

An isolated DCIA flap is marked with the patient in the standing position. Preoperative imaging of the perforator location is reviewed and confirmed on the skin over the flanks, which is superior and lateral to the ASIS. The inferior mark is made first. It is inferior and lateral to the ASIS and begins in the midaxial line. It is drawn transversely posteriorly to incorporate as much soft tissue as possible above the superolateral buttocks. The distance from the perforator to the end point is roughly between 10 and 15 cm. The line is brought onto the anterior abdominal wall for another 10 to 15 cm. A skin pinch is performed to determine maximal width to provide a tension-free closure.

When combined, the DIEP or SIEA flap is marked first, then extended into the zone of perfusion of the DCIA perforator with lateral markings as described above (**Fig. 4**).

Elevation of the flap begins with the anterior incision, whether in isolation or combination with the DIEP/SIEA flap. Incision is carried down to musculofascial wall and proceeds laterally. Careful dissection is performed around the ASIS, the location of the perforator based on skin Doppler mark. Perforators are identified and circumferential dissection is performed at the muscle level. The posterior incision is then made, and the flap is elevated medially. The external abdominal oblique is incised parallel to the axis of muscle orientation such as the DIEP flap. Careful intramuscular dissection is performed because the pedicle tends to take a tortuous course through each muscle layer. Self-retaining retractors are placed, and pedicle course is traced to the location it pierces the internal abdominal oblique. The muscle is incised, and the pedicle traced medially to the transversalis fascia. The transversalis fascia marks the end point of dissection. Care is taken to identify lateral nerve branches that run in the plane between the internal abdominal oblique and the transversus abdominis. Pedicle length at this point is on average 6 cm with arterial diameter greater than 1.5 mm.[16]

Stacked, hemiabdominal extended perforator flap

The stacked, hemiabdominal extended perforator flap (SHAEP) was introduced as a novel approach in 2018.[19] This included the standard DIEP flap with addition to a more laterally based blood supply—DCIA, SCIA, SIEA, lumbar artery perforator—to enhance perfusion and augment volume. This was previously described by Buchel with combinations of the DIEP, SIEA, and DCIA.[16]

Flap elevation is described as above. Occasionally a lumbar artery perforator is the source vessel to perfuse the lateral abdominal tissue. Regardless, the lateral pedicle (ie, DCIA perforator) is dissected through the abdominal wall for approximately 6 to 8 cm to the ASIS. The pedicle is ligated and then an intraflap anastomosis is performed under the microscope on a sterile back table (**Fig. 5**). The lateral pedicle, often DCIA perforator, is anastomosed either to the cephalic continuation of the deep inferior epigastric, or to a sizeable lateral branch. This creates a stacked hemiabdominal extended flap that can be inset as a single, conjoined unit.

Chest vessel exposure and anastomosis

The recipient vessels for microsurgical anastomosis are the internal mammary artery and vein. Exposure begins first with creation of the breast pocket. Based on preoperative markings, skin flaps are elevated until the desired pocket is achieved. If tissue expanders are present, the expander is removed with complete capsulectomy. This prevents internal scar and deformation of the breast pocket from capsular contracture. If the expander is in the subpectoral or dual-plane position, the pectoralis major muscle is delaminated from the skin flap and sutured back down to the chest wall before exposure of the vessels.

After the pocket is recreated, a closed suction drain is placed and pectoralis muscle blocks are performed.

The internal mammary vessels are exposed under loupe magnification. The second intercostal is the optimal space for vessel diameter and preferred location for microsurgical anastomosis. In nipple-sparing mastectomies, this space may be difficult or impossible to obtain, at which point the third intercostal space is usually accessible.

The pectoralis muscle is incised parallel to the fibers. The subpectoral plane is developed over the

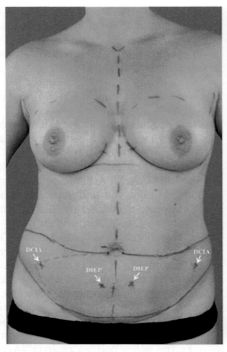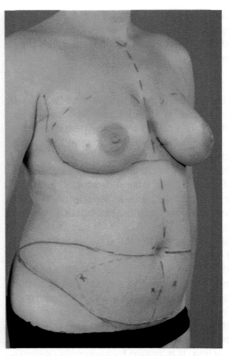

Fig. 4. Preoperative markings for an extended abdominal flap including DIEP (*dotted light blue*) and addition of DCIA flap (*solid dark blue*). (*From* Allen RJ et al. The Stacked Hemiabdominal Extended Perforator Flap for Autologous Breast Reconstruction. Plast Reconstr Surg. 2018;142(6):1424-34.)

second intercostal space as well as over the second and third rib costal cartilage. At this point, a decision is made regarding the amount of costochrondral rib resection. With a large interspace, the vessels may be accessible without removing any rib cartilage. More often, a portion of the cartilage is removed. Our preference is to remove half

of the width of the cartilage. This leaves half of the sternal articulation and maintains some stability to the chest wall.

Internal mammary perforator arteries and veins may be encountered during recipient vessel exposure. These should be evaluated to determine if they can be used as the recipient vessels, or at the very least if the perforating vein can be anastomosed to the flap superficial vein. The only caveat is that in nipple-sparing mastectomies, these perforators may be vital to nipple–areolar complex perfusion and, therefore, should be preserved (**Fig. 6**).

The fatty plane between the intercostals and the pleura is developed. This houses the internal mammary vessels, which lie within 2 to 3 cm of the sternal border. Venous anastomoses are performed with the venous coupler. Arterial anastomoses are performed with handsewn 9-0 nylon. If a superficial vein is being used, options are to perform a venous anastomosis at this time to the retrograde internal mammary vein, or to an intercostal perforating vein at the time of flap inset.

Internal Doppler implants are used in all buried flaps, and occasionally in flaps that have skin paddles for postoperative monitoring. The internal Doppler is placed around the postanastomotic artery (**Fig. 7**).

Fig. 5. Back table intra-flap anastomosis between DCIA and cephalic continuation of the DIEP. Asterisk denotes cephalic continuation of the deep inferior epigastric artery and vein. (*From* Allen RJ et al. The Stacked Hemiabdominal Extended Perforator Flap for Autologous Breast Reconstruction. Plast Reconstr Surg. 2018;142(6):1424-34.)

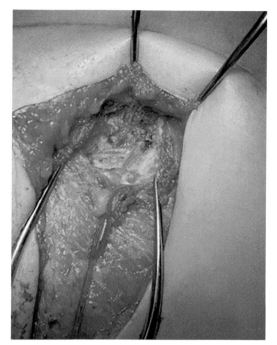

Fig. 6. Internal mammary vessel exposure with perforator in the second intercostal space.

Superficial inferior epigastric artery flap—delaying the flap

Despite having a lower donor site morbidity, the SIEA flap remains less popular. This is because studies have shown higher complication rates, as high as 14% overall, with arterial insufficiency, thrombosis or spasms being the most common causes, and reoperation rates between 6% and 20%.[7,20,21] The delay phenomenon, in which vessels surrounding the main pedicles are ligated to augment the pedicle's blood supply, has been well-acknowledged and recently applied and

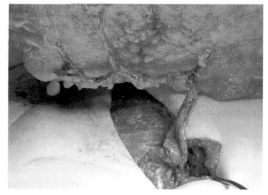

Fig. 7. DIEP flap anastomosis to internal mammary vessels.

described by the senior author and his colleagues.[22] The delay procedure, which was primarily performed for the SIEA flap, requires subtotal elevation of the flap. The flap is elevated in the standard fashion, the superficial inferior epigastric vessels are identified and dissected circumferentially for several centimeters. The remaining flap is elevated, ligating all deep perforators. The caveat is that the flap is kept in continuity inferiorly and laterally via skin bridges (Fig. 8). This maintains some additional perfusion and drainage because the choke vessels open and the SIEA adapts to perfuse the flap. A recent study by the senior author and his team showed that mean cross-sectional diameter of the SIEA increased by an average of 0.9 mm after delay, from 1.37 to 2.26 mm.[22] The time interval between the delay procedure and reconstruction ranged from 6 days to 14 months, depending on the oncologic management. At least 6 days between delay and flap reconstruction is recommended. The delay procedure is performed on an outpatient basis, and the complications rates among the 24 flaps were comparable to the literature, with an overall 12% complication rate and no anastomotic revisions or flap loss (Fig. 9).

Perforator exchange

Yet another advancement in modern abdominal-based flap reconstruction is the perforator-to-perforator anastomosis or "perforator exchange" technique. This was introduced in 2019 by Della-Croce and colleagues.[23] Occasionally multiple perforators are selected per flap. Often, there is intervening muscle between the perforators. Perforator exchange is intraoperative technique that further reduces abdominal muscle morbidity eliminating any muscle transection when multiple perforators are being selected. The flap is elevated, and the perforators are carefully dissected to their fullest extent until limited by the intervening muscle. At this point, the dominant perforator and pedicle are dissected in the standard fashion, and any additional perforators are ligated or "disassembled" from the pedicle. Afterward, the flap is brought to a sterile back-table and the perforator is reanastomosed to either its branch or a comparable branch off the pedicle. This reestablishes perforator perfusion to the flap and obviates muscle sacrifice.

Neurotization

Flap neurotization results remain elusive. Blondeel and colleagues[24] reported early on their experience with neurotization of breast flaps. Since then, there seems to be a trend toward both flap neurotization procedures, and several

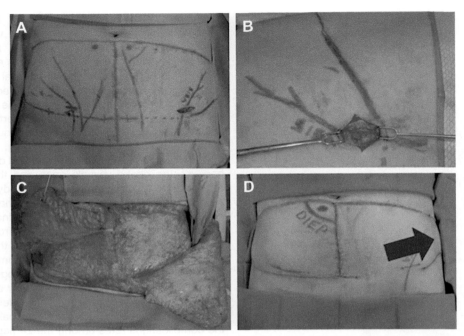

Fig. 8. Flap creation procedure for surgical delay of left SIEA flap and right DIEP flap. (*A*) Preoperative markings of abdominal flap design including the location and course of the SIEA, SIEV, and DIEA perforators bilaterally. (*B*) Incision over SIEA to verify arterial size intraoperatively. (*C*) Elevated left SIEA and right DIEP flaps. (*D*) Skin closure of delayed flaps, note the lateral skin and fascial attachment left during the delay procedure. (*From* Hoffman RD, Allen RJ et al. Surgical Delay-Induced Hemodynamic Alterations of the Superficial Inferior Epigastric Artery Flap for Autologous Breast Reconstruction. Ann Plast Surg. 2022;88(5 Suppl 5):S414-S21.)

studies have demonstrated efficacy at 12 months.[25,26] Neurotization is not routinely performed at the senior author's institution, instead they are considered on a case-by-case basis. The preferred technique for neurotization is to use an interposition allograft between the anterior intercostal nerve in the second or third intercostal space. The donor nerve is identified with the pedicle and preserved during flap elevation. The nerve is harvested at the level exiting the fascia at which point it is strictly sensory. Under the microscope on the back-table, a neurorrhaphy is performed between the donor nerve and a processed nerve allograft of equivalent caliber. A 9-0 Nylon is used for epineurial repair. The flap is transferred to the recipient site. The anterior intercostal nerve is easily identified crossing over the internal mammary vessels from medial to lateral at the inferior border of the costal cartilage. After arterial and venous anastomosis, neurorrhaphy is performed from the intercostal nerve to the allograft in a similar fashion.

Flap contouring and inset

In standard bilateral breast reconstruction with DIEP flaps, each hemiabdomen reconstructs the contralateral breast. The flap is oriented such that the lateral tail of the abdominal flap is the superior point of the breast at time of inset. This point is the most distal point of perfusion and often causes troublesome fat necrosis. Once the anastomosis has been performed, the entire flap is inspected for healthy dermal bleeding. Usually, this superior tail is resected before inset, weighing less than 50 g.

With immediate flap reconstruction, a thorough inspection and assessment of the mastectomy skin flaps is important. Indocyanine green angiography can aid microsurgeons in determining mastectomy flap viability. Skin deficits should be identified and transposed to the flap. This is often necessary in irradiated breasts. The remaining skin of the flap is deepithelialized, with preference to remove all the dermis to prevent contracture at the superficial surface of the flap. Any further debulking is performed to contour the breast. The ability to contour or cone the breast depends on fat thickness and quality. The flap is inset, secured with absorbable suture from the superficial fascia to the chest wall. The superficial vein is anastomosed to an internal mammary vein perforator during the inset. Alternatively, it can be anastomosed to the retrograde internal mammary vein before inset.

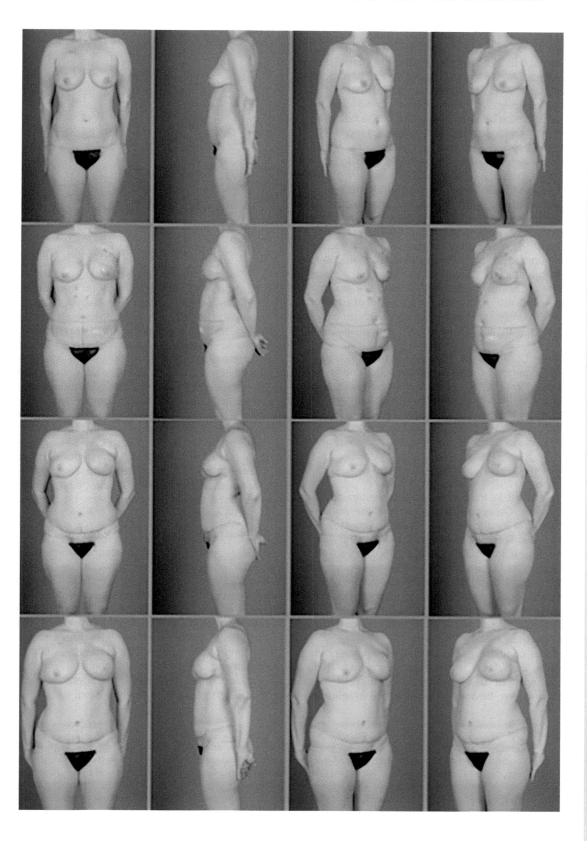

Donor site management

With a 2-team approach, the abdominal wall closure can be performed after the flaps have been transferred to the recipient sites. The abdominal skin flap is elevated such as in a traditional abdominoplasty. Undermining is confined to the medial rectus above the umbilicus. The fascial incisions are closed with a 2-layer running 0-PDS or barbed equivalent suture. The patient is placed in a reflex or "beach-chair" position to facilitate closure. One or 2 closed suction drains are placed above the fascia. Progressive retention sutures are used to reduce tension at the skin closure and help prevent seroma formation. The abdomen is closed in a layered fashion including 2-0 polydioxanone suture (PDS) or barbed suture for Scarpa fascia and running 2-0 barbed suture for the deep dermal and subcuticular layers. Before closure, the umbilical stalk is identified, transposed to the skin surface, and retrieved through an elliptical excision with circumferential defatting prior. The umbilicus is inset with absorbable deep dermal and skin sutures.

If the DCIA flap has been harvested, the internal and external oblique musculofascial units are repaired with a PDS or equivalent barbed suture. Abdominal flap closure is the same. Incisions are dressed with an adhesive surgical tape (eg, Prineo, Ethicon, LLC USA). An abdominal binder or compression girdle is placed at the end of surgery.

Postoperative monitoring and care

The patient is transferred to the postanesthesia care unit. On receiving the patient, the nurse is shown the location of skin paddle perforator signals, which are marked intraoperatively with a prolene suture. Internal implantable Dopplers are also checked for signals (Fig. 10). The nurse performs flap checks every 15 minutes for the first hour, then every 30 minutes for the second hour. By this time, the patient is transferred to one of the medical-surgical floors that routinely cares for postsurgical free flap patients.

Flaps checks are then performed every 4 hours. A foley catheter is left in place overnight. Arterial lines are not used during surgery. Sequential compressive devices stay in place throughout

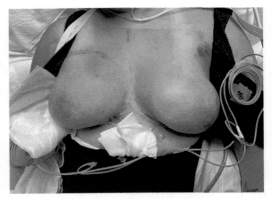

Fig. 10. Postoperative bilateral buried DIEP flaps monitored with internal Doppler. The internal Dopplers are placed around the post-anastomotic artery.

the hospital stay and deep veinous thrombosis (DVT) chemoprophylaxis is initiated after surgery.

Postoperative day one the foley catheter is removed, the diet is advanced to regular, intravenous fluids are discontinued, and the patient is mobilized up into a chair. Flap checks are performed every 4 hours. On average patients remain in the hospital for 3 nights. Internal Doppler devices are cut flush with the skin before discharge. Patients follow-up on a weekly basis until their drains are removed. By week 6, they may perform rigorous activities without restrictions. Second-stage revisions are routinely performed at 3 months after reconstruction. This typically includes balancing procedures, mastopexy, scar revisions of the breast and donor sites, fat grafting, and nipple creation.

Complications

Complications can generally be categorized as related to either the flap or the donor site.

Flap-related complications include venous insufficiency, arterial thrombosis, and fat necrosis. Venous complications are more common than arterial complications and more commonly result from extrinsic factors such as hematoma, kinking, or twisting of the vein. Arterial thrombosis is less common and can be a result of technical error, severe mismatch, intrinsic damage from radiation or extrinsic factors such as compression.

Fig. 9. Bilateral delayed SIEA reconstruction. First row: Preoperative images of 36-year-old woman with BRCA gene mutation and invasive ductal carcinoma of the left breast. Second row: images take 70 postoperatively after surgical delayed of bilateral SIEA flaps with concurrent bilateral nipple-sparing mastectomy and tissue expander placement. Third row: images 160 days after SIEA-based autologous breast reconstruction. Fourth row: Images 54 days after second stage with the removal of skin islands at inframammary fold and dog-ear excision. (From Hoffman RD, Allen RJ et al. Surgical Delay-Induced Hemodynamic Alterations of the Superficial Inferior Epigastric Artery Flap for Autologous Breast Reconstruction. Ann Plast Surg. 2022;88(5 Suppl 5):S414-S21.)

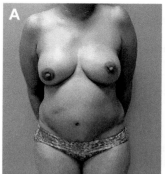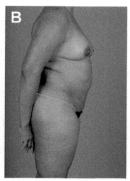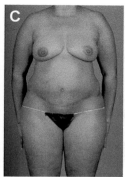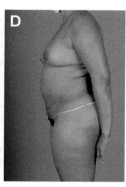

Fig. 11. (A) Preoperative image of a 63-year-old woman with history of BRCA gene mutation. (B–D) Images 12 months after bilateral prophylactic nipple sparing mastectomies with immediate DIEP reconstruction followed by second-stage revision including scar revisions and fat grafting.

The most common flap-related complication following autologous reconstruction is fat necrosis.[6] This is attributed to flap mal-perfusion and varies in predictability and extent of involvement. Many studies have demonstrated rates of fat necrosis between 6% and 40%.[6,27–30] Retrospective studies performed by the senior author and his institution have shown early complication rates including venous occlusion (3%), arterial occlusion (1%), and fat necrosis rates (12%) to be low and favorable when compared with alternative methods of reconstruction.[31–36]

Other complications following abdominal-based breast reconstruction include abdominal wall bulge/hernia, dehiscence, delayed wound healing, infection, hematoma, seroma. When compared with pedicled TRAM reconstruction, postoperative bulge following DIEP flap is reportedly lower (0.5% vs 9%).[31] Increased overall complication rates are associated with active smoking and postoperative radiation therapy. Uncontrolled hypertension, diabetes, and patient BMI greater than 40 are also associated with increased incidence in wound healing and infection complications.[31]

DISCUSSION

ABR has made great strides since the introduction of the DIEP flap in the early 1990s. Its adoption has been widespread and remarkable. Since then, advancements in microsurgical technique and preoperative imaging have helped to reduce surgical complexity and expedite flap reconstruction. Operating times, flap complications, and overall length of stay continue to decline. Surgical candidacy has increased. Emphasis is placed on immediate restoration of total breast volume that can be performed safely and with minimal abdominal wall morbidity. Therefore, modern abdominal-based breast reconstruction has evolved in the form of extended flaps (eg, DCIA), stacked flaps, and even delay procedures of the DIEP and SIEA flaps. Additionally, the field continues to experience innovation by flap neurotization and perforator exchange techniques to optimize sensory restoration and further minimize abdominal muscle morbidity. Immediate, completely buried bilateral ABR is no longer uncommon and represents the pinnacle of breast reconstruction.

SUMMARY

Now, more than ever, plastic surgeons are faced with increased demand in terms of bilateral and nipple-sparing reconstruction. The DIEP and SIEA flaps continue to produce excellent esthetic results with high patient satisfaction. The DCIA flap also has a niche in enhancing volume or acting as a secondary donor site when the DIEP is unavailable. Abdominal flaps are especially indicated for failure of prosthetic reconstruction and restoration of healthy, natural tissue in an irradiated breast. Autologous breast reconstruction requires the plastic surgeon to be well versed and adaptable in all aspects of abdominal-based breast reconstruction, applying multiple techniques to restore the breast to its natural shape and volume (Fig. 11).

CLINICS CARE POINTS

- Preoperative imaging (CTA or MRA) facilitates perforator mapping and surgical efficiency
- Volume disparities between breast and donor site may require extended or stacked flaps (eg, DCIA or PAP flaps)

- Supercharging with a superficial vein augments venous outflow and decreases risk of congestion and fat necrosis
- Consider a delay procedure in SIEA flap candidates when the artery is present but less than 1.5 mm
- ICG angiography can show intraoperative flap perfusion and aid in surgical decision-making
- Perform a perforator exchange to avoid sacrificing significant interposing rectus muscle
- Preserve motor nerves and limit abdominal flap undermining to reduce donor site morbidity and complications

DISCLOSURE

The authors declare that they have no relevant or material financial interests that relate to the information described in this article.

REFERENCES

1. Key statistics for breast cancer. American cancer society. 2022 [updated January 2022; cited 2022 1 July 2022]; Available at: cancer.org/cancer/breast-cancer.
2. Masoomi H, Hanson SE, Clemens MW, et al. Autologous breast reconstruction trends in the United States: using the nationwide inpatient sample database. Ann Plast Surg 2021;87(3):242–7.
3. Hartrampf CR, Scheflan M, Black PW. Breast reconstruction with a transverse abdominal island flap. Plast Reconstr Surg 1982;69(2):216–25.
4. Antia NH, Buch VI. Transfer of an abdominal dermo-fat graft by direct anastomosis of blood vessels. Br J Plast Surg 1971;24(1):15–9.
5. Taylor GI, Daniel RK. The anatomy of several free flap donor sites. Plast Reconstr Surg 1975;56(3):243–53.
6. Allen RJ, Treece P. Deep inferior epigastric perforator flap for breast reconstruction. Ann Plast Surg 1994;32(1):32–8.
7. Coroneos CJ, Heller AM, Voineskos SH, et al. SIEA versus DIEP arterial complications: a cohort study. Plast Reconstr Surg 2015;135(5):802e-7e.
8. Taylor GI, Townsend P, Corlett R. Superiority of the deep circumflex iliac vessels as the supply for free groin flaps. Plast Reconstr Surg 1979;64(5):595–604.
9. Elzinga K, Buchel E. The Deep Circumflex Iliac Artery Perforator Flap for Breast Reconstruction: un lambeau perforateur de l'artere iliaque circonflexe profonde pour la reconstruction mammaire. Plast Surg (Oakv) 2018;26(4):229–37.
10. Hutcheson HA, Hartrampf CR Jr. Breast reconstruction using abdominal tissue. Plast Surg Nurs 1986;6(3):97–104.
11. Milloy FJ, Anson BJ, McAfee DK. The rectus abdominis muscle and the epigastric arteries. Surg Gynecol Obstet 1960;110:293–302.
12. Hamdi H, Rebecca A. The deep inferior epigastric artery perforator flap (DIEAP) in breast reconstruction. Semin Plast Surg 2006;20:95–102.
13. Allen R, Chen C, LoTiempo M. Deep inferior epigastric artery perforator flap for breast reconstruction. In: Levine K, Vasile J, Chen C, et al, editors. Perforator flaps for breast reconstruction. New York: Thieme; 2016. p. 30–9.
14. Gagnon AB and Blondeell PN. Deep and superficial inferior epigastric artery perforator flaps and reconstructive surgery, Cirugia Plastica, 32 (4), 2006. p. 7-13.
15. Spiegel AJ. Superficial inferior epigastric artery flap for breast reconstruction. New York: Thieme: Perforator Flaps for Breast Reconstruction; 2016.
16. Buchel E. Deep circumflex iliac artery perforator flap for breast reconstruction. New York: Thieme: Perforator Flaps for Breast Reconstruction; 2016. p. 126–32.
17. Hendricks H, Ingianni G, Bohm E, et al. A microvascular peritoneal flap based on the deep circumflex iliac artery. Eur J Plast Surg 1995;18:88–90.
18. Bergeron L, Tang M, Morris SF. The anatomical basis of the deep circumflex iliac artery perforator flap with iliac crest. Plast Reconstr Surg 2007;120(1):252–8.
19. Beugels J, Vasile JV, Tuinder SMH, et al. The stacked hemiabdominal extended perforator flap for autologous breast reconstruction. Plast Reconstr Surg 2018;142(6):1424–34.
20. Park JE, Shenaq DS, Silva AK, et al. Breast reconstruction with SIEA flaps: a single-institution experience with 145 free flaps. Plast Reconstr Surg 2016;137(6):1682–9.
21. Selber JC, Samra F, Bristol M, et al. A head-to-head comparison between the muscle-sparing free TRAM and the SIEA flaps: is the rate of flap loss worth the gain in abdominal wall function? Plast Reconstr Surg 2008;122(2):348–55.
22. Hoffman RD, Maddox SS, Meade AE, et al. Surgical delay-induced hemodynamic Alterations of the superficial inferior epigastric artery flap for autologous breast reconstruction. Ann Plast Surg 2022;88(5 Suppl 5):S414–21.
23. DellaCroce FJ, DellaCroce HC, Blum CA, et al. Myth-busting the DIEP flap and an introduction to the abdominal perforator exchange (APEX) breast reconstruction technique: a single-surgeon retrospective review. Plast Reconstr Surg 2019;143(4):992–1008.
24. Blondeel PN, Demuynck M, Mete D, et al. Sensory nerve repair in perforator flaps for autologous breast

reconstruction: sensational or senseless? Br J Plast Surg 1999;52(1):37–44.

25. Momeni A, Meyer S, Shefren K, et al. Flap neurotization in breast reconstruction with nerve allografts: 1-year clinical outcomes. Plast Reconstr Surg Glob Open 2021;9(1):e3328.

26. Spiegel AJ, Menn ZK, Eldor L, et al. Breast reinnervation: DIEP neurotization using the third anterior intercostal nerve. Plast Reconstr Surg Glob Open 2013;1(8):e72.

27. Nahabedian MY, Tsangaris T, Momen B. Breast reconstruction with the DIEP flap or the muscle-sparing (MS-2) free TRAM flap: is there a difference? Plast Reconstr Surg 2005;115(2):436–44 [discussion: 45-6].

28. Chen CM, Halvorson EG, Disa JJ, et al. Immediate postoperative complications in DIEP versus free/muscle-sparing TRAM flaps. Plast Reconstr Surg 2007;120(6):1477–82.

29. Kroll SS. Fat necrosis in free transverse rectus abdominis myocutaneous and deep inferior epigastric perforator flaps. Plast Reconstr Surg 2000;106(3):576–83.

30. Wu LC, Bajaj A, Chang DW, et al. Comparison of donor-site morbidity of SIEA, DIEP, and muscle-sparing TRAM flaps for breast reconstruction. Plast Reconstr Surg 2008;122(3):702–9.

31. Gill PS, Hunt JP, Guerra AB, et al. A 10-year retrospective review of 758 DIEP flaps for breast reconstruction. Plast Reconstr Surg 2004;113(4):1153–60.

32. Weichman KE, Tanna N, Broer PN, et al. Microsurgical breast reconstruction in thin patients: the impact of low body mass indices. J Reconstr Microsurg 2015;31(1):20–5.

33. Levine SM, Snider C, Gerald G, et al. Buried flap reconhhstruction after nipple0sparing mastectomy: advancing toward single-stage breast reconstruction. Plast Reconstr Surg 2013;132(4). 489e-297e.

34. Broer PN, Weichman K, Tanna N, et al. Venous coupler size in autologous breast reconstruction–does it matter? Microsurgery 2013;33(7):514–8.

35. Weichman KE, Broer PN, Tanna N, et al. The role of autologous fat grafting in secondary microsurgical breast reconstruction. Ann Plast Surg 2013;71(1):24–30.

36. Tanna N, Broer PN, Weichman KE, et al. Microsurgical breast reconstruction for nipple-sparing mastectomy. Plast Reconstr Surg 2013;131(2):139e–47e.

Operative Efficiency in Deep Inferior Epigastric Perforator Flap Reconstruction
Key Concepts and Implementation

Sneha Subramaniam, MD, Neil Tanna, MD, Mark L. Smith, MD*

KEYWORDS

- Deep inferior epigastric perforator flaps • Microvascular breast reconstruction • Lean • ERAS
- Enhanced recovery • Operative efficiency

KEY POINTS

- Preoperative assessment should include imaging.
- Patient education is essential for timely discharge.
- Assess patients for risk factors: smoking, clotting disorders, prior surgeries, obesity, and comorbidities.
- Use LEAN techniques to enhance flow in the OR.
- Utilization of enhanced recovery pathways allow for increased operative efficiency, faster postoperative recovery, fewer complications, and reduced hospital stay.

INTRODUCTION

The deep inferior epigastric perforator flap (DIEP) was first introduced in breast reconstruction by Dr Robert Allen Sr. in the early 1990s and has since become one of the most popular approaches for breast reconstruction.[1] As with many new techniques, the first generation of DIEP flap surgeons had to develop, through trial and error, the most efficient and safe ways to carry out the procedure. Both operative time and hospital stay were frequently long and resource intensive. This could be attributed primarily to undeveloped process mapping, extended flap monitoring, dependence on opioids for pain control and delayed patient mobilization. However, as health care has become focused on value-based treatment and reducing the operative time, length of stay and complications after deep inferior flap reconstruction have become areas of focus in high-volume centers.[2] The goals of operative efficiency are to improve the quality and consistency of outcomes, decrease waste, prevent mistakes and complications, and optimize the surgical experience for both the patient and caregivers. In this article, we will examine key areas that contribute to operative efficiency and provide tips on how practitioners can integrate these protocols within their own practice and health systems.

PREOPERATIVE EFFICIENCY
Patient Risk Assessment

Proper patient selection helps to reduce complications, readmissions, and reoperations. Patients with breast cancer may have comorbidities that must be considered before surgery for appropriate preoperative planning. Studies analyzing preoperative risk factors for patients undergoing microvascular breast reconstruction show that the most important preoperative factors to consider are obesity, smoking, hypercoagulable conditions, prior radiation, hypertension, and chronic obstructive pulmonary disease.[3–6]

Smokers have been shown to have higher rates of partial flap loss. A study from Germany in 2020 noted that while total flap loss was not greater in 4577 free flaps (3926 women patients), there were a larger number of wound healing difficulties

Friedman Center, Northwell Health System, 600 Northern Boulevard, Suite 310, Great Neck, NY 11021, USA
* Corresponding author.
E-mail address: marksmithmd@gmail.com

Clin Plastic Surg 50 (2023) 281–288
https://doi.org/10.1016/j.cps.2022.11.002

and greater numbers with partial flap loss in the smoking cohort than in the nonsmoking cohort. Partial flap loss was seen in 3.2% of the smoking group versus 0.9% in the nonsmoking cohort, $P < .001$. Wound-healing disturbances requiring revision surgery in both donor sites and recipient sites were also significantly higher in smokers than in their nonsmoker counterparts.[7] Staging strategies have been used to mitigate some of the wound-healing risks and allow time for smoking cessation before surgery. These include delay procedures at the donor site to improve blood supply, putting off definitive microsurgical reconstruction by placing tissue expanders, or delaying reconstruction altogether.

Obesity and high body mass index have also been noted to be an important preoperative risk factor for DIEP outcomes.[8] Larger mastectomy specimens may lead to increased risk of skin flap necrosis while larger flaps make harvesting technically more challenging. In addition, seroma risk and donor site wound healing issues are both increased.

Frailty and age have also been recent areas of focus regarding preoperative risk assessment in microvascular breast patient candidates. Although older patients tend to be more frail, age alone should not preclude patients from undergoing microvascular breast reconstruction.[9] However, those who are considered to have higher frailty scores, tend to be at greater risk for postoperative complications and should have the appropriate preoperative planning and clearances before going to the operating room.[10,11]

Hypercoagulability is another concern in patients undergoing DIEP flap reconstruction. Although routine genetic testing for hypercoagulable conditions is discouraged due to low yield, those with a personal or family history of thromboembolic events or acquired risk factors for hypercoagulability may benefit from the evaluation by a hematologist preoperatively to assess the need for testing.[12] One study reported that approximately 80% of patients with hypercoagulable conditions still had successful flap reconstructions, with vascular events or flap loss in the other 20% usually occurring in the delayed postoperative period.[13] Studies have also shown that intraoperative vascular problems may lead to increased risk of subsequent vascular complication and flap losses. However, these postoperative vascular events do not seem to be affected by choice of anticoagulation.[14]

Preoperative Imaging

Preoperative imaging provides information on perforator location and size, communication with the superficial venous system, intramuscular course, and branching patterns, in addition to assessing potential disruption of the pedicle from prior surgeries, thus making it an essential step in surgical planning and efficienct decision making in the operating room. The most common imaging modalities are magnetic resonance angiography (MRA) and computed tomography angiography (CTA). Meta-analysis of the utility and evaluation of the accuracy of the different modalities of locating perforators for DIEP flaps indicate that MRA and CTA are usually better than ultrasound because they give you multiple cross-sectional views of the abdominal wall and its vasculature. By having a three-dimensional visualization of the perforators, surgeons are able to identify perforator location, diameter, and intramuscular anatomy in order to select the perforator(s) that will best perfuse the flap.[15]

CTA for preoperative DIEP planning has been shown to decrease operative times (mean operative reduction time of 58 minutes) and lower risk of partial flap failure (RR 15, $P < .001$)[16] specifically about perforator identification and selection. Surgeons who do not use CT angiogram for preoperative planning have been shown to include more perforators (2.3 vs 1.4, $P < .001$) in the flaps than those who did not, reducing efficiency and potential increasing morbidity to the abdominal wall.[17] Similar to any imaging modality, however, CTA imaging comes with its own set of drawbacks including exposure to ionizing radiation and higher incidence of contrast sensitivity and nephrotoxicity.[18] Our preference is to use MRA because it provides excellent visualization of the venous anatomy, which we believe to be an important consideration in perforator selection. We use prone positioning for the study, which limits motion artifact (from respirations) and puts the superficial venous system in a single plane against the table so on coronal viewing it allows the surgeon to topographically map the perforator locations and see the communication of the deep and superficial venous systems. The sagittal and axial views are useful in determining the intramuscular course of the perforating vessels. The primary determinants used in perforator selection are degree of communication with the superficial system, vessel caliber, and length of intramuscular course.[19–22]

Patient Education

A good relationship and open communication between surgical team and the patients aids in a successful and efficient perioperative course and leads to better outcomes in DIEP flap surgery. It is important that the patient has planned ahead for their surgery and recovery period.

Some centers provide standardized patient education classes for prospective breast reconstruction patients. The classes allow patients to think as though they are a part of the decision-making process and enable them to organize their questions before their individualized appointments.[23] These preoperative group classes also reduced individual preoperative appointment times (31.8 minutes vs 53 minutes) and allowed a 43% increase in new patient visit availability for the surgeons without diminishing patient satisfaction.[24,25]

OPERATIVE EFFICIENCY
Intraoperative Efficiency

Although preoperative planning sets a surgeon up for success, intraoperative organization is an important component to carrying out a successful procedure in an efficient manner. Intraoperative efficiency can be defined by the flow that allows surgeons to operate most productively, sharpening mental faculties and manifesting in optimized performance. The key to achieving flow is promotion of the environment. This is something that is not determined by just the surgeon but by the entire intraoperative team and by standardizing team roles and briefing team members on the operative plan to promote pride and autonomy.

Unnecessary prolonged OR times and postoperative stays can be harmful to patients and can also be wasteful from a financial and resource perspective. Duration of surgery is an independent risk factor for postoperative complications and should be minimized.[26] Bekeny and colleagues describe 2 theories in operations management that apply to throughput in the health-care arena.[27] The first is Little's law, the idea that throughput is maximized by increasing the capacity to host patients or reducing the time they spend in the system. The second is Lean management, a process of identifying and eliminating waste within the system. Simply put, to maximize the number of patients that can be treated, one can either increase the capacity of the system (ie, expand infrastructure) or become more efficient (ie, Lean) in moving patients through the system.[27] Because infrastructure expansion is often cost prohibitive, many health systems are using Lean management concepts that focus on identifying value, mapping the process, identifying bottlenecks, minimizing waste and performing continuous self-improvement. If we consider what is of value in surgery, there is great value in reducing operative time, reducing inefficiency and waste, and having an environment that is conducive to peak performance by the surgical team. By mapping the steps in an operation, one can begin to see where bottlenecks and wasted time and resources occur. Focusing on correcting these inefficiencies provides the best return on effort. Below we discuss some approaches we have used to improve intraoperative efficiency.

Multiple Surgeons

Although DIEP flap surgery can be performed by a single plastic surgeon, multiple studies have shown that having 2 plastic surgeons involved decreases operative time, hospital length of stay and donor site complications.[28,29] Considering that immediate reconstruction usually already entails that the plastic surgeon is working concomitantly with a breast surgeon, introducing a third surgeon requires additional coordination to maximize surgeon productivity. This may vary by breast surgeon and their willingness to perform surgery with an additional 1 or 2 plastic surgeons present and must be adjusted accordingly.

Surgical Instruments and Supplies

Unnecessary instruments on a surgical tray are a common source of waste and inefficiency during surgery. Unused instruments still need to be counted (wasted time), resterilized (additional processing and cost), and they clutter the surgical table (excess inventory).[30,31] In addition, fine microsurgical instruments are easily damaged during sterilization so keeping additional instruments on the tray often results in those instruments sustaining damage that goes unrealized until they are actually needed during the case. Instead, we prefer to keep additional instruments in a separate set or peel packed so that they are only used on an as-needed basis. One study examined a plastic surgery service line during the course of 3 months and noted that only 15.8% of instruments on plastic surgery trays and 23.5% of instruments on breast reconstruction trays were used intraoperatively. After review, it was determined 45% of instruments could be removed from a general plastic surgery tray and that approximately 37% could be removed from the breast reconstruction tray. This amounted to a reduction of approximately 81,696 instrument sterilization cycles annually, potentially saving US$163,800 in instruments costs and US$69,441 on sterilization.[31]

Having all sutures, equipment, and implantable materials readily available, either by using a specific room that is fully stocked for the procedure or by creating an equipment cart that contains these items so that they can be brought to the room on the day of surgery, are ways to reduce the time wasted retrieving these items during surgery.[32]

Operating Room Setup

An important contributor to surgical efficiency is how the operating room is set up for the case. Organizing the operating room in such a way as to minimize the need to move equipment and tables once the procedure starts is another way to reduce disruption during surgery. For example, on a bilateral mastectomy case, our breast surgeons typically prefer to operate on the noncancerous breast first. This reduces the need for a second set of breast instruments for the prophylactic mastectomy side. Traditionally, the nurse would set up their table on the side of the first mastectomy and when it was completed, would stay there and work across from the breast surgeon when he or she performed the opposite side mastectomy. However, this approach prevents the plastic surgery team from accessing and preparing the first mastectomy site for flap transfer (ie, wasted time and non-utilized talent). Instead, we now have the nurse set up across from the first mastectomy side, and once the mastectomy is completed, rather than taking additional time to get hemostasis, the breast surgeon moves to the opposite side where the nurse is already set up to work on the second breast while the plastic surgeon and their assistant come in to get hemostasis and begin preparing recipient vessels. In addition, the microscope is set up on the side of the first mastectomy so that once the recipient vessels are prepared the microscope can access the field for the flap transfer, even if the breast surgeon is still performing the second mastectomy. **Fig. 1** details how we have set up the operative room theater to optimize efficiency.

We have also found it helpful to set up a Mayo stand with all the instruments necessary to get hemostasis, prepare the recipient vessels, and do the microsurgical transfer, ahead of time. This allows the second surgeon to be relatively self-sufficient while the scrub nurse focuses on the surgeon performing the flap harvest and avoids the scrub nurse having to hand instruments across the harvesting surgeon's surgical field or behind the surgeon. **Fig. 2** shows a picture of the Mayo stand with instruments for recipient site preparation.

POSTOPERATIVE EFFICIENCY
Enhanced Recovery Pathways

Enhanced recovery after surgery (ERAS) pathways were originally introduced in colorectal surgery but have since expanded into other surgical disciplines, including plastic surgery[33–37] and efficient and effective patient discharge from the hospital postoperatively. Because the term ERAS is now

a registered trademark, we use ERP (enhance recovery pathway) as our abbreviation. There are various ERP protocols that exist; however, the one outlined here is used by our group and was based on the study published by Jablonka and colleagues[38] and involves a 2-day hospital stay.

This protocol incorporates the key elements that have been shown to decrease complications and length of stay after surgery. Invoking the idea behind the Paredo Principle (ie, 80/20 rule), which states that 80% of the effect is the result of 20% of the interventions, we have tried to hone in on the key elements that have demonstrated the most clinical benefit in our hands while eliminating the remaining 80% that have relatively minor impact on outcomes. The other 80% may provide an additional small potential benefit but at the expense of additional risk of untoward side effects, logistical hurdles, or added cost that mitigates that benefit.

Nonopioid Pain Control

Perhaps, the greatest influence on length of stay has been achieved by using a multimodal, nonopioid, pain management approach. Although many ERAS pathways use preoperative medications to decrease opioid use intraoperatively, our focus has been on avoiding opioid use after surgery. This begins with intraoperative nerve blocks using a combination of intermediate and long-acting local anesthetics. We typically prepare a mixture of 20 cc of 1.3% liposomal bupivicaine (Exparel - Pacira Biosciences, Inc, Tampa, FL), 30 cc of 0.25% bupivicaine, and 100 cc of injectable saline. Before flap transfer, we inject a total of 10 cc of the mixture directly into the pectoralis and intercostal muscles at the internal mammary recipient site and at the drain site. An additional 10 cc is injected in the serratus plane to block the lateral intercostal nerves. If axillary or inframammary incisions are used, an additional 5 cc is injected along those sites as well. After flap transfer, bilateral transversus abdominis plane blocks are performed under ultrasound guidance using 30 cc of the mixture on each side. Another 20 to 30 cc is injected along the lower abdominal incision and drain sites. At the end of surgery, the patient is given a 1-g dose of intravenous acetaminophen and 15 mg of IV ketorolac. This is continued every 6 hours postoperatively until the patient is taking food orally, at which time oral equivalents are used.[39] Narcotic use is reserved only for breakthrough pain. Multiagent antiemetic use is also given during surgery to avoid postoperative nausea. By avoiding narcotic use, patients have less nausea, constipation, and lethargy after surgery. Given that, in a

OR Setup

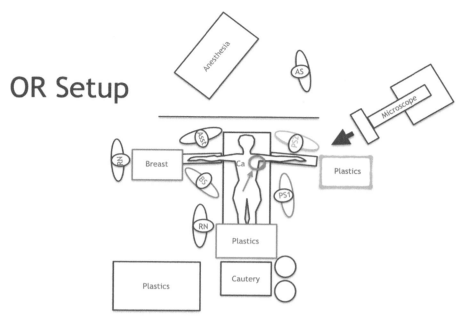

Fig. 1. Recommended DIEP flap operating room setup: Setup for second mastectomy showing breast surgeon (BS) on the side of the cancerous breast while the harvesting plastic surgeon (PS1) begins harvesting the second flap. The recipient site plastic surgeon (PS2) begins preparation of the recipient vessels and then does the microsurgical anastomoses. The red circle with the arrow marks the first mastectomy site. AS, anesthesiologist; Asst, Assistant; RN, Nurse.

recent study, 6% of opioid naive patients were still using opioids 3 to 6 months after even minor surgical procedures (compared with 0.4% of nonoperative controls), reducing opioid exposure helps reduce the risk of opioid dependency.[40]

Venous Thrombo-Embolic Prophylaxis

All patients receive Lovenox 40 mg or Heparin 5000 units given subcutaneously before surgery. Pneumatic compression wraps are placed on the lower extremities. Patients continue prophylactic dose anticoagulation throughout their hospital stay and wear the compression wraps while in bed. The length of postoperative venous thrombo-embolic prophylaxis depends on risk. Patient with a Caprini Score of 8 or more are continued on prophylactic Lovenox for 4 weeks postoperatively.[41]

Postoperative day 0

Depending on the facility and the nurse staffing, several postoperative monitoring environments have been used by our team for the first night after surgery, including overnight stay in the recovery room or transfer to an ICU, step-down, or regular floor bed. Ideally, patients are transferred to a private room on a regular floor to have a quieter environment. We usually use near-infrared spectroscopy-based tissue oximetry (Vioptix) or

implantable Doppler probes (Cook Medical, Bloomington, IN) to follow flap perfusion postoperatively. Ideally, a Doppler signal from the perforator is marked with a small suture on the flap skin island as a backup site for monitoring in case of device malfunction. Patients are typically allowed to take ice chips or small amounts of clear beverages the first night. Laboratory studies are usually not drawn unless there is a concern due to existing medical conditions or blood loss during surgery.

Postoperative day 1

Patients have their urinary catheter removed in the morning and are moved into a chair to eat breakfast. They are then ambulated several times the first day. Intravenous hydration is stopped once adequate oral intake is established and IV pain medications are changed to oral format. Patients are given instructions by the nurse on how to manage the drains.

Postoperative day 2

Flap monitoring is discontinued, and patients are discharged home with follow-up arranged within 1 week to assess surgical sites and to remove any drains with low output.

Although many surgeons remain concerned about the risk of flap loss if flap monitoring is

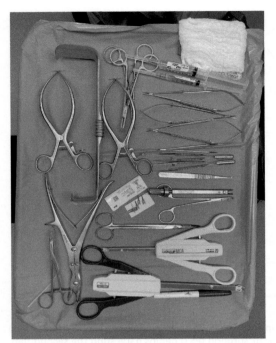

Fig. 2. Mayo stand with recipient site instruments for the second plastic surgeon. It is important for each team to develop its process map and to engage all team members in the discussion regarding intraoperative coordination to ensure optimal efficiency and integration. It is expected that things may change based on the surgeons' experience and speed, the introduction of new technologies and changes in staffing resources; however, it important to remember that Lean management is an iterative process that requires continuous reevaluation to incorporate change and to maintain optimal efficiency.

discontinued prematurely, a recent study by Jablonka and colleagues that looked at a series of 1813 patients and 2847 flaps showed that by postoperative day 2, the cost-utility of inpatient flap monitoring exceeds acceptable societal thresholds. This is because after postoperative day 2, both the likelihood of flap loss and flap salvage drop such that the odds of undertaking a successful flap salvage at this time point is less than 1 in 900.[40]

Our experience using this protocol during the last 5 years, for more than 500 patients and more than 1000 DIEP flaps, has demonstrated a mode length of stay of 2 days and a flap loss rate less than 0.3% demonstrating that short length of stay and high flap success rate are not mutually exclusive.

SUMMARY

As health care evolves to a more value-based approach, it is essential for surgeons doing resource intensive procedures to optimize efficiency and outcomes. Efficiency in DIEP flap breast reconstruction entails a multipronged approach that incorporates effective preoperative planning, patient education, operative efficiency and postoperative pathways to ensure successful outcomes while limiting resource consumption and waste.

CLINICS CARE POINTS

- Preoperative Assessment: Most complications can be managed but are greatly facilitated by preoperative counseling of the patient on what may be entailed. In patients who we identify as having an increased risk of complications, we discuss the relative risk of various reconstructive options and the management of their associated complications. For patients who are amenable to proceeding, we document the discussion and include the specific risks in our informed consent. For the highest risk patients, delayed reconstruction, with or without placement of an expander as an interim spacer, should be considered to make sure that cancer treatment is not impeded by surgical complications and to potentially allow more time for medical optimization of the patient (eg, smoking cessation, A1c optimization).

- Preoperative Imaging: In a high volume practice, it is useful to meet with your radiologist to discuss the intent of the study, how it should be reported and how incidental findings are communicated to physician and patients. This ensures optimal views of the anatomy and ensures that incidental findings, which may be present in more than 50% of studies, are not missed by the surgeon.[42]

- Patient Education: In our practice, we direct patients to our website where we provide them with information and a list of questions to consider. At their visit, we also provide a checklist and review key elements of the surgical process including time/date/location of their surgery, presurgical testing date, medications to avoid before surgery, presurgical cleansing instructions, nil per os instructions, what to bring to the hospital and what to leave home, how to prepare at home for after surgery, what to expect in the hospital including the anticipated length of stay, activity restrictions, bathing, sleeping position, prescription and over-the-counter medications that might be needed, drain care instructions, follow-up appointment time, and what to look out for after surgery. This helps patients understand and prepare for surgery, avoids miscommunication, and sets expectations for the recovery process. Patients who have expectations set for early discharge are more likely to go home on schedule than those who do not.[25]

- Intraoperative Efficiency: It is critical to review the efficiency goals with the entire team, including nursing, anesthesia, and hospital administration in advance of implementation in the operating room. Once the patient benefits and cost savings are understood, buy in for the process is usually much more enthusiastic.

- Enhanced Recovery Protocols: Similar to intraoperative efficiency measures, it is critical to in-service nurses on monitoring and recovery goals so that they understand the concepts behind enhanced recovery protocols. Nurses whos are not familiar with nonopioid pain management techniques may actually encourage patients to take opioid medications after surgery unnecessarily, anticipating that they will be in pain if they do not.

DISCLOSURE

There are no sources of outside support for this research and the authors have no conflicts of interest to disclose.

REFERENCES

1. Tanna N, Clayton JL, Roostaeian J, et al. The volume-outcome relationship for immediate breast reconstruction. Plast Reconstr Surg 2012;129(1):19–24.
2. Healy C, Allen RJ Sr. The evolution of perforator flap breast reconstruction: twenty years after the first DIEP flap. J Reconstr Microsurg 2014;30(2):121–5.
3. Roy M, Sebastiampillai S, Haykal S, et al. Development and validation of a risk stratification model for immediate microvascular breast reconstruction. J Surg Oncol 2019;120(7):1177–83.
4. Fischer JP, Sieber B, Nelson JA, et al. Comprehensive outcome and cost analysis of free tissue transfer for breast reconstruction: an experience with 1303 flaps. Plast Reconstr Surg 2013;131(2):195–203.
5. Depypere B, Herregods S, Denolf J, et al. 20 Years of DIEAP flap breast reconstruction: a big data analysis. Sci Rep 2019;9(1):12899 [published correction appears in Sci Rep. 2020 Jan 24;10(1):1398].
6. Palve JS, Luukkaala TH, Kääriäinen MT. Predictive risk factors of complications in different breast reconstruction methods. Breast Cancer Res Treat 2020;182(2):345–54.
7. Prantl L, Moellhoff N, Fritschen UV, et al. Impact of smoking status in free deep inferior epigastric artery perforator flap breast reconstruction: a multicenter study. J Reconstr Microsurg 2020;36(9):694–702.
8. Patterson CW, Palines PA, Bartow MJ, et al. Stratification of surgical risk in DIEP breast reconstruction based on classification of obesity. J Reconstr Microsurg 2022;38(1):1–9.
9. Walton L, Ommen K, Audisio RA. Breast reconstruction in elderly women breast cancer: a review. Cancer Treat Rev 2011;37(5):353–7.
10. Magno-Pardon DA, Luo J, Carter GC, et al. An analysis of the modified five-item frailty index for predicting complications following free flap breast reconstruction. Plast Reconstr Surg 2022;149(1):41–7.
11. Panayi AC, Foroutanjazi S, Parikh N, et al. The modified 5-item frailty index is a predictor of perioperative risk in breast reconstruction: an analysis of 40,415 cases. J Plast Reconstr Aesthet Surg 2022;S1748-6815(22):00231–5 [published online ahead of print, 2022 Apr 25].
12. Pannucci CJ, Kovach SJ, Cuker A. Microsurgery and the hypercoagulable state. Plast Reconstr Surg 2015;136(4):545e–52e.
13. Wang TY, Serletti JM, Cuker A, et al. Free tissue transfer in the hypercoagulable patient: a review of 58 flaps. Plast Reconstr Surg 2012;129(2):443–53.
14. Fosnot J, Jandali S, Low DW, et al. Closer to an understanding of fate: the role of vascular complications in free flap breast reconstruction. Plast Reconstr Surg 2011;128(4):835–43.
15. Kiely J, Kumar M, Wade RG. The accuracy of different modalities of perforator mapping for unilateral DIEP flap breast reconstruction: a systematic review and meta-analysis. J Plast Reconstr Aesthet Surg 2021;74(5):945–56.
16. Wade RG, Watford J, Wormald JCR, et al. Perforator mapping reduces the operative time of DIEP flap breast reconstruction: a systematic review and meta-analysis of preoperative ultrasound, computed tomography and magnetic resonance angiography. J Plast Reconstr Aesthet Surg 2018;71(4):468–77.
17. Haddock NT, Dumestre DO, Teotia SS. Efficiency in DIEP Flap breast reconstruction: the real benefit of computed tomographic angiography imaging. Plast Reconstr Surg 2020;146(4):719–23.
18. Rozen WM, Bhullar HK, Hunter-Smith D. How to assess a CTA of the abdomen to plan an autologous breast reconstruction. Gland Surg 2019;8(Suppl 4):S291–6.
19. Thiessen FEF, Vermeersch N, Tondu T, et al. Dynamic infrared thermography (DIRT) in DIEP flap breast reconstruction: a clinical study with a standardized measurement setup. Eur J Obstet Gynecol Reprod Biol 2020;252:166–73.

288

20. Gfrerer L, Carty MJ, Erdmann-Sager J, et al. Abstract 77: pre-operative DIEP flap patient education class helps decrease anxiety and increase excitement/preparedness around surgery. Plast Reconstr Surg Glob Open 2019;7(4 Suppl):54–5. Published 2019 Apr 29.

21. Kagen AC, Hossain R, Dayan E, et al. Modern perforator flap imaging with high-resolution blood pool MR angiography. Radiographics 2015;35(3):901–15.

22. Mohan AT, Saint-Cyr M. Advances in imaging technologies for planning breast reconstruction. Gland Surg 2016;5(2):242–54.

23. Henn D, Momeni A. A standardized patient education class as a vehicle to improving shared decision-making and increasing access to breast reconstruction. J Plast Reconstr Aesthet Surg 2020;73(8):1534–9.

24. Bamba R, Wiebe JE, Ingersol CA, et al. Do patient expectations of discharge affect length of stay after deep inferior epigastric perforator flap for breast reconstruction? J Reconstr Microsurg 2022;38(1):34–40.

25. Thorarinsson A, Fröjd V, Kölby L, et al. Blood loss and duration of surgery are independent risk factors for complications after breast reconstruction. J Plast Surg Hand Surg 2017;51(5):352–7.

26. Bekeny JC, Fan KL, Malphrus E, et al. Optimizing throughput in clinical practice: lean management and efficient care in plastic and reconstructive surgery. Plast Reconstr Surg 2021;147(3):772–81.

27. Weichman KE, Lam G, Wilson SC, et al. The impact of two operating surgeons on microsurgical breast reconstruction. Plast Reconstr Surg 2017;139(2):277–84.

28. Haddock NT, Kayfan S, Pezeshk RA, et al. Co-surgeons in breast reconstructive microsurgery: what do they bring to the table? Microsurgery 2018;38(1):14–20.

29. Stein MJ, Dec W, Lerman OZ. Lean and six sigma methodology can improve efficiency in microsurgical breast reconstruction. Plast Reconstr Surg Glob Open 2021;9(7):e3669. Published 2021 Jul 6.

30. Fu TS, Msallak H, Namavarian A, et al. Surgical tray optimization: a quality improvement initiative that reduces operating room costs. J Med Syst 2021;45(8):78.

31. Wood BC, Konchan S, Gay S, et al. Data analysis of plastic surgery instrument trays yields significant cost savings and efficiency gains. Ann Plast Surg 2021;86(6S Suppl 5):S635–9.

32. Janhofer DE, Lakhiani C, Song DH. Enhancing operative flow. Plast Reconstr Surg 2018;142(2):246e–7e.

33. Ljungqvist O, Young-Fadok T, Demartines N. The history of enhanced recovery after surgery and the ERAS society. J Laparoendosc Adv Surg Tech A 2017;27(9):860–2.

34. Liu VX, Rosas E, Hwang JC, et al. The kaiser permanente Northern California enhanced recovery after surgery program: design, development, and implementation. Perm J 2017;21:17–1003.

35. Batdorf NJ, Lemaine V, Lovely JK, et al. Enhanced recovery after surgery in microvascular breast reconstruction. J Plast Reconstr Aesthet Surg 2015;68(3):395–402.

36. Oh C, Moriarty J, Borah BJ, et al. Cost analysis of enhanced recovery after surgery in microvascular breast reconstruction. J Plast Reconstr Aesthet Surg 2018;71(6):819–26.

37. Offodile AC 2nd, Gu C, Boukovalas S, et al. Enhanced recovery after surgery (ERAS) pathways in breast reconstruction: systematic review and meta-analysis of the literature. Breast Cancer Res Treat 2019;173(1):65–77.

38. Jablonka Eric, et al. Transversus Abdominis Plane Blocks with Single-Dose Liposomal Bupivacaine in Conjunction with a Nonnarcotic Pain Regimen Help Reduce Length of Stay following Abdominally Based Microsurgical Breast Reconstruction. PlastReconstrSurg 2017;140(2):240–51. https://doi.org/10.1097/PRS.0000000000003508.

39. Jablonka EM, Lamelas AM, Kanchwala SK, et al. A simplified cost-utility analysis of inpatient flap monitoring after microsurgical breast reconstruction and implications for hospital length of stay. Plast Reconstr Surg 2019;144(4):540e–9e.

40. Brummett CM, Waljee JF, Goesling J, et al. New persistent opioid use after minor and major surgical procedures in US adults. JAMA Surg 2017;152(6):e170504 [published correction appears in JAMA Surg. 2019 Mar 1;154(3):272].

41. Bassiri-Tehrani B, Karanetz I, Bernik SF, et al. The timing of chemoprophylaxis in autologous microsurgical breast reconstruction. Plast Reconstr Surg 2018;142(5):1116–23.

42. Wagner RD, Doval AF, Mehra NV, et al. Incidental findings in CT and MR angiography for preoperative planning in DIEP flap breast reconstruction. Plast Reconstr Surg Glob Open 2020;8(10):e3159.

Modern Approaches to Alternative Flap-Based Breast Reconstruction
Profunda Artery Perforator Flap

Zack Cohen, MD[a,1], Saïd C. Azoury, MD[a,1], Evan Matros, MD, MMSc[a],
Jonas A. Nelson, MD, MPH[a], Robert J. Allen Jr, MD[a,*]

KEYWORDS

- Autologous free flap breast reconstruction • Profunda artery perforator flap • Thigh-based flaps

KEY POINTS

- Abdominal-based tissue is the gold standard for autologous free flap breast reconstruction.
- The profunda artery perforator (PAP) flap may be an option for those who are not candidates for abdominal tissue transfer.
- The PAP flap is based off perforators from the profunda artery, supplying the skin and subcutaneous tissue of the posteromedial thigh.
- Owing to low donor-site morbidity, reliability of the vascular supply, and excellent cosmetic outcomes, the PAP flap has emerged as a preferred alternate source.

 Video content accompanies this article at http://www.plasticsurgery.theclinics.com.

HISTORY

As microsurgical techniques are refined, autologous breast reconstruction will grow in popularity. Advances made in autologous breast reconstruction have reduced operative time, length of stay, and morbidity.[1,2] Abdominal-based flaps remain the gold-standard tissue source in breast reconstruction.[3–5] However, when an abdominal donor site is unavailable, alternate flaps, including thigh-based tissue, should be explored. Owing to the rich vascular supply of the thigh, several flaps have been designed from this anatomic region for the reconstruction of both locoregional and distant defects. A gluteal thigh flap was first described in 1980 in the setting of coverage and reconstruction of chronic wounds of the perineal and sacral area.[6] Song and colleagues[7] described the use of a posterior thigh-free flap based on perforators arising off the profunda artery. In their series of 15 lower extremity-based flaps, all were used for reconstruction of burn contractures of the head and neck. Only two of the 15 flaps were harvested as profunda artery perforator (PAP) flaps, whereas the rest were anterolateral or anteromedial thigh flaps. Angrigiani and colleagues[8] expanded on the posterior thigh flap and described the technical aspects of PAP flap harvest and perforator reliability using latex injection in cadaveric specimens. In 25 live patients, 14 had pedicled flaps for reconstruction of the

---

[a] Plastic and Reconstructive Surgery Service, Memorial Sloan Kettering Cancer Center, 321 East 61st Street, New York, NY 10065, USA
[1] Contributed equally as first author.
* Corresponding author.
E-mail address: allenr1@mskcc.org

Clin Plastic Surg 50 (2023) 289–299
https://doi.org/10.1016/j.cps.2022.10.001
0094-1298/23/© 2022 Elsevier Inc. All rights reserved.

ischial/perineal region, and 11 had free flaps for resurfacing of burn contractures in the head and neck or for the reconstruction of lower extremity defects.

Allen[9] was the first to expand the use of PAP flaps for autologous breast reconstruction. In his landmark paper, he detailed the harvest and transfer of 27 PAP flaps, including descriptions of the use of preoperative imaging, surgical technique and method of harvest, postoperative recovery, and complications. This study heralded a massive shift in the potential reconstructive options for breast cancer patients. With increasing familiarity and surgeon experience, the PAP flap has emerged as a popular alternate donor site when abdominal flaps are contraindicated or undesired.

The PAP flap addresses the disadvantages of gracilis flap variants. By nature of being a perforator flap, the PAP flap spares sacrifice of any muscle. In comparison to gracilis flaps, the PAP flap is larger in volume, has a longer and greater caliber pedicle, and its skin paddle design can be larger.[10] When compared with transverse upper gracilis (TUG) flaps, the dissection is more distant from draining lymphatics and avoids key structures in the femoral triangle, thus preventing potential dead space, and decreasing the subsequent risk of lymphedema/seroma and the potential associated morbidity.[10,11] The donor site scar for a PAP flap can be conveniently hidden in the inferior gluteal crease to create an esthetic donor site. Further, the tissue of the posterior thigh is favorable for creating a youthful breast, as it tends to contain firmer, yet moldable fat. The elliptical skin paddle design also allows for insetting and shaping into a natural, youthful breast mound. These factors likely contribute to the increasingly common utilization of PAP flaps as an alternative to abdominal-based tissue.

Indications and Patient Selection

PAP flaps are preferred for breast reconstruction in patients with contraindications to an abdominal-based donor site. This includes patients with scant abdominal tissue, prior failed abdominal flap/history of abdominoplasty, significant prior abdominal surgeries, or patients who are reluctant to have abdominal scarring. Young patients who desire future pregnancy may wish to avoid abdominal donor site harvest. We recommend avoiding PAP flap harvest in patients with significant burns/scars of the thigh region or those with the significant iliofemoral vascular occlusive disease.

It has been shown that in patients with a low body mass index (BMI) and/or minimal abdominal tissue, there is often an adequate volume of potential donor tissue in the posterior thigh region.[12–14] Several studies have been performed analyzing both patient and PAP flap characteristics.[10,12–20] The average PAP flap weight across these studies ranged from 242 to 425 g (g) (minimum 132 g, maximum 815 g), whereas the average patient BMI ranged from 23 to 27 kg/m². **Table 1** provides a detailed review of patient and PAP flap characteristics across studies specific to breast reconstruction.[10,12–20] PAP flaps can also be combined with a second free flap (eg, deep inferior epigastric perforator [DIEP] flap) in a "stacked" flap fashion, or augmented with implants and/or fat grafting when a larger breast size is desired than what the posterior thigh donor site can provide.[21] Nonetheless, similar to abdominal-based flaps, PAP flaps provide sufficient volume to reconstruct a wide volumetric range of mastectomy defects.[22]

Profunda Artery Perforator Flap Anatomy

The PAP flap is based on perforators branching off the profunda femoris (deep femoral) artery. The profunda femoris arises 3 to 4 cm distal to the inguinal ligament on the posterolateral aspect of the common femoral artery. The vessel then runs posterior to the femur in a lateral to medial direction. Coursing between the adductor magnus and semitendinosus muscles, it gives off several musculocutaneous and septocutaneous perforators supplying the fat and skin of the posteromedial thigh.[23] The first perforating vessel supplies the adductor magnus and gracilis muscles. The second branch supplies the semimembranosus, biceps femoris, and vastus lateralis muscles.[24] Typically, the perforator(s) selected for microvascular anastomosis arise 5 to 7 cm caudal to the inferior gluteal crease. The profunda artery consistently supplies at least two useable perforators, with some patients having five perforators in a single thigh.[24] These vessels have been shown to be of adequate caliber and size for microsurgical transfer and postoperative flap perfusion.[25–29] The arterial perforator averages 2.3 mm in diameter, with its associated vena comitans averaging 2.8 mm in diameter.[23] Pedicle length measures an average length of 11 to 13 cm across several studies.[15,17,20,23,24]

Preoperative Imaging

In the era of advanced imaging, modalities including magnetic resonance angiography (MRA) and computed tomography angiography (CTA) are increasingly used in the preoperative

Table 1
Review of patient and profunda artery perforator flap characteristics across 10 studies

Study, Year	Study Type	Mean Age (Years)	Number of Patients/ Number of Flaps	Mean BMI (kg/m²)	Mean Flap Weight Range (Grams)	Mean Pedicle Length (cm)	Mean Skin Paddle Size (cm)
Hunter et al,[10] 2015	PC	–	13/22	21.6	242 (132–455)	–	–
Haddad et al,[15] 2016	PC	–	30/30	–	301 (195–700)	9.88	–
Ito et al,[16] 2016	RR	41.6	5/7	23.5	257.1 (200–350)	9.4	24.6 × 6.1
Hupkens et al,[17] 2016	PC	44	30/40	23.3	372.4 (250–470)	11	32 × 12
Allen et al,[19] 2016	RR	48	96/164	22.5	367.4 (225–739)	10.2	27.2 × 6.3
Haddock et al,[12] 2017	RR	–	56/101	26.4	425 (170–815)	10.3	–
Fosseprez et al,[18] 2017	RR	–	15/17	–	–	–	–
Haddock et al,[20] 2019	RR	51.5	20/40	27.3	398.5 (170–600)	12.9	–
Haddock et al,[13] 2020	RR	–	138/265	26.5	403 (190–800)	11.2	–
Atzeni et al,[14] 2021	PC	47.56	86/116	24.72	251.3 (152–455)	–	–

Abbreviations: BMI, body mass index; cm, centimeters; min, minutes; PC, prospective cohort study; RR, retrospective review.

setting for assessment and confirmation of perforators (**Fig. 1**). We prefer preoperative MRA for the detailed anatomy and three-dimensional reprocessing techniques that it provides. This high-resolution imaging allows the surgeon to carefully plan the incisions sites and anticipated skin paddle. Unlike abdominal-based flap harvest, the inconsistent location of a dominant perforator in PAP flaps has many surgeons relying on preoperative imaging. However, newer modifications of the PAP, including a diagonal (dPAP) and vertical (vPAP) design to be discussed later in the text, allow for capture of more perforators along the course of the profunda artery, compared with flaps with a classical transverse (tPAP) orientation. Therefore, imaging may not be mandatory for diagonal and vertical flap designs.

Operative Technique

When possible, we prefer a split-leg bed or lithotomy for patient positioning and adequate exposure of the inner thigh (**Fig. 2**). When positioning patients in lithotomy, one should be cognizant to pad pressure points and properly position the

lower extremities to avoid potential nerve entrapment/compression. Both split-leg and lithotomy allow the surgeon to be situated in-between the patient's thighs and approach the operation from multiple angles, facilitating efficient and safe flap harvest. In addition, the nature and location of the PAP flap permits a two-team approach, allowing the mastectomy and recipient site to be prepared in conjunction with flap harvest. In stacked DIEP-PAP flap cases, the DIEP flap dissection can commence at the same time as the PAP flap. Similar to abdominal-based breast reconstruction, PAP flaps can be performed in an immediate or delayed fashion. In fact, single-stage breast reconstruction with PAP flaps offers comparable results to delayed reconstruction.[30,31]

After visualization of perforator status with advanced imaging modalities, the donor vessel(s) are confirmed with a Doppler probe and are marked for intraoperative reference (see **Fig. 2**). The adductor longus and gracilis muscles are highlighted as important landmarks, as is the inferior gluteal crease (see **Fig. 2**). The skin paddle is designed using the pinch test, such that the width of the flap is an estimate of the amount of tissue

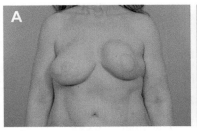
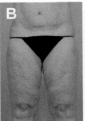
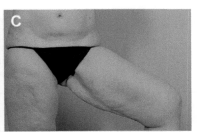

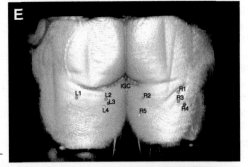

D

Perforator Flap Angiography Report (PAP)

Inferior Gluteal Crease (IGC): Se3, Im111

Note: All measurements are in mm.

Left Posterior Thigh Perforators:

#	Series: Image	Distance to IGC	Distance to Midline	Vessel Diameter
L1	3: 121	15.1(Inferior)	115.1	1.5
L2	3: 124	19.5(Inferior)	47.7	1.7
L3	3: 130	28.5(Inferior)	42.2	1.7
L4	3: 135	36.0(Inferior)	52.4	1.6

Right Posterior Thigh Perforators:

#	Series: Image	Distance to IGC	Distance to Midline	Vessel Diameter
R1	3: 115	6.1(Inferior)	118.8	2.0
R2	3: 124	19.5(Inferior)	35.9	1.8
R3	3: 129	27.0(Inferior)	119.0	1.6
R4	3: 134	34.5(Inferior)	132.4	1.6
R5	3: 148	55.4(Inferior)	28.9	2.1

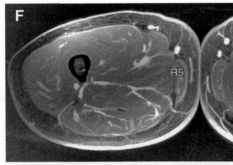
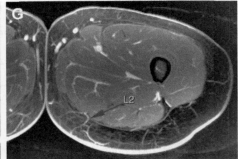

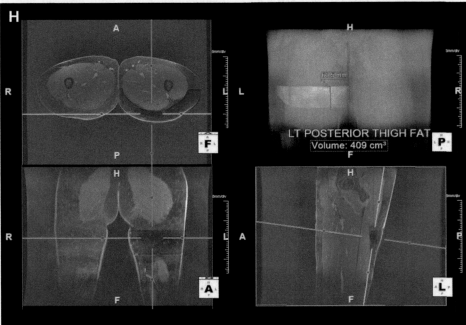

that can be excised while still allowing for a tension-free primary closure of the donor site. In the most classic orientation (tPAP), skin markings are typically made with the patient upright, to ensure the incision remains hidden in the inferior gluteal crease. The anterior incision is made and taken through the subcutaneous tissue. Electrocautery is used to proceed with dissection from anterior to posterior. The fascia investing the gracilis is entered and the muscle retracted anteriorly. The adductor magnus fascia is then exposed, incised, and dissected proximally in a subfascial manner until the perforators are identified. Intramuscular dissection of the perforators then proceeds in a standard fashion until adequate pedicle length is achieved or the profunda artery is encountered (see **Fig. 2**). When pedicle length and vessel caliber are deemed suitable for microsurgical transfer, the flap is divided and transferred to reconstruct the mastectomy defect. If additional time is needed for preparation of the recipient site, the perforating flap vessels can still be ligated given the fact that perfusion remains intact via posterior skin attachments and musculocutaneous perforators. When ready, the posterior attachments are divided, and the flap is harvested, weighed, and prepared on the back table for transfer.

Microsurgical anastomosis is then performed in a standard fashion, most often antegrade to the internal mammary artery and vein. Alternatively, the retrograde mammary or thoracodorsal vessels can be used as backup options.[32,33] We use SPY-PHY (Stryker Corp., Kalamazoo, MI; manufactured by Medical London LP, London, Ontario, Canada) angiography to visualize and confirm flap perfusion following microvascular anastomosis, and any tissue with questionable viability is excised. The flap is then inset with absorbable sutures. One should take time to ensure sufficient inferomedial pole fullness, as these areas tend to be difficult to augment during subsequent revisional

procedures[34] (see **Fig.** 2). Selective de-epithelialization is then carried out while maintaining an adequate skin paddle for postoperative monitoring. The skin paddle can be easily removed at the time of revision or staged nipple reconstruction.[35] The skin is approximated in layers over a closed suction drain placed in the mastectomy space.

Given the muscle-sparing nature inherent to the PAP flap, there is a decreased chance of dead space in the donor site. Nonetheless, care must be taken to ensure a tension-free, multilayered closure. This is achieved with a careful elevation of the inferior skin flap off the investing thigh fascia. Quilting sutures can further facilitate closure and decrease tension on the wound. The donor site is approximated in layers over a closed-suction drain (see **Fig.** 2). The lower extremity is placed in a compression garment, and patients are instructed to avoid strenuous activity for at least 6 weeks, at which time activities can be resumed as indicated.

Variations in Profunda Artery Perforator Flap Design: Transverse, Vertical, and Diagonal

Various derivations and modifications have been made to the original PAP flap used in breast reconstruction, which was designed with a transverse skin paddle (tPAP).[9] The tPAP has several limitations – namely, the width of the skin paddle is limited in size to about 6 to 8 cm. In addition, there is a great degree of tension on the donor site, increasing the risk of wound complications. The incision is also compressed when patients are in the sitting position, a factor that may potentiate wound complications and/or chronic posterior thigh paresthesia secondary to damage to the posterior cutaneous nerves.[36]

Hupkens and colleagues[17] described a geometric modification of the tPAP flap in which dissection was extended cranially to include additional

Fig. 1. Preoperative images of the (A) breasts and (B, C) lower extremities. Patient had a history of right breast cancer and underwent mastectomy with reconstruction using a deep inferior epigastric perforator (DIEP) flap. The left breast subsequently developed cancer and was reconstructed with a pedicled latissimus dorsi flap and implant. Note severe capsular contracture of left breast as well as laxity of tissue in the posteromedial thighs. Magnetic resonance angiography (MRA) of the bilateral lower extremities with and without intravenous contrast and three-dimensional (3D) postprocessing was performed. (D) Perforator flap angiography report detailing vessel caliber and location. IGC=inferior gluteal crease. (E) 3D perforator map showing perforator location on posterior thigh. (F) Axial view of the thigh showing a favorable R5 perforator located 55.4 mm inferior to the IGC, 28.9 mm to the right of midline, and 6.9 mm posterior to the posterior margin of gracilis. Vessel diameter is 2.1 mm. It travels 185.2 mm with an intramuscular course before joining the inferior gluteal artery. (G) Axial view of the thigh showing a favorable L2 perforator located 19.5 mm inferior to the IGC, 47.7 mm to the left of midline, and 39.5 mm posterior to the posterior margin of gracilis. Vessel diameter is 1.7 mm. It travels 185.2 mm with an intramuscular course before joining the inferior gluteal artery. (H) Fat volume of a 22 cm × 6 cm flap on posterior left thigh is 409.0 cc.

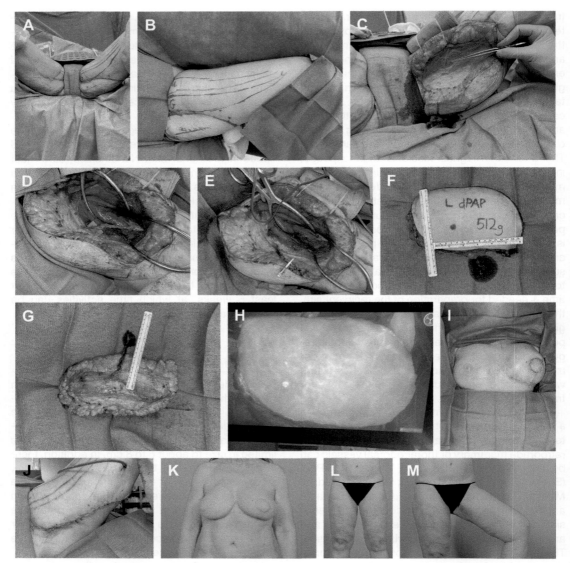

Fig. 2. Preoperative surgical site markings and patient positioning for a planned diagonal PAP. (*A*) Patient positioning in lithotomy. (*B*) Preoperative marking delineating the adductor longus (AL) muscle, gracilis (G) muscle, and a 22 cm × 10.5 cm anticipated diagonal skin paddle. (*C*) The anterior skin incision was made and carried down through the fascia investing the gracilis, at which point the gracilis was retracted anteriorly. Forceps identify the gracilis pedicle. (*D*) The investing fascia overlying the adductor magnus was incised and subfascial dissection proceeded. Meticulous posterior dissection of the adductor magnus fascia revealed a large perforator with two cutaneous branches. (*E*) A microvascular bulldog was then placed on the main perforator and its associated vena comitans, at which point the vessels were clipped and divided. (*F*, anterior; *G*, posterior). The posterior incision was completed to allow for flap harvest and weighing (512 g). Flap preparation proceeded on the back table and revealed a pedicle length of 10.5 cm. The flap was then transferred to the left mastectomy defect, and microvascular anastomoses were performed in a standard fashion to the internal mammary system. (*H*) SPY-PHI (Stryker Corp., Kalamazoo, MI; manufactured by Medical London LP, London, Ontario, Canada) angiography of the free flap revealed excellent tissue perfusion. (*I*) The flap was then selectively de-epithelialized and inset with absorbable sutures to recreate a youthful breast mound, and the wound was closed over a drain. (*J*) Layered closure of the donor site over a closed-suction drain. (*K*) Postoperative appearance of the breast and (*L*, *M*) lower extremities. Note improved contour of the left upper thigh with an inconspicuous donor site scar.

tissue from the inferior gluteal area, thus increasing the volume available for harvest. Similarly, others have described a vertical PAP (vPAP) flap in which a longitudinal skin paddle was delineated to maximize the number of larger, distal perforators that are harvested.[37,38] Tielemans and colleagues[39] then expanded on the "extended" PAP flap in 2021, citing similar complication profiles to "standard" PAP flaps and a 97.8% flap survival rate. The vertical incision avoids dissection near lower extremity nerves and lymphatics, and distributes tension in a circumferential manner around the thigh, thus decreasing the risk of potential wound complications/scar migration. The donor site remains well-concealed with a vPAP and resembles an inner thighplasty scar.

Dayan and Allen Jr. described the harvest of a diagonal PAP (dPAP) oriented along Langer's lines, which allows for a wider skin paddle and decreased tension on the donor site seen with traditional tPAP flaps.[36] The diagonal design captures more fat from the posteromedial thigh that is ideal for breast reconstruction. Similar to a vPAP, the incision with dPAPs is not compressed in a sitting position, thus decreasing potential wound sequelae and/or thigh paresthesia.

Lastly, a fleur-de-lis modification of the PAP flap in which both vertical and horizontal limbs are included allows for the harvest of the entire angiosome of perforators and maximizes flap volume from a single donor site.[40–42]

Specialized Profunda Artery Perforator Flaps: Expanded Use and Modifications

Since its introduction by Allen, the PAP flap has been refined and its use extended beyond breast reconstruction. Several techniques have been used that increase the potential reconstructive aspects of the PAP flap. For example, Mayo and colleagues[43] described the utilization of the PAP flap for reconstruction of lower extremity and head and neck defects.

A PAP flap can be harvested from both thighs and used in a "stacked" fashion for unilateral or bilateral breast reconstruction. The most common combination of stacked flaps used for reconstruction is a DIEP flap combined with a PAP flap.[20,44–48] This remains a viable option for patients with scant donor tissue who wish to avoid staged revision with implants or repeated attempts at fat grafting. The placement of a second flap into a mastectomy defect provides additional volume for body-specific reconstruction, with acceptable complication rates.[45] However, utilization of a second free flap necessitates an additional set of microvascular anastomoses, thus increasing operative time, technical difficulty, surgeon fatigue, and potential complications. However, recipient vessel options in this scenario are plentiful and include the antegrade and retrograde internal mammary systems, thoracodorsal, thoracoacromial, and branching vessels off of the primary flap pedicle.[33] Haddock and colleagues[49] noted an increase in the rate of flap loss when the retrograde internal mammary system is used, and for this reason they advocate for the use of intra-flap vessels for secondary recipient anastomoses. That being said, the retrograde system is our preferred second option if the antegrade mammary vessels are of poor quality.

The creation of a sensate flap for breast reconstruction remains a topic of debate.[50,51] Nonetheless, Dayan and Allen Jr. first described the successful transfer of a sensate PAP flap[36] in which neurorrhaphy was achieved by anastomosing the anterior branch of the obturator nerve to the lateral branch of the T4 intercostal nerve. In a recent study using cadaveric thigh dissection, Song and colleagues[52] described the feasibility and location of the posterior femoral cutaneous nerve and its potential for the transfer and creation of a sensate PAP flap.

Postoperative Care

Postoperatively, routine flap monitoring is carried out at the recipient site, typically with a pencil Doppler assessment of the skin paddle. Patients are instructed to wear lower body compression garments for 3 weeks to help decrease swelling and prevent potential scar widening/hypertrophy or seroma formation. Drain output is carefully monitored for volume and consistency. Patients are typically admitted for 1 to 3 days. When criteria for discharge are met, patients are educated on drain care and have reinforcement of activity restrictions until they follow-up in clinic. In addition, one should attempt to avoid pressure on the donor incision site.

Outcomes and Complications

Complication rates following PAP flap surgery are low and acceptable at both the recipient and donor sites. Donor site complications include seroma, hematoma, wound dehiscence, wound infection/cellulitis, and pain.[19] Allen and colleagues[19] reviewed 164 total flaps used in 96 patients. They noted a recipient complication profile of hematoma (1.9%), seroma (6%), fat necrosis (7%), and one instance of flap loss. Haddock and colleagues published the results of their PAP flap experience in 2017 and 2020.[12,13] Of 101 PAP

Table 2
Review of donor site complications across 10 studies

Study, Year	Study Type	Hematoma	Wound Dehiscence	Wound Infection	Seroma	Total Flap Loss
Hunter et al,[10] 2015	PC	–	4.50%	–	4.50%	9.09%
Haddad et al,[15] 2016	PC	–	–	–	6.67%	6.67%
Ito et al,[16] 2016	RR	–	–	–	–	–
Hupkens et al,[17] 2016	PC	–	10%	–	–	–
Allen et al,[19] 2016	RR	1.90%	3.60%	–	6%	0.61%
Haddock et al,[12] 2017	RR	–	10.89%	5.90%	–	1.98%
Fosseprez et al,[18] 2017	RR	5.8%[a]	–	–	35.30%	11.80%
Haddock et al,[20] 2019	RR	–	3%	–	–	–
Haddock et al,[13] 2020	RR	2.60%	6.80%	4.90%	4.50%	3%
Atzeni et al,[14] 2021	PC	1.70%	2.60%	–	2.60%	–

Abbreviations: PC, prospective cohort study; RR, retrospective review.
[a] Denotes recipient site complication.

flaps, there were two total flap losses (2%) and one case of fat necrosis. In 2020 they expanded their investigation to 265 PAP flaps and noted 8 flap losses (3%). A prospective review of 30 PAP flaps by Haddad and colleagues[15] noted two cases of flap loss (6.7%).

Patients should be educated on the nature of donor site complications, which are typically managed nonoperatively. Cho and colleagues[53] reported that higher donor site morbidity and complication rates were associated with increased BMI, with all of their complications localizing to the medial thigh. Donor complication rates noted by Haddock and colleagues[13] included seroma (4.5%), hematoma (2.6%), infection (4.9%), and significant wound issues (6.8%). Significant wounds were defined as those necessitating procedural intervention or negative pressure therapy. Qian and colleagues[54] performed a systematic review of 12 studies that included 516 PAP flaps in 327 patients in which the pooled success rate was 99%. Pooled donor complications included wound dehiscence (6%), seroma (2%), and hematoma (1%). The rate of partial flap loss was 2%, whereas total flap loss occurred at a pooled incidence of 1%. **Table 2** notes the rates of donor complications as well as total flap loss across the 10 studies that are cited in **Table 1**.

Enhanced recovery after surgery (ERAS) protocols exist across several surgical specialties and have been shown to be effective in breast reconstruction with abdominal-based tissue.[55] ERAS protocols in PAP flap-based breast reconstruction have been proven to lower hospital length of stay, operative time, and postoperative opioid consumption.[56] In addition, patient-reported outcome measures (PROMs) have been assessed for patients undergoing breast reconstruction with PAP flaps, and indicate high scores in all BREAST-Q domains.[13,14,57]

Case Example

We present a case of a 53-year-old woman with a history of bilateral breast cancer. She had right breast reconstruction with a DIEP flap and subsequently developed left breast cancer. The left side was reconstructed with a pedicled latissimus flap and silicone implant. Unfortunately, the patient developed capsular contracture of the left breast and desired implant removal and autologous reconstruction. The implant was removed, and an ipsilateral dPAP flap was harvested for left breast reconstruction (see **Figs. 1** and **2**, Video 1).

SUMMARY

PAP flaps have emerged as a leading alternative for autologous breast reconstruction when abdominal-based tissue is contraindicated or undesired. Several studies have cited excellent surgical and patient-reported outcomes with low, predictable recipient and donor site morbidity. The aforementioned modifications of the original PAP flap (eg, vPAP, dPAP, and fleur-de-lis PAP) increase the potential reconstructive capacity of this donor tissue. As techniques are refined and surgeon experience improves, we expect the clinical application and utilization of PAP flaps to expand accordingly.

CLINICS CARE POINTS

- Abdominal-based tissue is the gold standard for autologous free flap breast reconstruction.
- The profunda artery perforator (PAP) flap may be an option in those who are not candidates for abdominal tissue transfer.
- The PAP flap is based off perforators from the profunda artery, supplying the skin and subcutaneous tissue of the posteromedial thigh.
- Owing to low donor-site morbidity, reliability of the vascular supply, and excellent cosmetic outcomes, the PAP flap has emerged as a preferred alternate source.

FUNDING

This research was funded in part through the NIH/NCI Cancer Center Support Grant P30 CA008748, which supports Memorial Sloan Kettering Cancer Center's research infrastructure.

DISCLOSURE

The authors have no conflicts of interest to disclose.

SUPPLEMENTARY DATA

Supplementary data related to this article can be found online at https://doi.org/10.1016/j.cps.2022.10.001.

REFERENCES

1. Bonde C, Khorasani H, Eriksen K, et al. Introducing the fast track surgery principles can reduce length of stay after autologous breast reconstruction using free flaps: a case control study. J Plast Surg Hand Surg 2015;49(6):367–71.
2. Rozen WM, Ashton MW. Improving outcomes in autologous breast reconstruction. Aesthet Plast Surg 2009;33(3):327–35.
3. Tachi M, Yamada A. Choice of flaps for breast reconstruction. Int J Clin Oncol 2005;10(5):289–97.
4. Gurunluoglu R, Gurunluoglu A, Williams SA, et al. Current trends in breast reconstruction: survey of American society of plastic surgeons 2010. Ann Plast Surg 2013;70(1):103–10.
5. Pien I, Caccavale S, Cheung MC, et al. Evolving trends in autologous breast reconstruction: is the deep inferior epigastric artery perforator flap taking over? Ann Plast Surg 2016;76(5):489–93.
6. Hurwitz DJ, Walton RL. Closure of chronic wounds of the perineal and sacral regions using the gluteal thigh flap. Ann Plast Surg 1982;8(5):375–86.
7. Song YG, Chen GZ, Song YL. The free thigh flap: a new free flap concept based on the septocutaneous artery. Br J Plast Surg 1984;37(2):149–59.
8. Angrigiani C, Grilli D, Thorne CH. The adductor flap: a new method for transferring posterior and medial thigh skin. Plast Reconstr Surg 2001;107(7):1725–31.
9. Allen RJ, Haddock NT, Ahn CY, et al. Breast reconstruction with the profunda artery perforator flap. Plast Reconstr Surg 2012;129(1):16e–23e.
10. Hunter JE, Lardi AM, Dower DR, et al. Evolution from the TUG to PAP flap for breast reconstruction: comparison and refinements of technique. J Plast Reconstr Aesthet Surg 2015;68(7):960–5.
11. Dayan JH, Allen RJ Jr. Lower extremity free flaps for breast reconstruction. Plast Reconstr Surg 2017;140(5S):77S–86S. Advances in Breast Reconstruction).
12. Haddock NT, Gassman A, Cho MJ, et al. 101 consecutive profunda artery perforator flaps in breast reconstruction: lessons learned with our early experience. Plast Reconstr Surg 2017;140(2):229–39.
13. Haddock NT, Teotia SS. Consecutive 265 profunda artery perforator flaps: refinements, satisfaction, and functional outcomes. Plast Reconstr Surg Glob Open 2020;8(4):e2682.
14. Atzeni M, Salzillo R, Haywood R, et al. Breast reconstruction using the profunda artery perforator (PAP) flap: technical refinements and evolution, outcomes, and patient satisfaction based on 116 consecutive flaps. J Plast Reconstr Aesthet Surg 2021. https://doi.org/10.1016/j.bjps.2021.11.085.
15. Haddad K, Hunsinger V, Obadia D, et al. [Breast reconstruction with profunda artery perforator flap: a prospective study of 30 consecutive cases]. Ann Chir Plast Esthet 2016;61(3):169–76.
16. Ito R, Huang JJ, Wu JC, et al. The versatility of profunda femoral artery perforator flap for oncological reconstruction after cancer resection-Clinical cases and review of literature. J Surg Oncol 2016;114(2):193–201.
17. Hupkens P, Hameeteman M, Westland PB, et al. Breast reconstruction using the geometrically modified profunda artery perforator flap from the posteromedial thigh region: combining the benefits of its predecessors. Ann Plast Surg 2016;77(4):438–44.
18. Fosseprez P, Gerdom A, Servaes M, et al. [Profunda artery perforator flap: reliable secondary option for breast reconstruction?]. Ann Chir Plast Esthet 2017;62(6):637–45. Profunda artery perforator flap : quelle place dans la reconstruction mammaire par lambeau autologue ?

19. Allen RJ Jr, Lee ZH, Mayo JL, et al. The profunda artery perforator flap experience for breast reconstruction. Plast Reconstr Surg 2016;138(5):968–75.
20. Haddock NT, Cho MJ, Gassman A, et al. Stacked profunda artery perforator flap for breast reconstruction in failed or unavailable deep inferior epigastric perforator flap. Plast Reconstr Surg 2019;143(3):488e–94e.
21. Weichman KE, Broer PN, Tanna N, et al. The role of autologous fat grafting in secondary microsurgical breast reconstruction. Ann Plast Surg 2013;71(1):24–30.
22. Jo T, Jeon DN, Han HH. The PAP flap breast reconstruction: a practical option for slim patients. J Reconstr Microsurg 2022;38(1):27–33.
23. Saad A, Sadeghi A, Allen RJ. The anatomic basis of the profunda femoris artery perforator flap: a new option for autologous breast reconstruction–a cadaveric and computer tomography angiogram study. J Reconstr Microsurg 2012;28(6):381–6.
24. Ahmadzadeh R, Bergeron L, Tang M, et al. The posterior thigh perforator flap or profunda femoris artery perforator flap. Plast Reconstr Surg 2007;119(1):194–200.
25. DeLong MR, Hughes DB, Bond JE, et al. A detailed evaluation of the anatomical variations of the profunda artery perforator flap using computed tomographic angiograms. Plast Reconstr Surg 2014;134(2):186e–92e.
26. Wong C, Nagarkar P, Teotia S, et al. The profunda artery perforator flap: investigating the perforasome using three-dimensional computed tomographic angiography. Plast Reconstr Surg 2015;136(5):915–9.
27. Haddock NT, Greaney P, Otterburn D, et al. Predicting perforator location on preoperative imaging for the profunda artery perforator flap. Microsurgery 2012;32(7):507–11.
28. Agrawal MD, Thimmappa ND, Vasile JV, et al. Autologous breast reconstruction: preoperative magnetic resonance angiography for perforator flap vessel mapping. J Reconstr Microsurg 2015;31(1):1–11.
29. Largo RD, Chu CK, Chang EI, et al. Perforator mapping of the profunda artery perforator flap: anatomy and clinical experience. Plast Reconstr Surg 2020;146(5):1135–45.
30. Levine SM, Snider C, Gerald G, et al. Buried flap reconstruction after nipple-sparing mastectomy: advancing toward single-stage breast reconstruction. Plast Reconstr Surg 2013;132(4):489e–97e.
31. Tanna N, Broer PN, Weichman KE, et al. Microsurgical breast reconstruction for nipple-sparing mastectomy. Plast Reconstr Surg 2013;131(2):139e–47e.
32. Teotia SS, Cho MJ, Haddock NT. Salvaging breast reconstruction: profunda artery perforator flaps using thoracodorsal vessels. Plast Reconstr Surg Glob Open 2018;6(9):e1837.
33. Stalder MW, Lam J, Allen RJ, et al. Using the retrograde internal mammary system for stacked perforator flap breast reconstruction: 71 breast reconstructions in 53 consecutive patients. Plast Reconstr Surg 2016;137(2):265e–77e.
34. Allen RJ, Mehrara BJ. 36 - breast reconstruction. In: Farhadieh RD, Bulstrode NW, Mehrara BJ, et al, editors. Plastic surgery - principles and practice. New York, NY: Elsevier; 2022. p. 535–64.
35. Frey JD, Stranix JT, Chiodo MV, et al. Evolution in monitoring of free flap autologous breast reconstruction after nipple-sparing mastectomy: is there a best way? Plast Reconstr Surg 2018;141(5):1086–93.
36. Dayan JH, Allen RJ Jr. Neurotized diagonal profunda artery perforator flaps for breast reconstruction. Plast Reconstr Surg Glob Open 2019;7(10):e2463.
37. Rivera-Serrano CM, Aljaaly HA, Wu J, et al. Vertical PAP flap: simultaneous longitudinal profunda artery perforator flaps for bilateral breast reconstructions. Plast Reconstr Surg Glob Open 2017;5(2):e1189.
38. Scaglioni MF, Chen YC, Lindenblatt N, et al. The vertical posteromedial thigh (vPMT) flap for autologous breast reconstruction: a novel flap design. Microsurgery 2017;37(5):371–6.
39. Tielemans HJP, van Kuppenveld PIP, Winters H, et al. Breast reconstruction with the extended profunda artery perforator flap. J Plast Reconstr Aesthet Surg 2021;74(2):300–6.
40. Bourn L, Torabi R, Stalder MW, et al. Mosaic fleur-de-profunda artery perforator flap for autologous breast reconstruction. Plast Reconstr Surg Glob Open 2019;7(3):e2166.
41. Saussy K, Stalder MW, Delatte SJ, et al. The fleur-de-PAP flap for bilateral breast reconstruction. J Reconstr Microsurg Open 2017;02(01):e1–3.
42. Hunsinger V, Lhuaire M, Haddad K, et al. Medium-and large-sized autologous breast reconstruction using a fleur-de-lys profunda femoris artery perforator flap design: a report comparing results with the horizontal profunda femoris artery perforator flap. J Reconstr Microsurg 2019;35(01):008–14.
43. Mayo JL, Canizares O, Torabi R, et al. Expanding the applications of the profunda artery perforator flap. Plast Reconstr Surg 2016;137(2):663–9.
44. Blechman KM, Broer PN, Tanna N, et al. Stacked profunda artery perforator flaps for unilateral breast reconstruction: a case report. J Reconstr Microsurg 2013;29(9):631–4.
45. Mayo JL, Allen RJ, Sadeghi A. Four-flap breast reconstruction: bilateral stacked DIEP and PAP flaps. Plast Reconstr Surg Glob Open 2015;3(5):e383.

46. Haddock N, Nagarkar P, Teotia SS. Versatility of the profunda artery perforator flap: creative uses in breast reconstruction. Plast Reconstr Surg 2017; 139(3):606e–12e.

47. Haddock NT, Cho MJ, Teotia SS. Comparative analysis of single versus stacked free flap breast reconstruction: a single-center experience. Plast Reconstr Surg 2019;144(3):369e–77e.

48. Haddock NT, Suszynski TM, Teotia SS. Consecutive bilateral breast reconstruction using stacked abdominally based and posterior thigh free flaps. Plast Reconstr Surg 2021;147(2):294–303.

49. Teotia SS, Dumestre DO, Jayaraman AP, et al. Revisiting anastomosis to the retrograde internal mammary system in stacked free flap breast reconstruction: an algorithmic approach to recipient-site selection. Plast Reconstr Surg 2020; 145(4):880–7.

50. Weissler JM, Koltz PF, Carney MJ, et al. Sifting through the evidence: a comprehensive review and analysis of neurotization in breast reconstruction. Plast Reconstr Surg 2018;141(3):550–65.

51. Liew S, Hunt J, Pennington D. Sensory recovery following free TRAM flap breast reconstruction. Br J Plast Surg 1996;49(4):210–3.

52. Song B, Kumbla PA, Boyd C, et al. The feasibility of a sensate profunda artery perforator flap in autologous breast reconstruction: an anatomic study for clinical application. Ann Plast Surg 2020; 84(6S):S451–4.

53. Cho MJ, Teotia SS, Haddock NT. Classification and management of donor-site wound complications in the profunda artery perforator flap for breast reconstruction. J Reconstr Microsurg 2020;36(2):110–5.

54. Qian B, Xiong L, Li J, et al. A systematic review and meta-analysis on microsurgical safety and efficacy of profunda artery perforator flap in breast reconstruction. J Oncol 2019;2019:9506720.

55. Temple-Oberle C, Shea-Budgell MA, Tan M, et al. Consensus review of optimal perioperative care in breast reconstruction: enhanced recovery after surgery (ERAS) society recommendations. Plast Reconstr Surg 2017;139(5):1056e–71e.

56. Cho MJ, Garza R, Teotia SS, et al. Utility of ERAS pathway in nonabdominal-based microsurgical breast reconstruction: efficacy in PAP flap reconstruction? J Reconstr Microsurg 2021. https://doi.org/10.1055/s-0041-1733993.

57. Dickey RM, Garza R, Liu Y, et al. 4: four-flap breast reconstruction: assessing breast-q and donor site morbidity in bilateral stacked autologous breast reconstruction. Plast Reconstr Surg Glob Open 2021;9(7S):41.

Lumbar Artery Perforator Flaps in Autologous Breast Reconstruction

Steven M. Sultan, MD[a], David T. Greenspun, MD, MSc, FACS[b],*

KEYWORDS

- Breast reconstruction • Perforator flaps • Lumbar • DIEP • Microsurgery

KEY POINTS

- Lumbar artery perforator flaps are an ideal second option for autologous breast reconstruction in patients in whom the abdominal donor site is unavailable.
- Safe and reliable reconstruction using lumbar artery perforator flaps typically requires the participation of multiple skilled surgeons and is facilitated by the use of interposition arterial and venous grafts.
- The lumbar perforator flap has an analog in posterior body lift cosmetic surgery, and therefore harvest of this flap produces an excellent cosmetic result at the flap donor site.

INTRODUCTION

The abdominal donor site has been the most widely used source of tissue in autologous breast reconstruction since the introduction of the "free abdominoplasty flap" by Holmstrom in 1979.[1] The deep inferior epigastric perforator (DIEP) flap was introduced in 1994 and is now the accepted "gold standard" in autologous breast reconstruction.[2] In many instances, however, the abdominal donor site is inadequate for any number of reasons including a paucity of tissue, prior surgical procedures that have injured the inferior epigastric perforators, or prior failed abdominally based flap reconstruction. Several alternatives have been used for autologous reconstruction in such cases. The primary alternative donor site options can be categorized as follows: combination procedures that use two or more flaps to reconstruct a breast, gluteal-based flaps, thigh-based flaps, and lumbar artery perforator (LAP) flaps.

Although the buttock was a popular alternative donor site to the abdomen in the early era of perforator flap breast reconstruction, gluteal-based flaps have largely been abandoned in recent years, in no insignificant part due to deleterious effects on the appearance of the buttocks. Potential adverse effects on the buttock region associated with superior and inferior gluteal artery perforator flap harvest include loss of volume and fullness and disruption of normal anatomic contours and boundaries. Furthermore, the morbidity associated with possible sciatic or posterior femoral cutaneous nerve injuries that can occur during the harvest of the lower buttock based upon the inferior gluteal artery perforator has rendered this flap all but obsolete.[3,4]

At many centers, thigh-based flaps including profunda artery perforator flaps, transverse and diagonal upper gracilis flaps, and lateral thigh perforator flaps are now the preferred secondary options in autologous breast reconstruction when the abdominal donor site is not satisfactory.[5] It is the authors' opinion that for many women, the LAP flap is the most optimal

[a] Mount Sinai Hospital, 5 East 98th Street, 8th Floor, New York, NY 10029, USA; [b] The Plastic & Reconstructive Surgery Group, 2 Greenwich Office Park, Suite 210, Greenwich, CT 06831, USA
* Corresponding author.
E-mail address: dg@tprsg.com

Clin Plastic Surg 50 (2023) 301–312
https://doi.org/10.1016/j.cps.2022.11.005
0094-1298/23/© 2022 Elsevier Inc. All rights reserved.

secondary option for breast reconstruction—producing favorable results at both donor and recipient sites—and indeed this view is now shared by several high-volume centers around the world.[6,7]

In properly selected patients, aesthetically pleasing breasts can be reconstructed from tissue harvested from either the thigh or lumbar region. However, the harvest of thigh flaps can introduce unnatural contour at a flap's donor site. This is not entirely surprising, as the design of many thigh flaps does not adhere to the principles of aesthetic body contouring surgery. Although the DIEP flap has an analog in the tissue removed during an abdominoplasty, most thigh flaps used in breast reconstruction do not have analogs in body contouring surgery. The PAP flap, for example, is harvested from a portion of the posterior thigh deemed a "no-go" zone by Rohrich and colleagues in his seminal work on contouring by suction-assisted lipectomy.[8] To our knowledge, the so-called "saddle-bag" area of the lateral thigh—that many women find cosmetically objectionable and for which they seek cosmetic surgical body contouring—is seldom if ever treated by direct excision. A key reason that excision is not used to treat this area is that the natural silhouette of the lateral thigh is convex, and excision of a wedge of tissue down to the plane of the lateral thigh fascia would disrupt the normal convex contour and introduce undesirable concavity. Nevertheless, harvest of an lateral thigh perforator (LTP) flap involves excision of lateral thigh tissue at the level of the fascia; the procedure can thus create significant contour deformity at the flap donor site.[9] This is a significant enough issue that liposuction at the time of LTP flap harvest has been described as means of trying to address the secondary deformity associated with harvest of this flap.[9]

In contradistinction, harvest of tissue from the lumbar area of the lower back follows the principles of cosmetic body contouring. LAP flap design has its analog in the design of a lower body lift.[10] Just as a posterior body lift lifts the buttocks, narrows the waist and accentuates the lordotic curvature of the lower back, so too does harvest of LAP flaps. As a result, harvest of LAP flaps produces Callipygean contour at the donor site.

Major drawbacks to LAP flap breast reconstruction include the relatively high rate of flap failure (6% to 10%) reported for this procedure as well as a high incidence of donor site seroma.[11] Postoperative sensory changes at the donor site are also common. It is essential that patients considering LAP flap breast reconstruction be properly informed about the risks and benefits of this surgery.

History of Lumbar Artery Perforator Flaps

Pedicled flaps based upon the LAPs have been used in locoregional reconstruction of the lumbosacral region.[12,13] The first reported free flap harvested from this area for breast reconstruction was in 2003 by de Weerd and colleagues[14] Since that time, LAP flap breast reconstruction has slowly grown in popularity. Although the donor site is aesthetically ideal, the technical difficulty of the procedure and a comparatively high reported complication rate have likely contributed to a relative lack of widespread adoption of LAP flap breast reconstruction. Inherently, the procedure is technically challenging and best undertaken by microsurgeons who have significant experience with complex perforator flap microsurgery. We and others have found that refinements in execution have improved operative efficiency and outcomes.[11,15,16]

Anatomy

Several studies have delineated the vascular anatomy of the lumbar region and more specifically, that of the LAPs.[17,18] The dominant LAPs most commonly arise from the L4 posterior intercostal branches.[11,19] These perforators most commonly course between the quadratus lumborum and erector spinae muscles to enter the subcutaneous tissue approximately 7 to 10 cm lateral to the posterior midline. Alternatively and less commonly, these perforators can traverse through the erector spinae muscle fibers on their way to entering the fatty tissue of the lower back.[20] The ideal and most preferred anatomy of the perforator upon which to base an LAP flap is a sizable septo-cutaneous L4 perforator. L5 perforators are sometimes the largest; however, the intimate relation of the L5 perforator to the pelvic bone can present significant difficulty for the surgeon. L5 perforators can be adherent to the pelvic periosteum and thus dissection of the thin-walled veins off of the pelvis is tedious and unforgiving. Of course, the immobility of the pelvis can make exposure difficult and adds to the challenges of L5 perforator dissection. In addition, L5 perforators may originate on the iliolumbar vessels rather than the aorta. In such cases, the dissection may not be toward the spine but rather in a more lateral trajectory.

The Artery of Adamkiewicz typically arises between T8 and L1, and is thus easily avoided at the L4 to L5 level.[21] The Artery of Adamkiewicz supplies the lumbar and sacral spinal cord and must be preserved to avoid neurologic complications while harvesting lumbar flaps.[22]

Patient Selection, Preoperative Workup, and Surgical Planning

Any patient who requires autologous reconstruction but does not have a suitable abdominal donor site may be considered for LAP flap reconstruction. Many women have sufficient fatty tissue in the lumbar distribution and this can readily be assessed on clinical examination. Pinch testing and physical examination are used to determine if a sufficient amount of soft tissue is available to reconstruct a breast to the desired dimensions. The laxity of the lower back and buttock tissue are evaluated to ensure that donor site closure will be achieved with appropriate tension and contouring. Prior lower back surgery may or may not be a contraindication to LAP flap harvest, and discussion with a spine surgeon should take place when appropriate. In addition to the standard preoperative risk assessment done for a patient undergoing free flap breast reconstruction, careful attention should be paid to risk factors for hypercoagulability, as hypercoagulability is a relative contraindication.

The total surface area of skin that can be incorporated into an LAP flap is generally markedly less than can be harvested with the typical DIEP flap. The skin paddle of an LAP flap is typically elliptical in shape and measures 6 to 8 cm at the longest part of the short axis of the ellipse. The long axis of the LAP flap skin island typically measures between 22 and 27 cm. The fat lobules of the lower back are similar to those of the buttock region in that they are more taut and less malleable than the fatty lobules of the abdomen wall. LAP flaps thus have greater stiffness and turgor than do abdominal flaps. As a result, like an SGAP flap, the LAP flap produces excellent contour, but there is little ability to manipulate either the fatty component or the skin paddle when insetting these flaps. The surgeon essentially "sculpts" the breast at the time the flap is harvested, and the flap is simply "placed" into the recipient site defect. Women who require significant restoration of the skin envelope of the reconstructed breast may not be good candidates for LAP flap surgery.

Preoperative cross-sectional imaging with perforator mapping is essential (**Fig. 1**). In keeping with the recommendations of the American College of Radiology, to avoid exposing patients to unnecessary radiation when alternative testing modalities are available, we prefer magnetic resonance angiography (MRA). Use of MRA avoids the significant dose of radiation that is delivered to the abdominopelvic region when high-resolution CT scanning is used for perforator mapping.[23–25]

The LAP flap pedicle is short and the artery has a narrow caliber. Pedicle length tends to be in the range of 2 to 4 cm, and the arterial diameter in the rage of 0.8 mm to 1.2 mm. Without interposition grafts, microsurgical anastomoses of the pedicle vessels to the internal mammary vessels (our recipient vessels of choice) are extremely difficult. Size mismatch at the arterial anastomosis increases the risk of thrombosis owing to turbulent flow, and flap inset is complicated by a lack of freedom of movement attributable to the short pedicle. These issues have been mitigated with the use of arterial and venous interposition grafts.[26] Depending on individual circumstances, we harvest interposition grafts from either the deep interior epigastric system or the thoracodorsal system.

Markings

We use the lumbar region ipsilateral to the breast that is being reconstructed. Harvest of an LAP flap ipsilateral to the breast being reconstructed facilitates shaping of the breast, microsurgical anastomoses to mammary recipient vessels, and flap inset.

The flap is bounded anteriorly by the anterior superior iliac spine (ASIS) and posteriorly by the midline. The flap is centered vertically on the perforator/s that are selected based upon preoperative cross-sectional imaging. The vertical height of the skin island is determined by a pinch test and the skin island is designed as an ellipse (**Fig. 2**). It is important to avoid harvesting too large a skin paddle to avoid a closure under tension that can predispose to donor site wound breakdown.

Along the horizontal axis of the flap, the lumbar perforator/s generally enter the underside of the flap approximately 7 to 10 cm from the posterior midline.

The area of soft tissue to be included in the flap will extend well beyond the inferior border of the skin island. The fatty component of an LAP flap includes both lower back fat and gluteal fat. The surgeon should design the flap so that it will have a total vertical height of at least 13 to 16

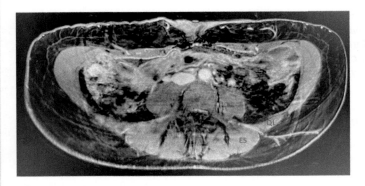

Fig. 1. Magnetic resonance angiogram showing a left septocutanous lumbar perforator (*highlighted in yellow*) passing between the quadrates lumborum (QL) and the erector spinae (ES) muscles. The relatively short distance between the surface of the thoracolumbar fascia (*red line*) and the tip of the transverse process (*asterisk*) can be appreciated on this representative image.

cm. The area of subcutaneous fat that will be incorporated into the flap from beneath undermined buttock skin is marked (see **Fig. 2**). We find it helpful to visualize harvesting a flap that ultimately takes the shape of an anatomic-shaped breast implant or inflated tissue expander.

Surgical Procedure

We always begin LAP flap reconstruction with preparation of the recipient site with the patient in supine position. Recipient vessels are dissected following the mastectomy in an immediate reconstruction or after the breast pocket has otherwise been prepared in a delayed reconstruction. We think it is most prudent to have the

recipient site ready before harvest of the flap and interposition grafts. The internal mammary vessels are the preferred recipients for lumbar flap reconstruction. The thoracodorsal vessels can be used as recipient vessels as well; however, they are less desirable than the mammaries given the geometry of the LAP flap and its pedicle.

If vascular grafts are to be harvested from the abdomen, we also dissect, but do not harvest, deep inferior epigastric vessels during the initial stage of surgery. To avoid prolonged ischemia of the grafts themselves, interposition graft ligation and harvest are done only after flap harvest is completed.

Once recipient site preparation is complete and we are ready to harvest the LAP flap, the chest is

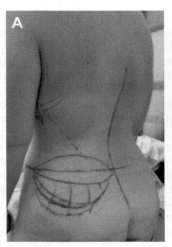
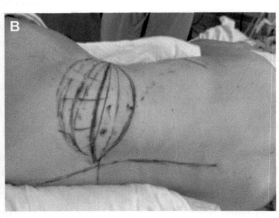

Fig. 2. LAP flap markings shown preoperatively (*A*) and on the operating room table with the patient positioned in lateral decubitus (*B*). The skin paddle is marked as a solidly outlined ellipse transected horizontally by a line corresponding to the level of the umbilicus. The ellipse measures roughly 6 to 8 cm vertically and 25 cm along its anterior-to-posterior axis. Along the vertical axis, the ellipse is centered on the identified perforators (marked as dots in image *B*). The dominant perforator is typically found approximately 7 to 10 cm anterior to the posterior midline. Other more anterior perforators may be identifiable with doppler, but these generally smaller vessels are not suitable for microvascular transfer of the flap. That portion of the flap that includes gluteal fat elevated subcutaneously is identified here with hash marks caudal to the skin island.

temporarily closed and covered with a sterile occlusive dressing. If abdominal grafts have been prepared, the graft donor site is similarly managed at this stage. The patient is then repositioned for the first time.

Positioning

The patient is positioned either in lateral decubitus position or prone position, depending on surgeon preference. There are pros and cons to each approach. It is often easier to identify the perforators when the patient is positioned prone; however, the deep inferior epigastric arteriovenous (AV) grafts can not be simultaneously harvested in this position. We sometimes use thoracodorsal grafts when the patient is placed prone for flap dissection. Although use of thoracodorsal grafts enhances efficiency in such situations, use of these grafts potentially eliminates a second set of recipient vessels as well as future latissimus dorsi flap harvest. Because the inferior epigastric grafts can be harvested with the patient in lateral decubitus position, operative efficiency is superior to prone positioning if flap dissection is done in lateral decubitus position when these grafts are used. Notably, an AV graft can be harvested from the thoracodorsal system in either the prone or lateral decubitus position.

Although the senior author has performed bilateral simultaneous LAP flap reconstruction, we generally favor staging bilateral LAP flap reconstructions. If bilateral LAP flap harvest is to be undertaken, prone positioning must be used.

Arteriovenous graft harvest

As described above, preparation—but not harvest—of an AV graft is typically completed before flap elevation. The inferior epigastric AV graft is harvested through a 5 cm groin incision. Dissection down to the rectus fascia is undertaken and the muscle fascia is split along the direction of the fascial fibers. The lateral border of the rectus muscle is identified and the muscle is reflected medially to expose the deep inferior epigastric pedicle on the underside of the rectus muscle (**Fig. 3**). The pedicle is dissected cranially and caudally as far as possible (typically 6 to 10 cm).

A thoracodorsal graft can be harvested in either prone or lateral position. A 5 to 8 cm incision is made along the bra strap line or within a relaxed skin tension line beginning just posterior to the anterior border of the latissimus muscle. The anterior border of the latissimus is exposed and reflected to allow access to the TD pedicle on the undersurface of the muscle. The vessel is identified and dissected cranially into the axilla and caudally toward the takeoff of the serratus branch (see **Fig. 3**). Prior axillary dissection or radiation are relative contraindications to use of the thoracodorsal pedicle as an AV graft, unless patency of the vessels is confirmed with preoperative imaging.

Flap elevation

Flap elevation is begun by incising along the skin paddle markings. The superior incision is then deepened and the dissection is beveled toward the upper limit of the flap. Only a small amount of subcutaneous fat beyond the edge of the skin island is captured along the superior border of the flap. Along the inferior border of the skin island, the flap is shaped by beveling into the gluteal fat and capturing a significant amount of gluteal fat in the flap (**Fig. 4**). This dissection occurs in nonanatomic tissue planes with the surgeon visualizing that, at this stage of the procedure, he or

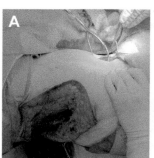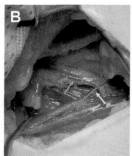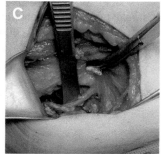

Fig. 3. AV graft harvest: An AV graft can be harvested from the deep inferior epigastric system with the patient in the lateral decubitus position (*A, B*). Deep inferior epigastric grafts are seen held in the surgeon's forceps (*A*) immediately after an LAP flap was harvested (LAP donor site is seen at the bottom of the photograph). A close-up view of the DIE graft (*green arrow*) with a preserved motor nerve (*yellow arrow*) crossing over the vessels is shown (*B*). Grafts can be harvested from the thoracodorsal system with the patient in lateral decubitus position as shown by the thoracodorsal (TD) vessels draped over the forceps (*C*).

CRANIAL ◄───► CAUDAL

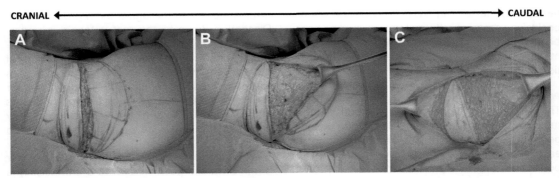

Fig. 4. Shaping the reconstructed breast during LAP flap harvest. The entirety of the flap skin island is incised (*A*). The flap is shaped by dissecting so as to capture a significant amount of gluteal fat along the caudal skin island incision (*B*, *C*). Along the cranial incision, surgical beveling is modest, and only a limited amount of fat is captured beyond the margin of the skin island (*C*).

she is sculpting the flap into the shape needed for the breast reconstruction (**Fig. 5**).

Care should be taken to avoid excessive dissection near the posterior midline lest an unsightly hollow result. However, care must also be taken not to undercut the flap in this area, as this portion of the flap will ultimately be needed to produce medial fullness of the reconstructed breast.

Once the superficial and peripheral flap borders have been defined by dissection with electrocautery, the flap is elevated from lateral to medial (lateral position) or from medial to lateral (prone position) until the lumbar perforators are identified piercing through the thoracolumbar fascia to enter the undersurface of the flap. The thoracolumbar fascia through which the perforators traverse is easily identified by its glistening white appearance. Notably, when raising the undersurface of the flap, dissection should be superficial to the gluteal fascia, and cluneal nerves should be preserved whenever possible (**Fig. 6**). If cluneal nerves must be divided, they should be repaired. Donor-site numbness, nerualgia and dysesthesia at the LAP donor site can be reduced with attention to

preservation, and when necessary, repair of cluneal nerves.

Once the perforator/s have been identified, the thoracolumbar fascia is opened and the perforator/s are dissected, ideally in the septal plane between the quadratus lumborum and the erector spinae muscles. A skilled assistant is essential at this stage of surgery to help with exposure. Dissection must be meticulous and bloodless. L5 perforators may be adherent to the boney pelvic margin and must be freed from the periosteum that sometimes encases them. Extreme care must be exercised during that dissection as bleeding from branches heading into the pelvis can be difficult to manage. Lumbar perforators are dissected toward their origin until the surgeon reaches the level of the tip of the transverse process associated with the vascular pedicle (see **Fig. 6**). Dissection is always terminated at this level to avoid injury to the dorsal sensory ganglion or injury to deep vessels that may be difficult to control safely. The pedicle is typically 2 to 4 cm on length. A sensate flap can be created by incorporation of a sensory nerve entering the underside of the flap.

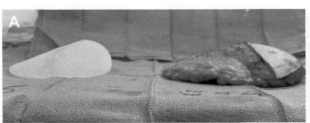
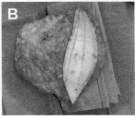

Fig. 5. Lateral (*A*) and anterior (*B*) views demonstrating the shape of the carefully elevated LAP flap. It is analogous to a form-stable implant as shown here (*A*).

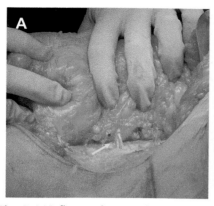
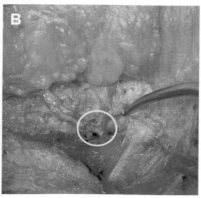
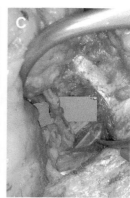

Fig. 6. LAP flap perforator identification and dissection. Once the superficial dissection of the flap has been completed, the deep surface of the LAP flap is elevated off of the underlying tissue and the lumbar perforators are identified and prepared. A large lumbar perforator is seen passing through the thoracolumbar fascia (*A*). Frequently two lumbar perforators coalesce just beneath the thoracolumbar fascia to form a larger single pedicle (*B*). The pedicle is dissected by opening the thoracolumbar fascia and following the perforator/s in the septocutanous plane to the level of the transverse process tip – a distance that is typically 2 to 4 cm (*C*). (*yellow arrow*) lumbar perforator; (*yellow circle*) two lumbar perforators coalesce into a single pedicle.

Flap harvest, donor site closure

Once the pedicle has been dissected and divided, flap elevation is completed using electrocautery to divide any remaining soft tissue attachments, and both the flap and the AV grafts are harvested. At this point in time, the flap is brought to the back table of the operating room where the AV grafts are anastomosed to the flap pedicle (**Fig. 7**). The arterial anastomosis is typically performed with a 1.0 to 1.5 mm coupler. If the arterial walls will not evert onto the tines of the coupler, the anastomosis is hand sewn with 10 to 0 nylon sutures. The venous anastomosis between the largest LAP pedicle venae comitant and that of the graft is completed with a coupler.

Except in circumstances when both prone positioning and deep inferior epigastric grafts are used, the LAP flap donor site is closed in layers while microsurgery is being done on the back table. Seromas occur frequently at the donor site, and we thus anticipate that a drain will be in place for up to 4 weeks. A 19 French round drain is placed in the donor site overlying the thoracolumbar fascia; it is brought out anteriorly near the ASIS so as to allow the patient to care for their drain without difficulty. We typically use a negative pressure dressing over the donor site suture line.

If interposition grafts are harvested from the thoracodorsal system, the upper back incision is closed over a drain before repositioning. If the grafts were harvested from the inferior epigastric system, the access incision is temporarily closed and covered with an occlusive dressing. Closure

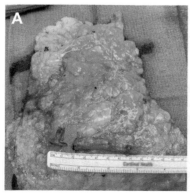
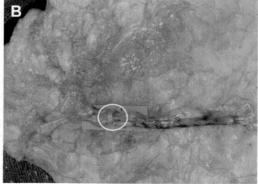

Fig. 7. LAP flap anstomoses to AV graft. A DIE graft, comprised of the deep inferior epigastric artery and two venae comitantes, is shown placed in proximity to the short lumbar artery pedicle on the undersurface of this LAP flap (*A*). Both the arterial and venous anastomoses are typically performed with couplers (*yellow circle*) (*B*).

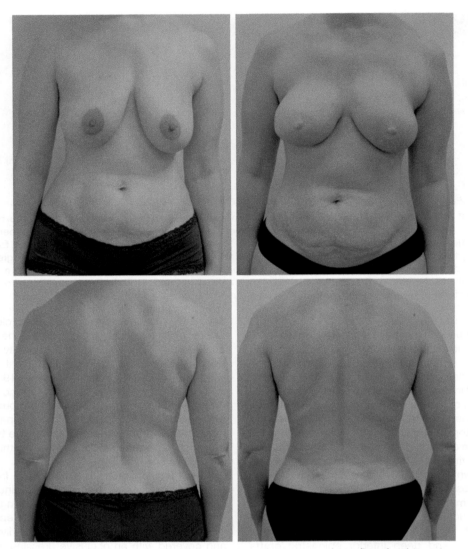

Fig. 8. Case 1: Bilateral LAP flap breast reconstruction achieved using staged LAP flaps for this patient with inadequate abdominal soft tissue for breast reconstruction. The patient's abdominal donor site was clearly inadequate to provide the volume necessary to reconstruct both breasts. She underwent bilateral mastectomies, immediate reconstruction of the left breast with an LAP flap and immediate reconstruction of the right breast with a prepectoral breast implant. Subsequently, the right breast implant reconstruction was replaced with an LAP flap. Deep inferior epigastric interposition grafts were used bilaterally.

of that site is then done after the patient is repositioned to supine.

Flap anastomosis, inset

The patient is repositioned to supine and the previously dissected mammary vessels are revealed by removing the temporary dressing. The flap and its anastomosed AV grafts are brought to the recipient site and heparinized saline is flushed through the flap. If the flap has been harvested from the ipsilateral donor site, the flap is rotated 180° so as to position the vascular pedicle medially and the "gluteal" fat superiorly. This configuration is ideal for performing microsurgery at the recipient site and for shaping the breast. Total vessel length from the undersurface of the flap to the open end of the vessels of the interposition grafts will be in the range of roughly 8 to 12 cm. With this total vessel length, and with the diameters of the grafts and recipient vessels reasonably matching, anastomoses to the chest vessels closely

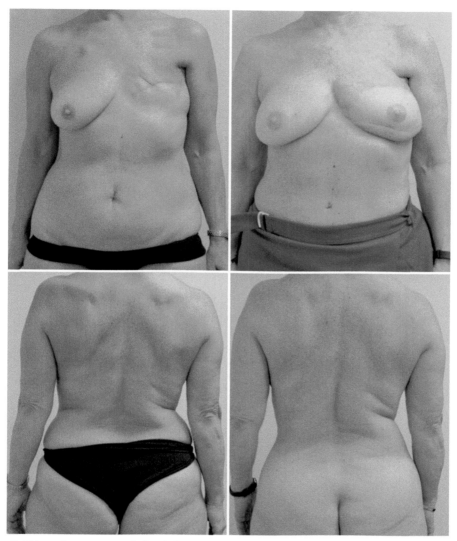

Fig. 9. Case 2: This patient presented after left mastectomy, axillary node dissection and post-mastectomy radiation. At the time of consultation, she sought right prophylactic mastectomy and bilateral autologous reconstruction. Her left breast was reconstructed with bipedicle conjoined DIEP flaps. The skin paddle of either an LAP flap
or a single DIEP flap would have been inadequate for the left reconstruction and thus both hemi-abdominal flaps
were used to reconstruct the left breast. Shortly thereafter, she underwent right prophylactic mastectomy and
immediate right LAP flap breast reconstruction. A contralateral excision of lumbar tissue was performed at a later
date for symmetry.

resembles microsurgery during DIEP flap breast reconstruction. After confirming patency of all anastomoses, the flap is inset.

The skin island will be oriented in the lower 1/3rd of the reconstructed breast, and that portion of the flap chiefly composed of gluteal fat forms the upper sloping portion of the reconstructed breast. This fat is tucked beneath the patient's own breast skin, and closure is done over a drain.

Revision Surgery

We find that most patients who undergo autologous breast reconstruction, regardless of the particular donor site used to harvest tissue, require a revisionary (so-called second stage) surgical procedure to optimize the results at both the donor and recipient sites. Our typical revisionary procedure is done on an outpatient basis 3 or more months following flap transfer surgery. These procedures include one or more

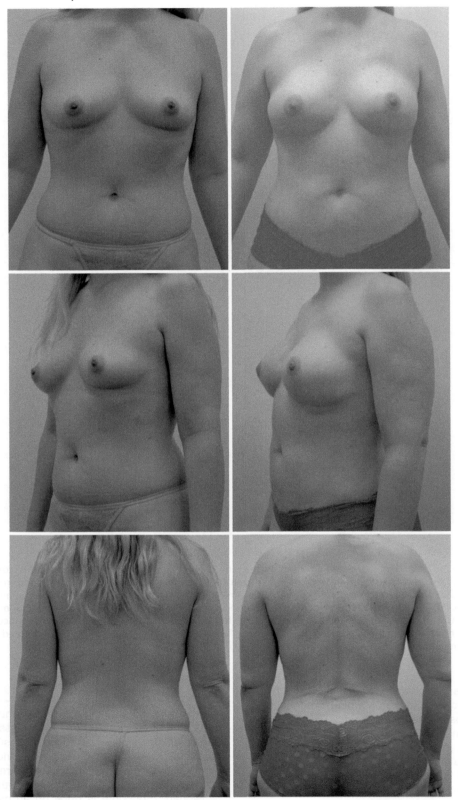

Fig. 10. Case 3: This patient is a 43-year-old woman who underwent staged bilateral prophylactic nipple-preserving mastectomies and LAP flap breast reconstructions. This patient's abdominal donor site was insufficient to achieve the desired volume and projection. Bilateral deep inferior epigastric interposition grafts were used. Autologous fat grafting was used at the time of revision surgery. Narrowing of the waistline that is achieved with lumbar artery perforator flaps is readily apparent.

of the following: revision of the reconstructed breast/s for shaping purposes and to reduce or eliminate flap skin island/s; nipple reconstruction; donor site scar revision; nipple reconstruction; contralateral breast reduction or mastopexy; symmetrizing procedure at the contralateral lower back for unilateral LAP flap reconstruction patients (**Figs. 8 to 10**).

SUMMARY

The LAP flap is an excellent option in autologous breast reconstruction when the abdominal donor site is unavailable. Performed correctly, elevation of this flap produces excellent contour at both the breast and the donor site. The callipygian contour that can be achieved at the donor site parallels the results of cosmetic body contouring procedures.

A major downside to LAP flap breast reconstruction is the relatively high rate of flap failure (6% to 10%) reported for this procedure. Donor site seroma and postoperative sensory changes at the donor site are also common issues. Size and position of the skin island limit the utility of the LAP flap in patients that require skin envelope restoration.

LAP flap surgery is an excellent choice for breast reconstruction in properly selected patients. In spite of certain limitations, the favorable attributes of LAP flap surgery make this approach our preferred nonabdominal flap for breast reconstruction.

CLINICS CARE POINTS

- Lumbar artery perforator (LAP) flap breast reconstruction is a technically challenging procedure with a relatively high reported failure rate. This procedure is best performed by experienced microsurgeons who routinely perform perforator flap surgery.

- Two microsurgeons are essential for efficient and safe execution of LAP flap breast reconstruction.

- Owing to the rigorous nature of this procedure and the complexity of the surgery, bilateral simultaneous LAP flap reconstruction should be reserved for surgeons already experienced with LAP flap surgery.

- A symmetrizing procedure is often performed several months after unilateral reconstructions to either directly excise or liposuction fat in the contralateral lumbar distribution.

- Donor site seromas are the most common complication of this procedure.

DISCLOSURE

The authors have no financial disclosures.

REFERENCES

1. Holmstorm H. The free abdominoplasty flap and its use in breast reconstruction. Scand J Plast Reconstr Surg 1979;13:423.
2. Allen RJ, Treece P. Deep inferior epigastric perforator flap for breast reconstruction. Ann Plast Surg 1994;32(1):32–8.
3. Guerra AB, Metzinger SE, Bidros RS, et al. Breast reconstruction with gluteal artery perforator (GAP) flaps: a critical analysis of 142 cases. Ann Plast Surg 2004;52(2):118–25.
4. LoTempio MM, Allen RJ. Breast reconstruction with SGAP and IGAP flaps. Plast Reconstr Surg 2010; 126(2):393–401.
5. Myers PL, Nelson JA, Allen RJ Jr. Alternative flaps in autologous breast reconstruction. Gland Surg 2021; 10(1):444.
6. Opsomer D, Stillaert F, Blondeel P, et al. The lumbar artery perforator flap in autologous breast reconstruction: initial experience with 100 cases. Plast Reconstr Surg 2018;142(1):1e–8e.
7. Haddock NT, Teotia SS. Lumbar artery perforator flap: initial experience with simultaneous bilateral flaps for breast reconstruction. Plast Reconstr Surg Glob Open 2020;8(5):e2800.
8. Rohrich RJ, Smith PD, Marcantonio DR, et al. The zones of adherence: role in minimizing and preventing contour deformities in liposuction. Plast Reconstr Surg 2001;107(6):1562–9.
9. Tuinder SM, Beugels J, Lataster A, et al. The lateral thigh perforator flap for autologous breast reconstruction: a prospective analysis of 138 flaps. Plast Reconstr Surg 2018;141(2):257–68.
10. Lockwood TE. Lower-body lift. Aesthet Surg J 2001; 21(4):355–69.
11. Vonu PM, Chopan M, Sayadi L, et al. Lumbar artery perforator flaps: a systematic review of free tissue transfers and anatomical characteristics. Ann Plast Surg 2022;89(4):10–97.
12. Roche NA, Van Landuyt K, Blondeel PN, et al. The use of pedicled perforator flaps for reconstruction of lumbosacral defects. Ann Plast Surg 2000;45(1): 7–14.
13. De Weerd L, Weum S. The butterfly design: coverage of a large sacral defect with two pedicled lumbar artery perforator flaps. Br J Plast Surg 2002; 55(3):251–3.

14. De Weerd L, Elvenes OP, Strandenes E, et al. Autologous breast reconstruction with a free lumbar artery perforator flap. Br J Plast Surg 2003;56(2):180–3.

15. Opsomer D, Vyncke T, Depypere B, et al. Lumbar flap versus the gold standard: comparison to the DIEP flap. Plast Reconstr Surg 2020;145(4):706e–14e.

16. Greenspun DT. Discussion: lumbar flap versus the gold standard: comparison to the DIEP flap. Plast Reconstr Surg 2020;145(4):715e–6e.

17. Kato H, Hasegawa M, Takada T, et al. The lumbar artery perforator based island flap: anatomical study and case reports. Br J Plast Surg 1999;52(7):541–6.

18. Lui KW, Hu S, Ahmad N, et al. Three-dimensional angiography of the superior gluteal artery and lumbar artery perforator flap. Plast Reconstr Surg 2009;123(1):79–86.

19. Bissell MB, Greenspun DT, Levine J, et al. The lumbar artery perforator flap: 3-dimensional anatomical study and clinical applications. Ann Plast Surg 2016;77(4):469–76.

20. Mujtaba B, Hanafy AK, Largo RD, et al. The lumbar artery perforator flap: clinical review and guidance on image reporting. Clin Radiol 2019;74(10):756–62.

21. Kiil BJ, Rozen WM, Pan WR, et al. The lumbar artery perforators: a cadaveric and clinical anatomical study. Plast Reconstr Surg 2009;123(4):1229–38.

22. Santillan A, Nacarino V, Greenberg E, et al. Vascular anatomy of the spinal cord. J neurointerventional Surg 2012;4(1):67–74.

23. Johnson PT, Mahesh M, Fishman EK. Image wisely and choosing wisely: importance of adult body CT protocol design for patient safety, exam quality, and diagnostic efficacy. J Am Coll Radiol 2015;12(11):1185–90.

24. Mayo-Smith WW, Morin RL. Image wisely: the beginning, current status, and future opportunities. J Am Coll Radiol 2017;14(3):442–3.

25. Vasile JV, Levine JL. Magnetic resonance angiography in perforator flap breast reconstruction. Gland Surg 2016;5(2):197.

26. Hamdi M, Craggs B, Brussaard C, et al. Lumbar artery perforator flap: an anatomical study using multidetector computed tomographic scan and surgical pearls for breast reconstruction. Plast Reconstr Surg 2016;138(2):343–52.

Modern Approaches to Alternative Flap-Based Breast Reconstruction
Transverse Upper Gracilis Flap

Jordan T. Blough, MD[a], Michel H. Saint-Cyr, MD, MBA, FRCSC[b],*

KEYWORDS

- Transverse myocutaneous gracilis • TMG flap • TUG • Breast reconstruction

KEY POINTS

- The transverse upper gracilis is a myocutaneous posteromedial thigh flap based on the medial circumflex femoral artery that is useful primarily as a secondary option for autologous reconstruction of small to moderate-sized breasts in women without a suitable abdominal donor site.
- Also known as the transverse myocutaneous gracilis (TMG), its advantages include consistent and reliable anatomy affording expeditious flap harvest, low donor site morbidity, and favorable cosmesis.
- The primary disadvantage of TMG reconstruction is the limited achievable breast volume, which often warrants further soft tissue or prosthetic augmentation.
- For surgeons comfortable with perforator flap dissection, the profunda artery perforator flap has largely supplanted the TMG in thigh-based breast reconstruction due to a longer pedicle (9.4 vs 6.4 cm), improved vessel size match, and microsurgical ergonomics.

BACKGROUND

Most microsurgeons agree that abdominally based free tissue transfer represents the gold standard in autologous breast reconstruction today. However, abdominally based reconstruction may be precluded by poor donor site availability (eg, previous abdominoplasty, prior surgical scars, or a paucity of tissue) or the desire to avoid abdominal scar or risk of abdominal bulge and core weakness. In addition to the trunk and buttock, the thigh is a useful alternative. The transverse upper gracilis (TUG), more broadly known as the transverse myocutaneous gracilis (TMG), as well as the profunda artery perforator (PAP) flaps are posteromedial thigh-based flaps with shared utilization in reconstructing small to moderate-sized breasts.

In its infancy, initial gracilis myocutaneous flap designs were unreliable, as they were longitudinally oriented and crossed distal to the mid-thigh. Yousif and colleagues[1] performed anatomic studies that showed the medial circumflex femoral artery and its major perforators to instead be transversely oriented at the superior aspect of the gracilis along the groin crease, thereby facilitating re-orientation of the flap transversely. Upon appreciating the consistent and reliable TMG perforasome, it was popularized in breast reconstruction by Schoeller and Wechselberger in the early 2000s, who report the largest experience (300 flaps).[2] The flap has since gained traction as one of the most popular alternatives in autologous breast reconstruction. Today, the TMG is largely being supplanted by the PAP flap for surgeons comfortable with perforator flap

[a] Division of Plastic and Reconstructive Surgery, Department of Surgery, Baylor Scott and White Health, Texas A&M College of Medicine, 2401 S. 31st Street., MS-01-E443, Temple, TX 76508, USA; [b] Plastic and Reconstructive Surgery, Banner MD Anderson Cancer Center, 2946 E. Banner Gateway Dr, Gilbert, AZ 85234, USA
* Corresponding author:
E-mail address: michel.saint-cyr@bannerhealth.com

Clin Plastic Surg 50 (2023) 313–323
https://doi.org/10.1016/j.cps.2022.11.001
0094-1298/23/© 2022 Elsevier Inc. All rights reserved.

dissection; however, it remains an important and reliable secondary and tertiary option.[3–5]

CLINICAL CONSIDERATIONS

The ideal candidate for TMG reconstruction desires small to moderate-sized breasts and is not a good candidate for abdominally based flaps. Typical patients include thinner or athletic patients, massive weight loss patients, or those with relatively higher thigh rather than abdominal tissue availability. Although most patients are normal BMI, obese patients are also reasonable candidates. Patients should be clearly accepting of size limitation, otherwise, an implant or autologous augmentation will be required to satisfy patient expectations.[2,5–7]

Contraindications to surgery include desire for large breasts, previous donor site injury, lower extremity lymphedema, desire to avoid a high medial thigh scar, or patient factors precluding major reconstructive surgery.[2,6] Previous medial thigh liposuction is not an absolute contraindication.[8]

Advantages of the TMG are manifold: consistent and reliable anatomy, affording expeditious dissection; no prerequisite for preoperative imaging; ability for harvest in lithotomy or frog-leg position, permitting a two-team approach and immediate reconstruction; inconspicuous scarring with benefits of a medial thigh lift; soft and pliable tissue that can be coned into a breast mound with immediate nipple-areolar reconstruction; expendable donor muscle; and low donor site pain.[2,5–7]

Disadvantages principally include lower flap volume versus abdominal and gluteal donor sites, shorter pedicle length, and donor-site risks like lymphedema and scar migration.[2,5–7,9]

Flap size limitations led to modifications to augment the bulk harvested, including more posterior dissection, beveling to capture more subcutaneous fat, including a vertical limb to form an "L flap" or trilobed "Fleur-de-lis" skin paddle (extended TUG flaps), conjoined Conjoined Transverse Upper Gracilis and Profunda Artery Perforator (TUGPAP) flap, flap stacking, or fat grafting.[2,6,7,10–12]

VASCULAR ANATOMY

The TMG is a type II myocutaneous flap based on the medial circumflex femoral artery as the dominant source vessel, originating from the profunda femoral artery in a majority of cases (57%), followed by common femoral artery (39%), and superficial femoral artery (2.5%).[13] The dominant pedicle enters the deep surface of the gracilis 8.6 cm from the pubis (range, 7.6 to 9.8 cm).

Pedicle length is on average of 6.7 cm, with mean arterial and venous diameters of 2.2 cm and 2.3 cm, respectively. Venous outflow is based on paired venae comitantes of similar diameter. There are a median of four cutaneous perforators per flap.[1,5–7]

As discussed, Yousif and colleagues[1] elucidated the vascular orientation. They showed that the medial circumflex femoral artery divides into three to six musculocutaneous branches just before entering the deep surface of the gracilis at the muscular hilum. Typically, a main perforator courses through at this level to the overlying skin, and the other perforators course both anteriorly to the skin overlying the adductor longus and sartorius, or posteriorly to the midline of the posterior thigh.[1] Perfusion to the skin paddle is preferentially posterior (eccentric), rather than centered on gracilis. In fact, perforator branches were shown to traverse at least 5 cm beyond the posterior margin of the muscle.[1,7] In less than 50% of thighs, a septocutaneous perforator may arise from the more proximal pedicle, coursing along the intermuscular septum of the adductor longus and gracilis. Thus, the skin paddle of the TMG was determined to be transversely oriented to capture the true angiosome of the major pedicle.[1] The skin paddle can also be dissected in perforator flap fashion based on these perforators (MCFAP); however, a gracilis-sparing approach is not necessary as the morbidity is of negligible consequence.[14]

The minor pedicle to the gracilis originates from smaller branches of the profunda femoral artery or superficial femoral artery, entering the distal half of the muscle on average 23.3 cm from the pubis (range, 21.8 to 26.0 cm). It typically shares an arterial input with a large pedicle of the sartorius.[7] Its angiosome can be recruited with an inferior extension off of the standard TUG flap as a trilobed "fleur-de-lis" skin paddle or fat over the gracilis through maintaining the interpedicle intramuscular anastomosis after minor pedicle ligation.[7,15] This inferiorly perfused tissue is confined directly over the gracilis.

The senior author's perfusion studies support previous vascular studies, demonstrating that posterior thigh perfusion extends up to a mean of 65% of thigh width (ie, past the posterior thigh midline).[7] This is advantageous, as the posterior thigh tissue exhibits greater bulkiness and is less morbid to excise than anteriorly. Despite success with extending flaps past the posterior thigh midline, the midline is generally considered the posterior extent of dissection, as clinically there is risk of marginal fat necrosis beyond the midline in our experience. In contrast, mean anterior thigh perfusion does not reach the anterior midline

(38%). Anterior dissection should be limited and superficial regardless due to less bulk availability and to avoid lymphatic disruption. Mean tissue perfusion weight was 573 g (range, 313 to 812 g) and volume 617 mL (range, 330 to 850 mL), larger than typically able to be harvested clinically with primary closure.[7]

SURGICAL TECHNIQUE
Preoperative Imaging

Unlike the PAP flap, pre-operative imaging is not necessary when harvesting the TMG flap.

Markings (Traditional Transverse Upper Gracilis)

In general, the flap is harvested from the thigh *contralateral* to the mastectomy site for favorable anastomosis to the internal mammary vessels, the preferred recipient system. The patient is marked in the standing position, beginning with a medial mid-axial line from pubic tubercle to the medial condyle of the femur, overlying the adductor longus muscle, which is the palpable and visible muscle band along the superomedial thigh best observed with forceful thigh adduction. A parallel line 2 cm posteriorly is then drawn to mark the mid-axis of the gracilis. The gracilis muscle can also be confirmed via palpation while abducting the thigh in simultaneous knee extension. It is also useful to mark the posterior thigh midline as the most posterior extent of dissection.

Next, the skin paddle superior border is marked transversely in similar fashion to a medial thigh lift along the inferior gluteal fold, but 2 cm inferior to the groin to mitigate the risk of wound healing issues and labial spreading. As discussed, the skin paddle is eccentrically positioned posteriorly over the proximal third of the gracilis to capture the best vascularized and bulkiest tissue while minimizing lymphatic disruption. Anteriorly, the maximal extension of the skin paddle is brought roughly 5 cm anterior/lateral to the gracilis to minimize lymphatic disruption and scar visibility. Posteriorly, although the flap can be carried to the posterior thigh midline based on perfusion studies, it is generally stopped midway between the medial midaxial line and the posterior thigh midline to reduce the risk of fat necrosis and scar discomfort while sitting. A pinch test is then performed to determine vertical skin paddle height, and the inferior incision marked, forming a crescentic skin paddle. Typical flap height is 5 to 10 cm, based on skin laxity and body habitus. Pinch test is again confirmed in thigh abduction, where tension is maximized. We do not routinely use handheld Doppler ultrasound during flap design, as the TMG flap reliability is excellent.

Flap Harvest (Traditional Transverse Upper Gracilis)

Flap dissection is rapid based on the predictable and reliable anatomy present, often less than 30 minutes per flap. The patient is positioned supinely in lithotomy position for dissection. First, the superior incision is made from the anterior extent to the medial midaxial line. Dissection is carried through subcutaneous fat until the septum between the adductor longus and the gracilis is located, and dissection brought inferiorly to rapidly identify the pedicle and obturator nerve. The obturator nerve enters the deep surface of the gracilis muscle just immediately superior to the vascular pedicle, running obliquely and superiorly divergent from the pedicle. The obturator nerve is divided. The skin paddle can be adjusted and confirmed as needed based on pedicle location.

Thereafter, tailor tacking is performed to adjust the inferior incision as needed to prevent undue tension after closure. The inferior incision is made and the skin paddle developed to the gracilis first anteriorly and then posteriorly. Flap dissection anterior/lateral to the adductor longus is kept superficial to Scarpa's fascia, minimizing lymphatic disruption over the femoral triangle. Likewise, the greater saphenous vein and its accessory veins are preserved and not incorporated into the flap, as they are associated with the vertical group of superficial inguinal lymph nodes; supercharging is also practically never required. Posterior flap elevation is performed with care to leave the deep fascia intact and to capture the fat over the hamstring muscles. Branches of the posterior femoral cutaneous nerve are spared as dissection approaches the midline. After skin paddle dissection, the gracilis muscle is isolated with its investing fascia intact to preserve musculocutaneous perforators. The gracilis is located posteriorly to the adductor longus and should not be confused with the sartorius, which crosses medially anterior to the adductor longus muscle more distally in the thigh.

The adductor longus is retracted anterolaterally, and the medial circumflex femoral artery is then isolated and dissected proximally until the profunda femoris artery (**Fig. 1**). Branches to the adductor longus and magnus muscles are divided to increase pedicle length. Prominent branches of the pedicle can be dissected a distance before ligation in stacked thigh flap cases for potential "in series" anastomosis if needed. The minor pedicle is ligated. Finally, the gracilis is divided

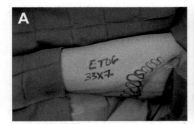 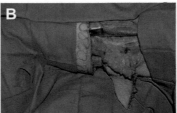 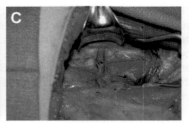

Fig. 1. TMG flap dissection (*A*). Incisions; (*B*) and (*C*). Flap with pedicle dissection of medial circumflex femoral artery between the gracilis and adductor longus to its origin at the profunda femoral artery).

as distally as possible under direct visualization with careful cauterization to maximize bulk and then proximally near its origin. Approximately 50% of the muscle bulk can be expected to persist after atrophying, and the muscle provides a useful lipofilling recipient site.[2]

Extended Transverse Upper Gracilis Modification

The Extended TUG (E-TUG) incorporates supplementary flap volume through a beveled dissection away from the skin paddle incision for a few centimeters, thereby capturing additional subscarpal fat (see **Fig. 1**).[6,7,16] Note that this undermining is preferentially posterocaudal in the thigh, where there is greater subcutaneous volume available and closing tension is lower. Subcutaneous fat can also be reliably incorporated over the gracilis muscle itself. Beveling to increase flap size should be performed judiciously, particularly at the area of maximal tension, as excessive undermining renders the donor site skin ischemic and high risk for wound healing complications. Additionally, overaggressive resection can lead to contour deformities.

Vertical Extended Transverse Upper Gracilis (Fleur-de-lis or L-Flap) Modification

A vertically oriented extension of the skin paddle recruits extra flap volume in patients with significant horizontal donor site laxity who do not mind a more conspicuous vertical medial thigh scar, creating a trilobed "Fleur-de-lis" skin paddle (**Fig. 2**).[6] The vertical limb is centered over the gracilis to maximize vascularity, as perforators tend to course along the anterior border of the gracilis and within the septum between the gracilis and adductor longus; it is not continued distal to the thigh midline, where vascularity becomes unreliable. A further modification is the L-flap, for which the anterior limb is omitted, as it contributes little volume and adds a more visible anterior scar.[5,6]

Diagonal Upper Gracilis and S-Transverse Upper Gracilis flap (S-TUG) Modifications

To overcome the size deficiency and tension-related donor site morbidity of traditional TUG flaps, authors Dayan and Allen further re-oriented the skin paddle diagonally along the resting skin tension lines, formulating the diagonal upper gracilis (DUG).[4,17] This increases flap width along the line of lowest tension and simultaneously avoids dissection over the lymphatics anteriorly; however, it does introduce a more conspicuous scar.

Similarly, the senior author redesigned the skin paddle as an "S-TUG," whereby the incision is also re-directed across the resting skin tension lines as the inferior S-shaped incision is brought into the axis of the gracilis (**Fig. 3**). This takes advantage of not only the vertical laxity, as in the standard TUG, but also the horizontal laxity that many patients have. The vertical extent can be increased in patients with greater horizontal laxity. The S-TUG also avoids creating the ischemic T-junction closure of the trilobed flap. The drawback to this technique is a more visible scar distally; however, it is hidden mid-axially.

Deciding on Skin Paddle Design

For women with mostly vertical laxity who have good upper thigh adiposity, or those concerned about scarring, the E-TUG is our design of choice. For women with greater horizontal laxity, especially with a history of massive weight loss, who are less concerned with conspicuous scarring, the S-TUG is used.

Donor Site Closure

There is significant potential for seroma, dehiscence, or other donor site issues after medial thigh harvest. Ultimately, avoiding an overaggressive dissection is the most efficacious strategy to minimize complications; however, meticulous closure is also paramount. Before closure, a long-acting local anesthetic agent is infiltrated with a blunt tip canula into the subcutaneous areas of dissection.

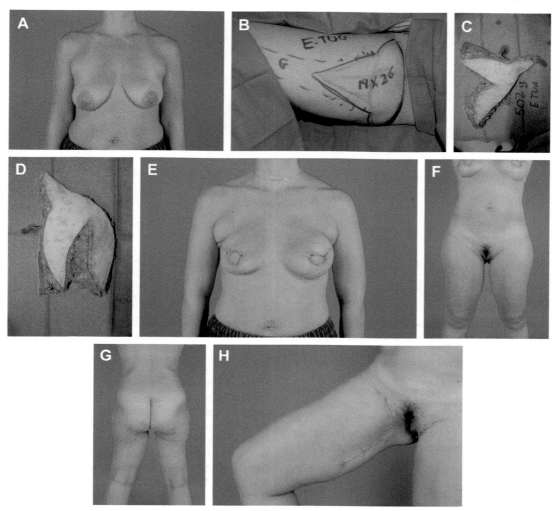

Fig. 2. Bilateral vertical extended trilobed TMG flaps for moderately large reconstruction (*A*). Preoperative; (*B*). Vertical E-TUG design; (*C* and *D*). 507 g flap from right thigh coned for left breast reconstruction; (*E–H*). Postoperative).

We prefer an efficacious and cost-effective analgesic cocktail of 60 mL of 0.25% bupivacaine, 50 mcg dexmedetomidine, 30 mg ketorolac, and 4 mg dexamethasone mixed in 250 mL of normal saline.[18] Thereafter, a 15 french Blake drain is placed, followed by progressive tension sutures to obliterate empty space. The superficial fascial system is then closed including suspension to Colles fascia, followed by deep dermal and running subcuticular layers. The thighs are dressed with compression wraps.

Breast Mound Shaping and Immediate Nipple Areolar Reconstruction

One of the significant advantages of the TMG flap over abdominally based flaps is the ability to truly "cone" the flap like a breast to create projection (Fig. 4). The limbs and shaping of the flap can be tailored to the reconstructive needs. Typically, this entails rotating the limbs together to form a teardrop shape folding superior to inferior aspect on itself. The anterior limb of a trilobed flap can be tucked deep or beside the flap to improve projection or medial fullness. Flap shaping will result in a standing cone deformity centrally at the apex, permitting excellent immediate nipple reconstruction. The surrounding areas of skin to be buried are de-epithelialized, optimally leaving a skin paddle to reconstruct the areola and allow for flap monitoring. Of note, the skin paddle is frequently a color mismatch from the surrounding mastectomy flap; for this reason, pre-flap breast tissue expansion can be useful to create a full skin brassiere and confine the skin paddle to the reconstructed areola only. The authors have found this to significantly enhance the overall cosmesis of autologous breast reconstructions. The skin paddle also

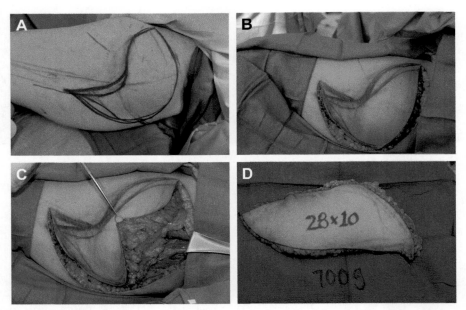

Fig. 3. (A-C) S-TUG flap design with vertical extension along the axis of the gracilis to take advantage of both horizontal and vertical laxity and (D) yield a large flap (28 cm × 10 cm; 700 g).

frequently transplants pubic hair, which can be treated with a laser.

Nipple reconstruction is performed in similar fashion to the C-V flap technique, with transposition of V-shaped flaps from the standing cone deformity. A piece of costal cartilage is placed as a graft beneath the flaps to preserve projection as needed.

Microsurgical Anastomosis

Typically, the coned flap is brought to the contralateral breast, positioned centrally at the appropriate position within the mastectomy pocket, and temporarily fixed with sutures. The authors' preferred recipient vessels are the internal mammary vessels at the third or often the fourth intercostal interspace for optimal size match, and due to the relatively short pedicle length. A rib-sparing approach is generally avoided due to the less forgiving pedicle length and ergonomics. The artery is spatulated as needed to ameliorate any mismatch. If the internal mammary system is not available, the serratus branch of the thoracodorsal artery, or the thoracodorsal artery proper are dissected and mobilized medially. Interposition vein grafting is reserved as a bailout option. Other authors successfully used the internal mammary vessels in 92% of cases and their mean venous coupler diameter was 2.5 mm (1.5 to 3.5 mm, range).[2] After confirming perfusion, a 15 french blake drain is placed in each breast pocket and the recipient sites closed in layers.

Fat Grafting

For patients with mild–moderate volume deficiency after a single flap, immediate and/or delayed autologous multilayered fat grafting can be used to augment volume and improve contour.[12,19] In the immediate setting, the distal gracilis muscle itself as well as the pectoralis muscle can be lipofilled. In delayed settings after at least 3 months, the flap, pectoralis, and mastectomy flaps can be grafted.

Flap Stacking, Implant Placement, and Conjoined TUGPAP

Patients are counseled extensively and selected judiciously for thigh-based breast reconstruction due to inherent limitations on reconstructed breast volume. Flap stacking can be planned for women who desire larger breasts or have limited volume at their donor sites (Fig. 5).[20,21] The authors' threshold for adjunctive augmentation is low, as over-aggressive flap dissection yields increased donor site complications and unsightly contour deformities. For unsatisfied patients with significant volume deficiency after flap transfer, occasionally small implants can be placed. Finally, the conjoined TUGPAP was described based on the overlapping perforasomes of the TMG and PAP flaps to yield a larger flap; however, the increased flap volume has to be weighed against the added flap dissection, second anastomosis and larger donor site created.[10]

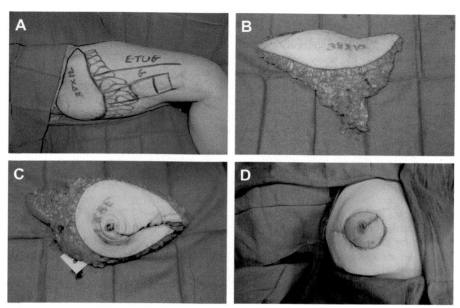

Fig. 4. Extended TUG (E-TUG) flap dissection (*A*). Design; (*B*). Supramuscular and caudal fat beveling; (*C* and *D*). Coning of the flap and immediate nipple-areolar reconstruction).

Postoperative Considerations

Patients participate in an enhanced recovery after surgery protocol, beginning with pre-operative education and protein supplementation. We work with our anesthesia colleagues to avoid excessive intraoperative narcotics and optimize fluid resuscitation. Thigh donor sites are infiltrated with an analgesic

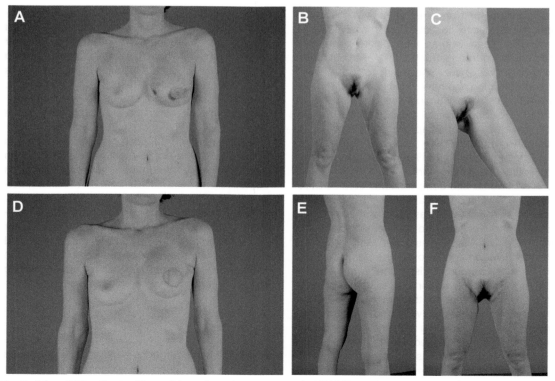

Fig. 5. A low BMI patient with small breasts undergoes extended TUG (E-TUG) reconstruction (*A–C*). Preoperative; (*D–F*). Postoperative, before future revision surgery).

cocktail as discussed.[18] Patients are placed on a clear liquid diet immediately following surgery, and switched to a regular diet the following morning. On the first postoperative day, the foley catheter is removed and intravenous fluids weaned if urine output is adequate. Multi-modal analgesia, thrombo-prophylaxis, stool softeners, and 24 h of intravenous antibiotic prophylaxis are prescribed. Flaps are monitored clinically and by handheld doppler hourly for 24 h, and every 4 h thereafter. Patients are expected to ambulate on the first day postoperatively. Positionally, patients are encouraged to sleep supinely, and to avoid hip flexion and abduction to prevent undue tension on donor sites. Patients follow our standard postoperative ERAS (enhanced recovery after surgery) protocol and are usually discharged by the second postoperative day. Compressive thigh wraps are continued for 4 weeks, and the drains removed once collecting minimal output (less than 30 cc over 24 h, over two consecutive days, one drain per site remove at a time).

DISCUSSION
Clinical Outcomes

The TMG flap continues to be a consistent and reliable alternative to abdominally -based flaps for autologous breast reconstruction that microsurgeons should be comfortable with. Owing to flap size constraints, it remains primarily a secondary option, particularly for low BMI, massive weight loss, or athletic women who desire a small to medium-sized reconstruction.[2,5-7] Patient satisfaction scores have shown it to be a well-accepted option and have been validated through BREAST-Q.[22] Microsurgical outcomes are comparable to abdominally based reconstruction, with low rates of total flap failure—2% to 6%; in comparison, partial flap loss and fat necrosis occur less frequently (<5%) in part due to lower flap volumes requiring perfusion.[2,3,11]

Overall donor-site complications have been reported at 26% in pooled analysis.[10] Lymphedema represents the most devastating of these complications, and was reported on occasion before refinements in flap dissection to be more conservative anteriorly over the femoral triangle.[2,3,5-7,23] Lymphatic disruption is obviated by keeping dissection superficial to the superficial fascia while anterior to the gracilis and leaving the greater saphenous vein and its accessory veins in situ, or omitting the anterior limb altogether as in an "L" shaped flap. In their extensive experience with 300 flaps for breast reconstruction, Weitgasser and colleagues reported no lymphedema; Jo and colleagues corroborated this in a systematic review of over 600 flaps.[2,3]

Overaggressive flap harvest increases the risks of donor site complications and poor cosmesis of the thigh, but cautious flap design and donor site management result in low morbidity and an aesthetic improvement in the thigh silhouette.[9] Rates of dehiscence, infection, fluid collection, and other issues were reported to occur as high as 86%.[9] Risk is significantly mitigated through avoiding undue tension during design; limiting beveling, which can also create contour irregularities; placing greater attention on closure including progressive tension sutures; lowering the incision slightly below the inguinal crease, also reducing labial spreading; and re-orienting the incision along resting skin tension lines, as in the DUG or S-TUG orientation.[4,17]

The medial thigh is a favorable donor site from an aesthetic standpoint, lifting and tightening the thigh as in a medial thigh lift. Post-bariatric patients are excellent candidates for this reason, as they benefit from the lift and there is significant volume and skin laxity available.[24] For patients with significant horizontal laxity, the vertical extended flap, DUG, and senior author's preference, the S-TUG, address this laxity to improve thigh contour and simultaneously increase flap size. The scar is also fairly inconspicuous with standard transverse designs; however, it is typically visible while wearing undergarments. Craggs and colleagues showed that 94% of patients were moderately to very happy with scar positioning, and experienced surgeons have noted just a 1% scar revision rate.[2,9] When revision is needed due to widening or inferior migration, the tissue is anchored to Colles fascia or periosteum. Increased scar visibility is also the primary disadvantage of reorienting the skin paddle as in DUG, S-TUG, or other vertical extensions.[2,4,6,17]

Regarding motor function, the gracilis muscle is a favorite donor for microsurgeons due to its expendability. Hip adductor strength has been objectively measured to decrease 11% after gracilis sacrifice; however, patients do not subjectively note a diminution in strength, particularly long-term.[4] Sensory disturbances around the donor site scar and paresthesias around the mediodorsal thigh have also been reported up to 75% in the short-term, which can be minimized by leaving the posterior cutaneous nerves undisrupted.[11,23]

Transverse Myocutaneous Gracilis versus Profunda Artery Perforator Flap

For many microsurgeons performing thigh-based breast reconstruction today, including the senior author, the PAP flap has largely superseded the TMG flap.[25] In a recent systematic review, authors compared 613 TUG versus 475 PAP flaps, noting multiple advantages of the PAP flap. Despite increased technical demands of perforator dissection, the PAP flap's primary benefit over the TMG flap is attributed to the increased pedicle length (9.4 cm vs 6.4 cm) and often larger arterial caliber (2.0 mm vs 1.5 mm).[3] In the authors' experience, the microsurgical anastomosis is notably more favorable with the PAP flap due not only to increased pedicle length and superior caliber match, but also ergonomically with less medial flap volume obstructing the microsurgical anastomosis in the chest. The pedicle length limitation is further shown in stacked thigh flap reconstruction, whereby the thoracodorsal vessels are the predominant recipient choice for the second TMG flap, whereas the second PAP flap's longer pedicle length affords more successful utilization of the retrograde internal mammary system.[3,20,21,26]

Microsurgical outcomes do not differ between the PAP and TMG flaps in terms of total or partial flap loss, fat necrosis, or other recipient site issues.[3] Regarding the donor site, several studies have shown comparable morbidity; however, recent pooled analysis suggests slightly higher risk of wound dehiscence (9.7% vs 7.6%) and sensory disturbance (7.8% vs 1.6%) for the TMG flap, but no significant differences in wound-related complications, seroma, and hematoma formation.[3] No cases of lymphedema were noted with TMG harvest in comparison to 1% in the PAP group.[3]

Despite a more technically demanding PAP flap harvest, pooled analysis showed no difference in operative time for unilateral reconstruction in comparison with the TMG flap, possibly somewhat counteracted by more favorable microsurgical ergonomics.[3] In addition to more tedious dissection, the other primary disadvantage of the PAP flap is the requirement for pre-operative CT angiography; however, a suitable perforator may be present in up to 99% of thighs.[27] Flap dissection in lithotomy rather than prone positioning also significantly mitigates procedure duration by eliminating position change.

Although the average PAP flap size may be slightly larger than the TMG (348 g vs 328 g) depending on the patient and surgeon, in practice they are comparable and their smaller size continues to be the primary limitation of thigh-based reconstruction.[3]

Flap Size, Volume Augmentation, and Flap Design Algorithm

The inherent flap size limitation of the TMG ushered in a host of design modifications to increase flap size including extended flaps (E-TUG) with beveling to increase subcutaneous fat, vertically extended "L flap" or trilobed "Fleur-de-lis" skin paddle extensions, the DUG, conjoined TUGPAP, and the senior author's own S-TUG modification.[2,6,7,10–12] Typical flap weight ranges 250 to 450 g in the literature for the standard TUG design, but the senior author has previously published larger flaps—386 g (range, 181 to 750 g) for the E-TUG and 470 g (range, 380 to 605 g) for vertically extended flaps, comparable to smaller DIEP flaps.[2,3,6] If adequate horizontal laxity is present and the patient accepts a more conspicuous scar, the S-TUG is the senior author's preferred design to maximize size while limiting morbidity. As discussed, adjunctive means of augmentation include immediate and delayed autologous fat grafting, flap stacking, or even placement of an implant, all of which are also frequently required even in abdominally based reconstruction.[12,20,21] In fact, Weitgasser and colleagues[19] showed in their experience needing fat grafting in 38% of abdominally based flaps versus 65% in TUG reconstruction. We have a low threshold to augment the flap through adjuncts rather than a more aggressive flap dissection that increases tension and ischemia, empty space, and donor site morbidity. Ultimately, patient selection and setting realistic expectations are key to attaining satisfactory reconstructive breast volume.

SUMMARY

The TMG flap is a reliable alternative in the armamentarium of breast reconstruction for women desiring small to moderate-sized breasts who are not candidates for abdominally based reconstruction. Although the PAP flap is superseding the TMG, microsurgeons should remain familiar with the technique.

CLINICS CARE POINTS FOR TRANSVERSE MYOCUTANEOUS GRACILIS RECONSTRUCTION

- The ideal candidate for transverse myocutaneous breast reconstruction has a favorable medial thigh rather than abdominal donor site and desires small to moderate-sized breasts.
- Lithotomy positioning permits a two-team approach, immediate reconstruction, and maximizes operative efficiency.

- The anterior skin paddle dissection over the groin is limited to the supra-scarpal plane and the greater saphenous and its accessory branches are left *in situ* to minimize disruption of inguinal lymphatics.
- Flap volume can be increased judiciously through beveling to recruit more posterocaudal fat and/or including a vertical limb to form an "L flap" or trilobed "Fleur-de-Lis" skin paddle (extended transverse upper gracilis [TUG] flaps), or through the modified S-TUG skin paddle design; however, undue tension and excessive flap beveling are avoided to limit donor site morbidity and contour deformity.
- During flap shaping, the limbs are folded together to cone the breast, and the resulting dog ear permits immediate nipple reconstruction.

DISCLOSURE

The authors have nothing to disclose.

REFERENCES

1. Yousif NJ, Matloub HS, Kolachalam R, et al. The transverse gracilis musculocutaneous flap. Ann Plast Surg 1992;29(6):482–90.
2. Weitgasser L, Mahrhofer M, Schwaiger K, et al. Lessons learned from 30 Years of transverse myocutaneous gracilis flap breast reconstruction: historical appraisal and review of the present literature and 300 cases. J Clin Med 2021;10(16). https://doi.org/10.3390/JCM10163629.
3. Jo T, Kim EK, Eom JS, et al. Comparison of transverse upper gracilis and profunda femoris artery perforator flaps for breast reconstruction: a systematic review. Microsurgery 2020;40(8):916–28.
4. Dayan JH, Allen RJ. Lower extremity free flaps for breast reconstruction. Plast Reconstr Surg 2017;140(5S Advances in Breast Reconstruction):77S–86S.
5. Vega SJ, Sandeen SN, Bossert RP, et al. Gracilis myocutaneous free flap in autologous breast reconstruction. Plast Reconstr Surg 2009;124(5):1400–9.
6. Saint-Cyr M, Wong C, Oni G, et al. Modifications to extend the transverse upper gracilis flap in breast reconstruction: clinical series and results. Plast Reconstr Surg 2012;129(1). https://doi.org/10.1097/PRS.0B013E31823620CB.
7. Wong C, Mojallal A, Bailey SH, et al. The extended transverse musculocutaneous gracilis flap: vascular anatomy and clinical implications. Ann Plast Surg 2011;67(2):170–7.
8. Saint-Cyr M, Shirvani A, Wong C. The transverse upper gracilis flap for breast reconstruction following liposuction of the thigh. Microsurgery 2010;30(8):636–8.
9. Craggs B, Vanmierlo B, Zeltzer A, et al. Donor-site morbidity following harvest of the transverse myocutaneous gracilis flap for breast reconstruction. Plast Reconstr Surg 2014;134(5):682e–91e.
10. Karir A, Stein MJ, Zhang J. The conjoined TUGPAP flap for breast reconstruction: systematic review and illustrative anatomy. Plast Reconstr Surg Glob Open 2021;9(4). https://doi.org/10.1097/GOX.0000000000003512.
11. Siegwart LC, Fischer S, Diehm YF, et al. The transverse musculocutaneous gracilis flap for autologous breast reconstruction: focus on donor site morbidity. Breast Cancer 2021;28(6):1273–82.
12. Russe E, Kholosy H, Weitgasser L, et al. Autologous fat grafting for enhancement of breast reconstruction with a transverse myocutaneous gracilis flap: a cohort study. J Plast Reconstr Aesthet Surg 2018;71(11):1557–62.
13. Al-Talalwah W. The medial circumflex femoral artery origin variability and its radiological and surgical intervention significance. Springerplus 2015;4(1). https://doi.org/10.1186/S40064-015-0881-2.
14. Hallock GG. The gracilis (medial circumflex femoral) perforator flap: a medial groin free flap? Ann Plast Surg 2003;51(6):623–6.
15. Peek A, Müller M, Ackermann G, et al. The free gracilis perforator flap: anatomical study and clinical refinements of a new perforator flap. Plast Reconstr Surg 2009;123(2):578–88.
16. Fattah A, Figus A, Mathur B, et al. The transverse myocutaneous gracilis flap: technical refinements. J Plast Reconstr Aesthet Surg 2010;63(2):305–13.
17. Dayan E, Smith ML, Sultan M, et al. The diagonal upper gracilis (DUG) flap. Plast Reconstr Surg 2013;132:33–4.
18. Lombana NF, Falola RA, Zolfaghari K, et al. Comparison of liposomal bupivacaine to a local analgesic cocktail for transversus abdominis plane blocks in abdominally based microvascular breast reconstruction. Plast Reconstr Surg 2022;150(3). https://doi.org/10.1097/PRS.0000000000009398.
19. Weitgasser L, Schwaiger K, Medved F, et al. Bilateral simultaneous breast reconstruction with diep- and tmg flaps: head to head comparison, risk and complication analysis. J Clin Med 2020;9(7):1–13.
20. Werdin F, Haug DM, Amr A, et al. Double transverse myocutaneous gracilis free flaps for unilateral breast reconstruction. Microsurgery 2016;36(7):539–45.
21. Park JE, Alkureishi LWT, Song DH. TUGs into VUGs and Friendly BUGs: transforming the gracilis territory into the best secondary breast reconstructive option. Plast Reconstr Surg 2015;136(3):447–54.

22. Jessica AS, Zhao J, Mackey S, et al. Transverse upper gracilis flap breast reconstruction: a 5-year consecutive case series of patient-reported outcomes. Plast Reconstr Surg 2022;150(2):258–68.

23. Siegwart LC, Bolbos A, Tapking C, et al. Safety and donor site morbidity of the transverse musculocutaneous gracilis (TMG) flap in autologous breast reconstruction-A systematic review and meta-analysis. J Surg Oncol 2021;124(4):492–509.

24. Schoeller T, Meirer R, Otto-Schoeller A, et al. Medial thigh lift free flap for autologous breast augmentation after bariatric surgery. Obes Surg 2002;12(6):831–4.

25. Saad A, Sadeghi A, Allen RJ. The anatomic basis of the profunda femoris artery perforator flap: a new option for autologous breast reconstruction–a cadaveric and computer tomography angiogram study. J Reconstr Microsurg 2012;28(6):381–6.

26. Schoeller T, Huemer GM, Wechselberger G. The transverse musculocutaneous gracilis flap for breast reconstruction: guidelines for flap and patient selection. Plast Reconstr Surg 2008;122(1):29–38.

27. Haddock NT, Greaney P, Otterburn D, et al. Predicting perforator location on preoperative imaging for the profunda artery perforator flap. Microsurgery 2012;32(7):507–11.

Modern Approaches to Alternative Flap-Based Breast Reconstruction
Stacked Flaps

Nicholas T. Haddock, MD*, Sumeet S. Teotia, MD

KEYWORDS

- Stacked flap • Conjoined flap • Double DIEP • PAP flap • LAP flap • Four flap
- Breast reconstruction • Microsurgery

KEY POINTS

- Stacked flaps are safe and an excellent adjunct to armamentarium of the reconstructive breast surgeon.
- Stacked flaps can come in multiple varieties and should be tailored to the individual's anatomy.
- Stacked flaps provide ample volume and skin in thin individuals or those with a significant recipient need, such as patients with delayed reconstruction and/or radiation.
- Expertise with single flaps is required before embarking on stacked flaps.

INTRODUCTION

Autologous tissue is the gold standard option for many patients seeking breast reconstruction. The fact that this option provides natural and permanent breast reconstruction cannot be overstated in all patients seeking breast reconstruction following mastectomy. That said, there is an overall concern in autologous breast reconstruction related to available donor sites. These concerns are especially true in thin patients and in the setting of large tissue needs, such as following radiation or delayed reconstruction.

Multiple donor site locations have been described for breast reconstruction[1–5] and typically work well in providing ample tissue for single breast reconstruction. There are situations, though, when a single donor site is not sufficient for a single breast reconstruction and multiple flaps are required for a single breast reconstruction. In many situations, the outcome will be compromised to limit the donor sites, and thus, anticipated morbidity. This is a reasonable balance between the pros and cons of autologous breast reconstruction in most situations; but in others, patients require more tissue, and thus, multiple donor sites are indicated for a single breast reconstruction.

Breast reconstruction with multiple flaps has been shown to be safe[6,7] and indicated in specific situations.

History

The initial use of stacked flaps for breast reconstruction came as double-pedicle transposed abdominally-based flaps.[8–10] This technique helped recruit additional perfusion from the typically unilateral pedicled rectus abdominis flap but had the known limitations of pedicled transverse rectus abdominis myocutaneous flaps (TRAM flaps).[11] In modern times, most reconstruction surgeons would consider this technique too morbid to justify a single breast reconstruction. Turbo-charging[12] and super-charging[13] of the tissue were also described to augment perfusion,

There are no financial disclosures.
Department of Plastic Surgery, University of Texas Southwestern, 1801 Inwood, Dallas, TX 75390, USA
* Corresponding author.
E-mail address: Nicholas.haddock@utsouthwestern.edu

plasticsurgery.theclinics.com

with the ipsilateral pedicle or contralateral pedicle, respectively.[14] The free TRAM flap[15–17] allowed for more freedom with inset, and in unique settings involving midline scars, a bi-pedicled free flap was introduced.[18] It was soon after noted that in thin patients stacking two flaps could provide sufficient volume and surface area to optimize aesthetic breast reconstruction.[19] To increase the flexibility with recipient vessel choice, a "parasitic" approach was described,[20] allowing one flap to be perfused by another, and this was later defined with multiple options using various abdominal pedicles in unilateral breast reconstruction.[21] It was not until more alternative perforator-based flaps were described that non-abdominal non-conjoined flaps were used.[22] This addition of donor site options[2–5,23] also allowed for the use of stacked flaps in bilateral breast reconstruction.[6,24,25]

Definitions

Unilateral breast reconstruction performed with more than one flap donor site is often referred to as breast reconstruction with stacked flaps. The term "stacked" typically refers to placing one object over another, but in breast reconstruction, this is not always what is performed. One of the most common multi-flap options for breast reconstruction is a conjoined, or double-pedicle, deep inferior epigastric artery perforator flap (DIEP). In this situation, the flaps are not separated, and thus, are not technically stacked.[26] We define multiple-flap breast reconstruction as

- Conjoined flaps: Double-pedicle flaps from the same donor site (eg, a double-pedicle DIEP flap or a profunda artery perforator flap (PAP flap) with an additional medial femoral circumflex pedicle)
- Stacked flaps: Two separate flaps with separate pedicle from separate donor sites (eg, two separate PAP flaps for a single breast or a single breast reconstruction with a DIEP flap and PAP flap)

Background

There are multiple descriptions for the ideal breast shape[27] and optimizing breast reconstruction esthetics.[28] The ultimate premise is that the skin envelope and volume cannot be compromised. Although a single breast following a skin sparing mastectomy, without radiation, can typically be reconstructed with a single flap, this is not always the situation, and sometimes, more tissue is required than provided with a single flap. The benefit of stacked, or conjoined, flaps is that when used appropriately, they nearly always provide all required aspects of breast reconstruction.

Patients with a significant skin deficit to provide breast shape, such as those undergoing delayed reconstruction, often require a significant portion of a single flap to be exposed at the lower half of the breast. This can provide the skin envelope needed to provide breast projection and ptosis, but the compromise is a more caudal inset of the flap, and ultimately, a loss of tissue in the upper pole of the breast. Although some argue that fat grafting can solve this problem, in the authors' experience, fat grafting resorption rates are high in patients who do not have adequate scaffold for fat revascularization. Additionally, the assumption that large-volume liposuction for fat harvest is a benign procedure is misleading to the patient as this approach often requires more surgery in the long run than an initial stacked flap breast reconstruction.

Ultimately, the use of multiple flaps for a single breast allows for a tailored approach based on patient-centric factors and provides all aspects required for total breast reconstruction. Revisionary surgery is much more predictable when excess tissue is present as a lift or reduction is straightforward in most reconstructive surgeon's hands. The currently available methods of adding tissue, such as fat grafting, additional secondary flaps, or the addition of implants can all have success in specific settings but are still less predictable and not without significant concern and potential morbidity.

DISCUSSION
Indications

As with any three-dimensional structure, total breast reconstruction requires multiple components to achieve superior aesthetic and natural results. The natural aesthetic breast must have a stable foundation on the chest wall, with volume in all quadrants providing three-dimensional projection, and adequate skin to allow natural ptosis. Although adjunct procedures, such as fat grafting, can be used to add volume, this does not provide increased projection and will not easily change the base of the breast on the chest wall. Although implants can provide projection, they do come with concerns that many patients are not willing to accept. Ideally, all of these components of aesthetic breast reconstruction are accomplished with the primary reconstruction.

In some patients, total breast reconstruction cannot be accomplished with a single flap. The most obvious, but extreme indication for multiple flaps is a delayed reconstruction following radiation. In this patient population, a larger amount of skin and volume is always required, and thus, multiple flaps should optimally be considered at the initial microvascular reconstruction. The other patient population that often benefits from multiple flaps is patients with a low body mass index (BMI). In many of these patients, one donor site does not provide adequate volume for desired breast reconstruction using autologous tissue.

Preoperative Planning

In our practice, there are three common donor site locations for autologous breast reconstruction.[29] In patients seeking autologous breast reconstruction, we consider the DIEP flap as our first choice followed by both the PAP flap[30] and the lumbar artery perforator flap (LAP flap).[31] A computed tomography angiogram (CTA) is completed in all patients, which helps guide the discussion with the patient providing shared decision-making over the balance between vascular anatomy, donor site volume, and patient preference.

When performing multiple flaps to a single breast two vascular recipient sources are required. Although the cranial and caudal internal mammary vessels are often a good choice,[32] there are situations when a side branch or extension from the primary flap pedicle is used. The left caudal internal mammary vein can sometimes be very small and not suitable as a recipient vessel. This is especially true in a delayed reconstruction following radiation. As an alternative, the flap pedicle can provide additional recipient sites. Preoperative imaging should always be used to evaluate for potential alternative recipient sites within the flap and can help identify flap pedicle extensions or side branches.[33] Ultimately, intra-operative confirmation of vessel flow is still required. Constant communication in the operating room between team members in different surgical sites helps with coordination and planning for recipient vessel selection.

Surgical Techniques: Conjoined Deep Inferior Epigastric Artery Perforator Flap

Conjoined DIEP flaps are the most common variant of multiple-flap breast reconstruction. Most breast microsurgeons are comfortable with DIEP flap harvest so this falls into the typical armamentarium. The conjoined DIEP flap is similar in dissection, but there are specific nuances related to managing the vascular pedicles[21] and inset. The DIEP vascular pedicle often provides multiple recipient vessel options for the secondary pedicle. The benefit of using a side branch or cranial

extension is it provides more freedom with inset, but in the event of primary vascular compromise, both flaps can be lost. Ultimately, this decision is made based on the individual case needs.[33]

The greatest benefit of the conjoined DIEP flap is the abundant skin provided by maintaining the entire abdomen as one segment. Depending on the needs, this can be inset horizontally, obliquely, or vertically. The horizontal and oblique insets provide the most skin and the vertical inset allows rolling a portion of the flap under itself to augment projection (Fig. 1).

Surgical Techniques: Stacked Profunda Artery Perforator Flap

The stacked PAP flap is most commonly employed in low BMI patients or potentially in patients with previous abdominal surgery limiting the availability of the DIEP flap.[22] Flap harvest is the same as previously described,[30,34] but more care must be taken to evaluate for any usable side branches on the vascular pedicle. The pedicle should be taken to the origin to provide maximum length and the chance of having a side branch with a suitable size. The distal branches are nearly never of adequate caliber. It is possible to perform a dual pedicle PAP and medial femoral circumflex (MFC) flap, but this does not provide a large augmentation to the skin paddle or volume of fat harvested. In our experience, this option is only used when the PAP perforator is small and the MFC perforators are dominant for the anterior aspect of the harvested tissue (Fig. 2).

Many patients seeking unilateral breast reconstruction with PAP flaps prefer to undergo a stacked PAP flap instead. The use of similar flaps from each leg allows for better symmetry of the thigh donor sites and less aggressive flap harvest, which could limit thigh wound complications[35] (Figs. 3 and 4).

Surgical Techniques: Stacked Lumbar Artery Perforator Flap

LAP flaps are a relatively new flap for breast reconstruction, but in centers of excellence are quickly gaining popularity. The stacked LAP flap is not a frequent option but in the right setting can be used. The difficult aspect of the LAP flap is the short vascular pedicle and the need for an additional composite graft (artery and vein graft) to safely complete the operation. In some settings, a composite graft can have multiple branches that allow two flaps to be connected to one recipient site on the chest. In other situations, two composite grafts are required and a cranial-caudal inset is used. Coordination and planning are

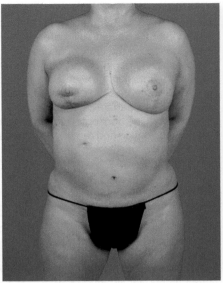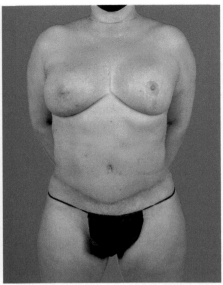

Fig. 1. A 59-year-old woman with a history of right breast cancer treated with mastectomy and radiation. She underwent implant reconstruction at an outside hospital and presented for autologous conversion secondary to capsular contracture. She underwent a right double-pedicle conjoined DIEP flap with left symmetry procedure.

required for the preparation of the chest and harvest of composite grafts.[36]

Surgical Techniques: Stacked Deep Inferior Epigastric Artery Perforator and Profunda Artery Perforator Flap

The stacked DIEP and PAP flap was the initial combination of the four-flap breast reconstruction.[6] The benefit of this approach is that all surgical sites can be approached simultaneously instead of in sequence and there is no position change required. The natural curve of the PAP

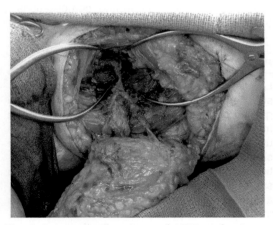

Fig. 2. Intra-operative photo of MFC perforator as part of a conjoined double-pedicle inner posterior thigh flap (PAP flap).

flap is suited well for inset at the inframammary fold while the DIEP flap is similar to the tapered upper portion of a natural breast. Shape-wise, this is the ideal positioning; however, the larger, or dominant, flap is routinely connected to the cranial inflow source as this is thought to typically be superior. The DIEP vascular pedicle also more commonly provides a side branch or cranial extension that can allow parasitic perfusion via the DIEP flap connected to a set of dominate cranial mammary vessels.

As with most multi-site surgeries, the complication rate is increased by more surgical sites being involved. That said, it is not an additive increase as in these situations usually each flap harvest site can be non-extensive allowing less tension on the closure (**Figs. 5** and **6**).

Surgical Techniques: Stacked Deep Inferior Epigastric Artery Perforator and Lumbar Artery Perforator Flap

The combination of DIEP flaps and LAP flaps would be considered ideal by many from a body contouring standpoint.[25] This procedure provides a similar result to the trunk that a circumferential body lift would provide and uses two of the most abundant options for breast reconstruction. Although there are clear benefits to this approach, there are very significant difficulties related to the vascular pedicles and the sequencing. All LAP flaps have an insufficient vascular pedicle to perform safely, and thus, require composite

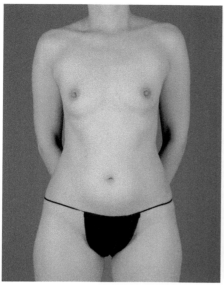
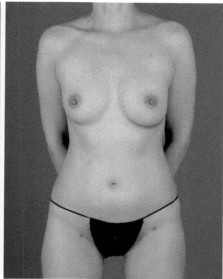

Fig. 3. A 45-year-old woman with left breast cancer treated with delayed immediate stacked PAP flaps and symmetry fat grafting to the right breast (anterior view).

arterial and venous grafts. With the typical donor site being the deep inferior epigastric artery and vein, this creates a unique circumstance. To augment the length of the LAP flap vascular pedicle, the surgeon borrows from the DIEP flap vascular pedicle, and in doing so, compromises the vascular pedicle length for the DIEP flap itself. Although this is certainly manageable, in a four-flap situation, a short vascular pedicle of any flap makes the flap inset more challenging.

Additionally, the timing of performing each flap harvest must be considered. If the DIEP flaps are harvested and anastomosed to the mammary vessels at the same time as harvesting the composite grafts for the LAP flap, then one must be comfortable repositioning into a prone position with multiple fresh anastomosis. This can be done safely but requires significant expertise. As an alternative, the DIEP flap harvest can be delayed until after the LAP flaps are harvested, the back is closed,

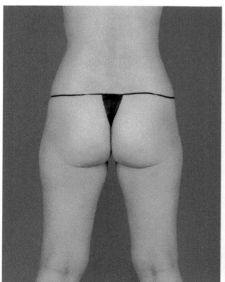
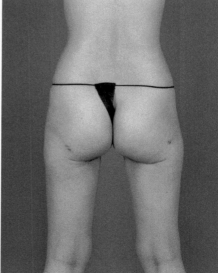

Fig. 4. A 45-year-old woman with left breast cancer treated with delayed immediate stacked PAP flaps and symmetry fat grafting to the right breast (posterior view).

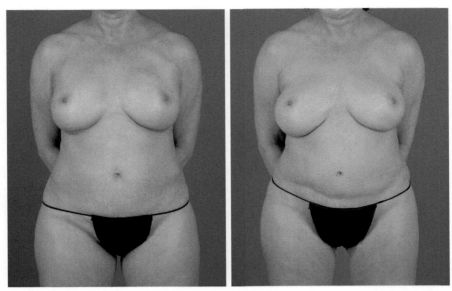

Fig. 5. A 58-year-old female with a history of breast cancer treated with bilateral mastectomy and implant reconstruction at an outside hospital. She presented for autologous conversion and underwent bilateral stacked DIEP and PAP flaps (anterior view).

and the flaps are re-perfused on the chest. This will add to the length of the total operation and leave the DIEP flaps partially perfused with a superior non-dominant flow during the multiple position changes. Either way, compromises must be made and a team approach with an efficient process is paramount during this operation (**Figs. 7 and 8**).

Surgical Techniques: Stacked Profunda Artery Perforator and Lumbar Artery Perforator Flap

The stacked PAP flap and LAP flap is a unique option, typically used in those that do not have enough tissue in a single donor site and have had a previous abdominoplasty. The PAP flaps can either be harvested first and anastomosed

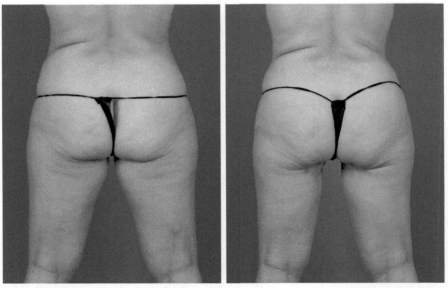

Fig. 6. A58-year-old woman with a history of breast cancer treated with bilateral mastectomy and implant reconstruction at an outside hospital. She presented for autologous conversion and underwent bilateral stacked DIEP and PAP flaps (posterior view).

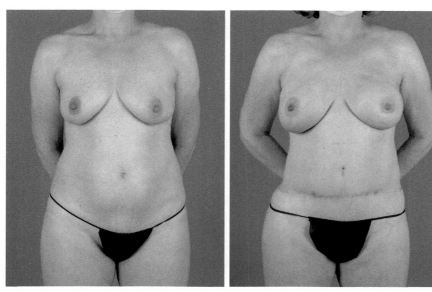

Fig. 7. A 56-year-old woman with a genetic predisposition to breast cancer treated with prophylactic nipple-sparing mastectomy and tissue expanders. This was followed by autologous reconstruction with bilateral stacked DIEP and LAP flaps (anterior view).

to the chest or delayed until after the LAP flaps. The benefit of harvesting the PAP flaps first is that this does allow for easier partial closure while in a prone position during the LAP flap harvest. Otherwise, the nuances of this combination are very similar to each on its own (**Figs. 9–12**).

Safety

There are many nuances to stacked flap breast reconstruction and as surgical complexity increases, the potential for complications increases. In a direct comparison of stacked flaps to single flaps, it was noted that these patients have increased deep venous thrombosis rates.[7] In our

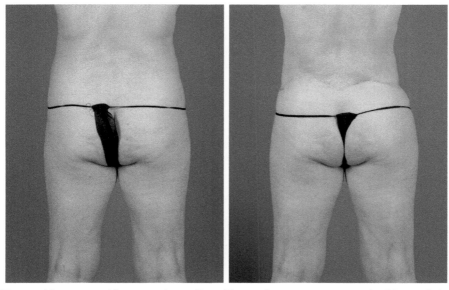

Fig. 8. A 56-year-old woman with a genetic predisposition to breast cancer treated with prophylactic nipple-sparing mastectomy and tissue expanders. This was followed by autologous reconstruction with bilateral stacked DIEP and LAP flaps (posterior view).

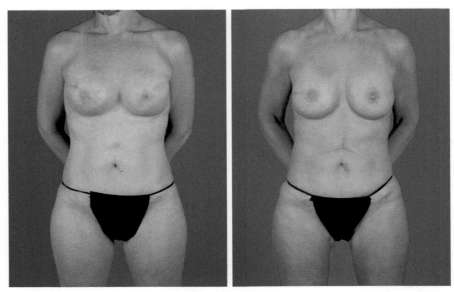

Fig. 9. A 56-year-old woman with a genetic predisposition to breast cancer treated with prophylactic nipple-sparing mastectomy and implant-based reconstruction at an outside hospital. She presented for autologous conversion and underwent bilateral stacked LAP and PAP flaps (anterior view).

practice, we routinely treat our stacked flap patients with extended anti-coagulation. The other finding in this report was that these patients have a higher return to the operating room, but this did not also confer an increased flap loss rate. With stacked flaps, it is often that a single flap is buried, and thus, despite the use of implantable Dopplers, subtle changes result in a negative exploration to confer viability. Patients should be counseled accordingly. Additionally, given the multiple surgical sites and the potential increase in problems requiring troubleshooting, we strongly

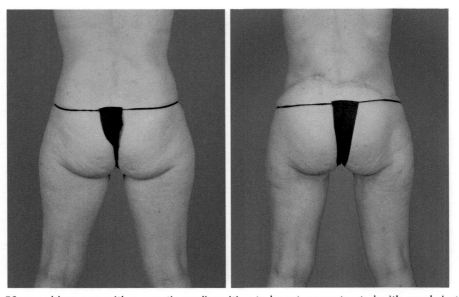

Fig. 10. A 56-year-old woman with a genetic predisposition to breast cancer treated with prophylactic nipple-sparing mastectomy and implant-based reconstruction at an outside hospital. She presented for autologous conversion and underwent bilateral stacked LAP and PAP flaps (posterior view).

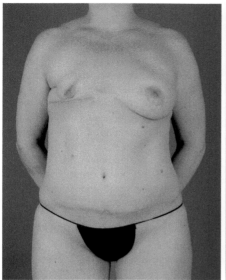
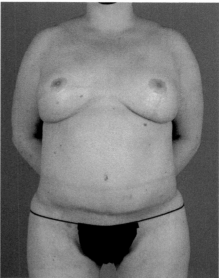

Fig. 11. A 48-year-old woman with a history of breast cancer treated with bilateral nipple-sparing mastectomy and tissue expander-based reconstruction at an outside hospital. Her right breast reconstruction was complicated by mycobacterium infection, and ultimately, the expander was lost. She had undergone a previous abdomino-plasty. She presented for autologous reconstruction and underwent bilateral stacked LAP and PAP flaps (anterior view).

encourage a co-surgery approach.[37] Before considering multi-flap breast reconstruction, the surgical team should be proficient with individual flap reconstruction and have high success rates.

Additionally, when multiple flaps are involved, a mindset focused on efficiency is paramount to avoid extended procedures and the related increased morbidity.[38]

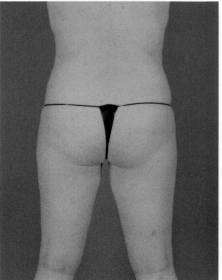
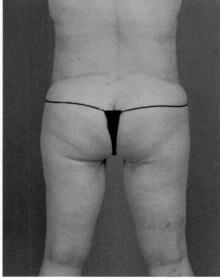

Fig. 12. A 48-year-old woman with a history of breast cancer treated with bilateral nipple-sparing mastectomy and tissue expander-based reconstruction at an outside hospital. Her right breast reconstruction was complicated by mycobacterium infection, and ultimately, the expander was lost. She had undergone a previous abdomino-plasty. She presented for autologous reconstruction and underwent bilateral stacked LAP and PAP flaps (posterior view).

SUMMARY

Stacked flaps are an excellent adjunct to the armamentarium for breast reconstruction surgeons. In our practice, including all variants described, multiple flap-based breast reconstruction accounts for one-third of all breast reconstructions with autologous flaps. In some patients, stacked flaps are the only way to accomplish total breast reconstruction in a single setting and without the addition of an alloplastic device.

CLINICS CARE POINTS

- Stacked flaps require significant preoperative planning including the use of preoperative imaging. This can help with decision-making on flap choice as well as secondary recipient vessel selection if a caudal mammary vessel is not available. There are often side branches or flap pedicle extensions that can be used.

- When there is a large skin need, the double DIEP flap is typically the best option. This option will typically allow total reconstruction with a single patch. The other available options often result in two skin paddles and less favorable cosmesis.

- When performing a four-flap breast reconstruction, optimization of the team via co-surgery is paramount. Ideally, the team has extensive experience with standard bilateral reconstructions and communicates well. Any additional measures that enhance operative efficiency can improve the safety of these multi-step operations.

- Patient counseling is always important in microvascular breast reconstruction, but this cannot be overstated for stacked flaps. When multiple donor sites are used for a single breast many surgical wounds have to heal. Patients should have a good understanding of the real risks related to these surgeries.

REFERENCES

1. Allen RJ, Treece P. Deep inferior epigastric perforator flap for breast reconstruction. Ann Plast Surg 1994;32(1):32–8.
2. Allen RJ, Haddock NT, Ahn CY, et al. Breast reconstruction with the profunda artery perforator flap. Plast Reconstr Surg 2012;129(1):16e–23e.
3. Tuinder SMH, Beugels J, Lataster A, et al. The lateral thigh perforator flap for autologous breast reconstruction: a Prospective analysis of 138 flaps. Plast Reconstr Surg 2018;141(2):257–68.
4. Allen RJ, Tucker C Jr. Superior gluteal artery perforator free flap for breast reconstruction. Plast Reconstr Surg 1995;95(7):1207–12.
5. de Weerd L, Elvenes OP, Strandenes E, et al. Autologous breast reconstruction with a free lumbar artery perforator flap. Br J Plast Surg 2003;56(2):180–3.
6. Haddock N, Suszynski TM, Teotia S. Consecutive bilateral stacked breast reconstruction using abdominally-based and posterior thigh free flaps. Plast Reconstr Surg 2021;147(2):294–303.
7. Haddock NT, Cho MJ, Teotia SS. Comparative analysis of single versus stacked free flap breast reconstruction: a single-Center experience. Plast Reconstr Surg 2019;144(3):369e–77e.
8. Marino H Jr, Dogliotti P. Mammary reconstruction with bipedicled abdominal flap. Plast Reconstr Surg 1981;68(6):933–6.
9. Ishii CH Jr, Bostwick J 3rd, Raine TJ, et al. Double-pedicle transverse rectus abdominis myocutaneous flap for unilateral breast and chest-wall reconstruction. Plast Reconstr Surg 1985;76(6):901–7.
10. Wagner DS, Michelow BJ, Hartrampf CR Jr. Double-pedicle TRAM flap for unilateral breast reconstruction. Plast Reconstr Surg 1991;88(6):987–97.
11. Boyd JB, Taylor GI, Corlett R. The vascular territories of the superior epigastric and the deep inferior epigastric systems. Plast Reconstr Surg 1984;73(1):1–16.
12. Yamamoto Y, Nohira K, Shintomi Y, et al. Turbo charging" the vertical rectus abdominis myocutaneous (turbo-VRAM) flap for reconstruction of extensive chest wall defects. Br J Plast Surg 1994;47(2):103–7.
13. Pernia LR, Miller HL, Saltz R, et al. Supercharging" the rectus abdominis muscle to provide a single flap for cover of large mediastinal wound defects. Br J Plast Surg 1991;44(4):243–6.
14. Harashina T, Sone K, Inoue T, et al. Augmentation of circulation of pedicled transverse rectus abdominis musculocutaneous flaps by microvascular surgery. Br J Plast Surg 1987;40(4):367–70.
15. Holmstrom H. The free abdominoplasty flap and its use in breast reconstruction. An experimental study and clinical case report. Scand J Plast Reconstr Surg 1979;13(3):423–7.
16. Friedman RJ, Argenta LC, Anderson R. Deep inferior epigastric free flap for breast reconstruction after radical mastectomy. Plast Reconstr Surg 1985;76(3):455–60.
17. Arnez ZM, Smith RW, Eder E, et al. Breast reconstruction by the free lower transverse rectus abdominis musculocutaneous flap. Br J Plast Surg 1988;41(5):500–5.

18. Arnez ZM, Scamp T. The bipedicled free TRAM flap. *Br J Plast Surg* Apr 1992;45(3):214–8.

19. Spear SL, Travaglino-Parda RL, Stefan MM. The stacked transverse rectus abdominis musculocutaneous flap revisited in breast reconstruction. Ann Plast Surg 1994;32(6):565–71.

20. Berrino P, Casabona F, Adami M, et al. The "parasite" TRAM flap for autogenous tissue breast reconstruction in patients with vertical midabdominal scars. Ann Plast Surg 1999;43(2):119–26.

21. Hamdi M, Khuthaila DK, Van Landuyt K, et al. Double-pedicle abdominal perforator free flaps for unilateral breast reconstruction: new horizons in microsurgical tissue transfer to the breast. J Plast Reconstr Aesthet Surg 2007;60(8):904–12 [discussion: 913-4].

22. Haddock NT, Cho MJ, Gassman A, et al. Stacked profunda artery perforator flap for breast reconstruction in Failed or Unavailable deep inferior epigastric perforator flap. Plast Reconstr Surg 2019;143(3): 488e–94e.

23. Hartrampf CR Jr, Noel RT, Drazan L, et al. Ruben's fat pad for breast reconstruction: a peri-iliac soft-tissue free flap. Plast Reconstr Surg 1994;93(2):402–7.

24. Bostwick J 3rd, Vasconez LO, Jurkiewicz MJ. Breast reconstruction after a radical mastectomy. Plast Reconstr Surg 1978;61(5):682–93.

25. Haddock NT, Kelling JA, Teotia SS. Simultaneous circumferential body lift and four-flap breast reconstruction using deep inferior epigastric perforator and lumbar artery perforator flaps. Plast Reconstr Surg 2021;147(6):936e–9e.

26. Haddock NT, Teotia ST. Discussion: the stacked Hemiabdominal extended perforator flap for autologous breast reconstruction. Plast Reconstr Surg 2018;142(6):1435–6.

27. Mallucci P, Branford OA. Population analysis of the perfect breast: a morphometric analysis. Plast Reconstr Surg 2014;134(3):436–47.

28. Wagner RD, Hamilton KL, Doval AF, et al. How to maximize aesthetics in autologous breast reconstruction. Aesthet Surg J 2020;40(Suppl 2):S45–54.

29. Haddock NT, Suszynski TM, Teotia SS. An Individualized patient-centric approach and Evolution towards total autologous free flap breast reconstruction in an Academic setting. Plast Reconstr Surg - Glob Open 2020. https://doi.org/10.1097/gox.0000000000002681.

30. Haddock NT, Teotia SS. Consecutive 265 profunda artery perforator flaps: Refinements, Satisfaction, and Functional outcomes. Plast Reconstr Surg Glob Open 2020;8(4):e2682.

31. Haddock NT, Teotia SS. Lumbar artery perforator flap: initial experience with simultaneous bilateral flaps for breast reconstruction. Plast Reconstr Surg Glob Open 2020;8(5):e2800.

32. Teotia SS, Dumestre DO, Jayaraman AP, et al. Revisiting Anastomosis to the Retrograde internal mammary System in stacked free flap breast reconstruction: an Algorithmic approach to recipient-site selection. Plast Reconstr Surg 2020; 145(4):880–7.

33. Cho MJ, Haddock NT, Teotia SS. Clinical decision making using CTA in conjoined, bipedicled DIEP and SIEA for unilateral breast reconstruction. J Reconstr Microsurg 2020;36(4):241–6.

34. Haddock NT, Gassman A, Cho MJ, et al. 101 Consecutive profunda artery perforator flaps in breast reconstruction: Lessons Learned with our Early experience. Plast Reconstr Surg 2017;140(2): 229–39.

35. Cho MJ, Teotia SS, Haddock NT. Classification and Management of donor-site wound complications in the profunda artery perforator flap for breast reconstruction. J Reconstr Microsurg 2020;36(2):110–5.

36. Cho MJ, Haddock NT, Gassman AA, et al. Use of composite arterial and venous grafts in microsurgical breast reconstruction: Technical Challenges and Lessons Learned. Plast Reconstr Surg 2018; 142(4):867–70.

37. Haddock NT, Kayfan S, Pezeshk RA, et al. Co-surgeons in breast reconstructive microsurgery: what do they bring to the table? Microsurgery 2018; 38(1):14–20.

38. Haddock NT, Teotia SS. Efficient DIEP flap: bilateral breast reconstruction in less than four Hours. Plast Reconstr Surg Glob Open 2021;9(9):e3801.

Hybrid Microsurgical Breast Reconstruction: HyFIL® & HyPAD™ Techniques

Neil Tanna, MD, MBA[a,b,*], Sarah L. Barnett, BA[a], Emma L. Robinson, BS[b], Mark L. Smith, MD[a,b]

KEYWORDS

- Hybrid breast reconstruction • Breast reconstruction • Postmastectomy reconstruction
- Autologous reconstruction • Implant reconstruction • DIEP flap • Reconstructive surgery

KEY POINTS

- Patients who desire autologous reconstruction but lack adequate donor site volume to match the necessary or desired breast volume present a reconstructive challenge that can be solved with hybrid breast reconstruction.
- In hybrid breast reconstruction, acellular dermal matrix and/or implants are used in conjunction with various tissue flaps, most notably the deep inferior epigastric perforator flap, to provide superior clinical and esthetic outcomes for both the breast and donor site.
- The HyFIL® technique is a hybrid breast reconstruction that augments the flap volume with lipofilling and the use of a prepectoral direct-to-implant reconstruction.
- The novel HyPAD™ technique augments the flap volume with the use of stacked prepectoral acellular dermal matrix in lieu of an implant.

INTRODUCTION
Background

Postmastectomy breast reconstruction has been steadily increasing in the United States, with a 75% increase since 2000.[1] Most patients will pursue implant-based breast reconstruction. Reconstruction options used to be strictly limited by body habitus. However, in the last decade, advancements in microsurgery, the introduction of acellular dermal matrices (ADMs) and meshes, and the increasing use of alternative donor sites have greatly increased the scope of autologous reconstruction. Today, almost every breast can be reconstructed using either autologous or heterologous techniques, influenced by the goals and preferences of the patient.[2] Plastic surgeons must consider factors such as the breast dimensions, patient preference, and patient body habitus when considering which reconstructive option is best.

Implant Reconstruction

Implant-based breast reconstruction is the simplest and most common form of breast reconstruction. Implants are used in the majority of immediate breast reconstructions[1] and are particularly well-suited for thin women.[2] A major advantage of implant reconstruction is the relative simplicity of the procedure—it can be completed by most plastic surgeons reliably with a straightforward

Financial Disclosures: None of the authors has any financial interest in any of the products, devices, or drugs mentioned in this article.
[a] Division of Plastic and Reconstructive Surgery, Northwell Health, Great Neck, NY, USA; [b] Divsion of Plastic & Reconstructive Surgery, The Donald and Barbara Zucker School of Medicine at Hofstra/Northwell, Hempstead, NY, USA
* Corresponding author. Division of Plastic and Reconstructive Surgery, Northwell Health, 600 Northern Blvd., Suite 310, Great Neck, NY 11021.
E-mail address: ntanna@gmail.com

Clin Plastic Surg 50 (2023) 337–346
https://doi.org/10.1016/j.cps.2022.10.006
0094-1298/23/© 2022 Elsevier Inc. All rights reserved.

recovery. However, patients with implants may be prone to infection, seroma, rupture, capsular contracture, implant visibility, palpability, and rippling.[3] These complications are more likely in patients undergoing radiation as part of their cancer treatment. Finally, with limited implant longevity, implants likely necessitate 1 or 2 additional surgeries in a woman's lifetime.

Autologous Reconstruction

Breast reconstruction using natural tissue, however, is a more invasive procedure with longer operative times and recovery periods. In addition, there is a risk profile and recovery associated with a second surgical site, the flap donor site. Nonetheless, failure rates remain low across all autologous procedure types.[4] With the use of women's own tissue, the autologous-reconstructed breast has the appearance and feel of a soft natural breast, which responds to changes in body habitus similarly to natural breasts.

There are a variety of types of autologous reconstruction methods, with donor tissue originating from different parts of the body (**Fig. 1**). The most common method of autologous reconstruction is the deep inferior epigastric perforator (DIEP) Flap. In DIEP flap reconstruction, the flap is harvested in an elliptical shape extending across the entire lower abdomen. Small incisions are made in the rectus abdominis muscle for vessel access but no muscle or fascia is removed (**Fig. 2**). The major disadvantages of DIEP flap

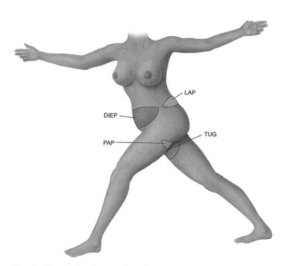

Fig. 1. Possible donor sites for autologous reconstruction. The most common source of autologous reconstruction is the DIEP flap. Alternative donor sites include the lumbar artery perforator (LAP) flap, profunda artery perforator (PAP) flap, TUG flap, and the gluteal artery perforator (GAP) flap.

reconstruction are the prolonged recovery and significant donor scar. Additionally, because the DIEP flap donor site can only be used once, many women choosing DIEP flap breast reconstruction often consider bilateral mastectomies. Alternative donor sites include tissue from the flanks in the lumbar artery perforator flap, the thighs with the profunda artery perforator flap or a transverse upper gracilis (TUG) flap, or the buttocks with the gluteal artery perforator flap.[5-9]

Comparison of Implant and Autologous Reconstruction

Although implant-based breast reconstructions typically require less operating time, leave fewer scars, and avoid the risk of donor site morbidity, many patients prefer the permanence, esthetics, and texture of flap-based breast reconstructions.[10,11] Unlike implant-based reconstruction, autologous methods rarely require additional surgeries for maintenance after the initial set of surgeries required for reconstruction and are associated with greater long-term satisfaction and improved health-related quality of life.[10,11] Additionally, reconstruction failure rates are lower following autologous reconstruction: total flap loss rates are reported to be 0.3% to 1.2%, whereas failed prosthetic reconstruction rates and implant infection range from 1.9% to 2.7%, and up to 44% following radiation.[2]

Clinical Challenge: Breast and Flap Volume Discordance

Although there are many benefits to microsurgical flap reconstruction, this is not a viable option for all patients. Namely, patients who desire autologous breast reconstruction but lack adequate flap volume to match the necessary or desired breast volume present a reconstructive challenge. Lacking adequate flap volume can severely compromise the functional and esthetic outcome of breast reconstruction. To address this, alternative reconstructive methods may be considered, including fat grafting of autologous flaps, stacked flaps, and hybrid breast reconstruction (HBR).

FAT GRAFTING

The volume of free flaps can be augmented secondarily via fat grafting. This method has many advantages because it may subvert the need for an implant, and correct contour deformities, asymmetries, and volume deficiencies, all-in-one short outpatient procedure.[12] However, limitations to fat transfer exist including variable fat retention and fat necrosis.[2] Additionally, fat

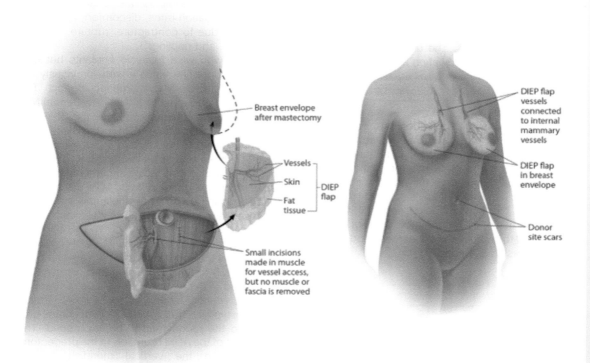

Breast envelope
after mastectomy

Vessels

Skin
                    ⎱DIEP
Fat ⎰flap
tissue

Small incisions
made in muscle
for vessel access,
but no muscle or
fascia is removed

DIEP flap
vessels
connected
to internal
mammary
vessels

DIEP flap
in breast
envelope

Donor
site scars

Fig. 2. DIEP flap breast reconstruction.

transfer donor sites may lack adequate volume for fat grafting.

Alternative and Stacked Flaps

Stacked flaps are the combination of multiple flaps to reconstruct the breasts. In unilateral reconstruction, the stacked DIEP is the most commonly used approach, whereby the abdominal flap is used to reconstruct one breast. In bilateral breast reconstructions or those situations where the abdominal donor site is not available, alternative donor sites, with or without stacked flaps, can be used. However, these options are technically more complex, often requiring multiple microvascular anastomoses, longer operative duration, and potentially additional donor-site morbidity.[13,14]

Hybrid Breast Reconstruction

An innovative solution to the discordance between desired breast reconstruction volume and available donor flap volume is the use of alloplastic and bioprosthetic materials to augment the flap volume in a single-stage hybrid approach. Historically, the latissimus dorsi flap has been used concurrently with an implant. However, this technique requires the sacrifice of a major muscle, which often leads to weakness, reduced mobility,

and contour deformity at the donor site.[15] In 2018, Momeni and Kanchwala pioneered a new approach that combines a prepectoral implant secured with ADM along and covered with an abdominal free flap in a single-stage procedure.[16] Similar to previous techniques, this allowed for control of both the soft tissue envelope as well as the size and projection of the breast mound. The novelty of this technique lies in the ability to eliminate the downside of submuscular placement (ie, increased risk of bleeding, pain, and animation deformity) while also reducing the tissue demands on the donor site allowing a more esthetic abdominal closure.[16,17] Alleviating the need to harvest the entire reconstruction volume at the abdomen allows the donor site scar to be lower, well-hidden, and less tight. There is also greater flexibility as surgeons can select an implant size that best meets patient needs. Esthetically, soft tissue coverage over the implant decreases implant palpability, visibility, and rippling.[18,19] Unlike the aforementioned alternative treatment options, the hybrid technique does not significantly increase the duration or complexity of the reconstruction.[2]

Other less established yet possible flap options for HBR include the thoracodorsal artery perforator, transverse rectus abdominus musculocutaneous, TUG, and inframammary adipofascial flaps.[20] Across all types of HBR, the flap provides vascularized soft tissue coverage to optimize appearance, feel, and minimize alloplastic-related complications. The underlying implant or ADM provides core projection and volume.

Types of Hybrid Breast Reconstruction

HyFIL®: Hybrid Flap, implant, lipofilling

The HyFIL technique combines flap, prepectoral implant, and fat transfer into one integrated procedure (**Fig. 3**). In this technique, a small silicone or saline round implant is inserted in the prepectoral position, secured to the anterior chest wall with ADM, and the flap is placed over the construct. The implant helps enhance the size and projection of the reconstructed breast. Lipofilling is used to improve the appearance and contour of the breasts as needed.

HyPAD™: Hybrid Flap, Prepectoral Acellular Dermal Matrix

There is a growing community of women who wish to avoid an implant in breast reconstruction, citing concerns related to breast implant-associated-anaplastic large cell lymphoma and breast implant

illness. Further, implants are associated with higher complication rates, discomfort, and repeat procedures due to contracture, rupture, seroma, malposition, and rippling.[21]

Patients who wish to avoid implants but lack adequate donor site volume were previously left without a suitable reconstruction option. The Hybrid Flap and Prepectoral Acellular Dermal Matrix (HyPAD™) technique combines the DIEP flap with stacked prepectoral ADM in the place of an implant (**Fig. 4**). The stacked ADM serves the similar purpose as a small implant, but to a lesser degree, providing soft tissue augmentation of the flap and core projection (**Fig. 5**). ADM has a variety of sizes and thickness levels; the authors preferentially use the rectangular 16 cm × 20 cm extra thick perforated sheet, which can add 75 to 140 mL of additional volume to the breast. The ADM is simply folded 3 or 4 time onto itself to create a rectangular pad that is 6 to 8 layers thick. More recently, we have used a more complex folding pattern to create a rounder shaped pad of ADM. These pads can typically add a 1.5 to 2 cm of central projection to the reconstructed breast mound. The placement of the ADM is entirely in the prepectoral region, along the vertical meridian at the

Breast Reconstruction

Fig. 3. The HyFIL® (hybrid flap, implant, lipofilling) technique combines flap, prepectoral implant, and fat transfer into one integrated procedure.

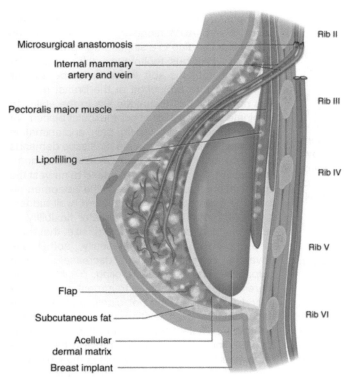

Microsurgical anastomosis

Internal mammary artery and vein

Pectoralis major muscle

Lipofilling

Flap

Subcutaneous fat

Acellular dermal matrix

Breast implant

Rib II

Rib III

Rib IV

Rib V

Rib VI

Breast Reconstruction

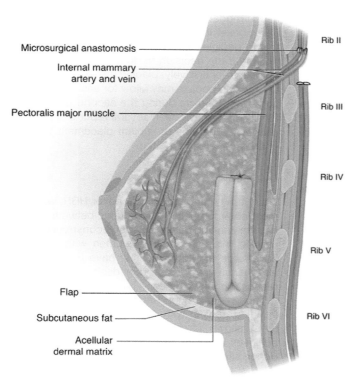

Microsurgical anastomosis

Internal mammary artery and vein

Pectoralis major muscle

Rib II

Rib III

Rib IV

Rib V

Flap

Subcutaneous fat

Acellular dermal matrix

Rib VI

Fig. 4. The HyPAD™ (hybrid flap, prepectoral acellular dermal matrix) technique combines flap reconstruction with stacked prepectoral ADM to provide additional volume augmentation and core projection.

inframammary fold. This allows for optimal breast projection. Furthermore, the ADM serves as a barrier to protect the flap and vascular pedicle should patients decide to further augment the reconstruction with an implant at a later stage of reconstruction.

ADM is commonly used across multiple surgical disciplines, including implant-based reconstruction and has been shown to have multiple advantages.[22,23] ADM improves control over the inferior pole and implant position and provides additional soft tissue coverage.[24-28] Biologically, ADM has been shown to incorporate the recipient tissue, undergoing processes of revascularization and recellularization with minimal complications.[22] It is particularly well-suited for breast reconstruction because it comes in different thicknesses, sizes, and shapes, so it can be customized to fit the specific needs of a patient. Reported complications from ADM include hematoma, infection, and seroma.[26] Given the benefits of ADM in breast reconstruction, it has now routinely been

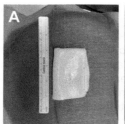 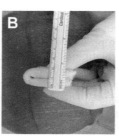 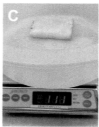 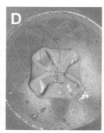 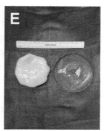

Fig. 5. In the HyPAD® (hybrid flap, prepectoral acellular dermal matrix) technique, the stacked ADM serves the similar purpose as a small implant, but to a lesser degree, providing soft tissue augmentation of the flap and core projection. Various angles (*A-D*) of the stacked ADM construct are shown. The stacked ADM is compared to a silicone breast prosthesis (*E*).

incorporated into hybrid reconstruction. It is important to note that the use of ADM in breast reconstruction is off label and all patients are counseled about this during the informed consent process.

Evaluation

When assessing a patient's candidacy for receiving an autologous flap reconstruction, surgeons may consider the volume of the flap available at the donor site relative to the desired breast reconstruction volume. Patients fall into 1 of 3 categories based on this relationship, with implications for the course of treatment. The volume of the donor site flap may be (1) greater than, (2) equal to, or (3) less than the volume of the desired breast reconstruction. Patients in the first or second category may be treated with traditional autologous reconstruction. Patients in the third category are considered for possible HBR. Alternatively, these patients can be considered for alternative/stacked flaps or traditional implant-based reconstruction.[17] Careful preoperative assessment of a patient's desired breast volume, existing native breast dimensions, and body habitus can help guide the surgeon and patient's expectations of treatment options and esthetic outcome.[29]

One pertinent consideration for HBR is timing. Immediate, delayed, and delayed-immediate with tissue-expander placement HBRs have all been completed successfully.[20] Conceptually, placing the implant and acellular dermis at the time of the flap placement allows layering of the multiple lamellae (breast skin, flap, ADM, implant) as the surgeon dictates. If an implant is placed secondarily, the scar between each of these layers must stretch to accommodate the implant and there may be some restriction to pocket expansion.

However, single-stage, immediate reconstruction has the highest risk of implant-induced pedicle compression and the greatest restriction on implant size from both the mastectomy skin and flap pedicle.[20] In practice, we have not found this to be a major issue. Conversely, delayed implant insertion allows for less pressure on the mastectomy skin flaps but requires additional procedures, adding an anesthetic burden on the patient and increasing the difficulty of pocket dissection for the surgeon.[19] Delayed implant placement cases have a mean of 4, and as many as 6, total procedures to obtain the final result.[30] In addition, delayed implant placement may be difficult in the patient who receives postoperative radiation. Generally, we have chosen to use smaller implant in the 120 to 200 cc range for

most patients. In the rare setting where a patient wants additional volume, it is much simpler at a second surgery to release an existing pocket to accommodate a larger implant than to create a new pocket in a scarred plane in close proximity to the pedicle or to dissect a new submuscular pocket. If the decision to do a delayed implant is made intraoperatively, placing a sheet of ADM under the flap pedicle may allow for easier preservation of the pedicle during the second procedure. Finally, there have been several reports of pedicle division at the time of implant placement without undue sequelae to the flap.

DISCUSSION

There are numerous indications for HBR, with the most common being discordance between donor flap volume and desired breast reconstruction volume.[16] This can occur in women who are thin, have large or ptotic breasts, have had previous abdominal surgeries, and/or desire larger breast reconstruction volumes.

The use of a hybrid approach with concurrent free flap transfer with implant and/or ADM placement allows for a single-stage procedure that achieves a desirable look and feel while limiting donor site morbidity and postoperative implant-related problems including palpability, rippling, capsular contracture, and reconstructive failures.[2] HBR poses unique advantages and limitations as a reconstructive technique.

HBR offers an augmented flap volume while maintaining the look and feel of a natural breast.[17,31] HBR avoids the pitfalls of other alternative reconstruction techniques, including the technical complexity of stacked flaps and the additional morbidity of alternative donor flaps. For some women, a primary benefit of autologous reconstruction is the avoidance of an implant, and the monitoring and subsequent procedures that come with it. To this end, the use of an implant in the HyFIL technique may seem counterproductive. The novel HyPAD technique presents a possible solution to achieve additional tissue augmentation without an implant.

Compared with implant-based reconstruction, the advantages of HBR include restoration of the natural breast contour, adaptation to changes in body weight, and a lower complication rate.[20] Benefits of HBR are even more significant for patients with irradiated breasts including fewer complications and better cosmesis.[2] The main disadvantage of HBR is the additional cost compared with implant or tissue reconstruction performed alone. However, the initially high surgical and financial costs are offset in the long term as the soft tissue coverage reduces the need for secondary procedures due to implant complications.[32-34]

DIEP flap reconstruction is often advertised on the Internet as a "tummy-tuck" reconstruction. However, this may be misleading because the need to harvest enough volume for breast reconstruction often means that the resulting scar is higher and less esthetically pleasing than in abdominoplasty patients.[17]

In select HBR cases, the entire reconstruction volume does not need to be harvested from abdominal tissue because alloplastic material is used to augment the free flap volume. This can result in a lower, less tight, and more esthetically pleasing scar.

Even volume ratios of 1:5 between the implant and flap provide significant cosmetic benefit through improved core projection.[35] This ratio allows the soft tissue of the flap to adequately camouflage the implant. Additionally, mastectomy skin flap necrosis is more easily managed in patients who undergo HBR, without the need for additional surgeries.[16] The addition of an implant to stacked-DIEP procedure for unilateral reconstruction in patients with inadequate donor site volume for single-flap DIEP also showed improved volume and projection to the autologous procedure alone.[36]

The complexity of breast reconstruction contributes to a high rate of revisionary procedures. HBR has been shown to significantly increase the success of these adjunct procedures, including autologous fat grafting and nipple reconstruction when compared with implant methods alone.[17] Autologous fat grafting is a treatment option for volume deficiencies and implant palpability and/or rippling. However, fat grafting to an implant-reconstructed breast, which only has a thin skin envelope, often leads to unsatisfactory results because most of the fat is reabsorbed. In HBR, fat can be deposited directly into well-vascularized flaps, leading to a greater volume and better take of the grafts.[17]

Following skin-sparing mastectomy, nipple reconstruction and micropigmentation can be performed to create a realistic-looking nipple–areolar complex. However, projection, which is a key hallmark of the natural nipple, is inevitably lost over time.[37] This is especially true for pure-implant reconstruction but also presents a challenge in autologous reconstruction. HBR, however, alleviates this difficulty with ample soft tissue and projection from the implant underneath.[17]

Flap reconstruction is often recommended over implant reconstruction in women with irradiated breasts. HBR provides a reasonable alternative for these patients who also need the additional volume from alloplastic material. The flap coverage from HBR protects the implant, minimizing the risk of capsular contracture, implant exposure, and wound breakdown.[17] In a series of 1000 irradiated breasts, HBR cases had significantly lower rates of implant loss (5% vs 30.3%) and reconstructive failure (15.2% or 10.0% vs 42.2%, respectively) than implant-only reconstructions.[38]

Reported postoperative complications from HBR include fat necrosis, mastectomy skin necrosis, flap loss, and venous congestion. The rates of nonimplant-related complications in HBR are in line with autologous reconstruction rates.[17] With implants in HBR, complications relating to the use of implants in the short term include hematoma, infection, and malposition.[17,39] The rates of implant-related complications and revisions for size are lower in HBR compared with implant-only reconstruction.[17] The use of ADM is associated with a further decrease in implant complication rates.[26]

A significant limitation of the HyFIL technique is the introduction of implant-associated complications and monitoring. The novel HyPAD technique addresses these concerns by replacing the small implant with a piece of stacked ADM for flap projection and augmentation. However, the thickest ADM sheets can still only provide about 90 to 140 mL of additional volume, whereas implants range in volume from 120 to 800 cc, depending on manufacturer. Therefore, A HyFIL approach may be preferable to the HyPAD technique in patients who need greater than 140 mL of additional core projections of the breast.

Another disadvantage of the HyPAD technique is the initial high cost associated with ADM. However, ADM reconstruction is associated with lower costs compared with non-ADM implant reconstruction at 2 years postoperatively, likely in part to fewer complications and reoperations.[32-34] Additionally, the food and drug administration (FDA) recommends that patients with prosthetic implants obtain screening breast MRIs 5 years after implantation and every 2 to 3 years after to evaluate for rupture. This contributed to total health-care costs of more than US$33 million in 2010.[40,41] Costs continue to increase for implants that rupture or expire and require surgical correction.[42] Thus, while initial costs of the ADM-based reconstruction may be similar or slightly higher than prosthetic implant use, the decrease in complications and screening makes their use at least cost-effective, if not advantageous to the patient and the surgeon. Finally, as a relatively new technique, there is a paucity of long-term outcome studies evaluating HBR complications and patient satisfaction. Future prospective, long-term studies are essential to optimize the clinical and esthetic outcomes of this technique. The use of ADM in breast reconstruction, although widespread, remains off label under current FDA guidelines.

SUMMARY

In breast reconstruction, discrepancies between the donor site flap volume and the desired breast reconstruction volume can pose a significant challenge.[43–47] HBR serves to address this concern with the addition of a prepectoral implant and/or ADM to a flap reconstruction. Prosthetic implants used in conjunction with various tissue flaps, most notably the DIEP flap, provide superior outcomes for both the breast and abdomen. With a HyFIL® technique, the use of vascularized soft tissue camouflages the implant while the implant provides the desired core projection and volume. However, the excess costs, follow-up screenings, and complication rates of the implant itself warrant consideration. The novel HyPAD™ technique augments the flap volume with the use of stacked prepectoral ADM, thus potentially avoiding many of the issues related to implants. Overall, HBR techniques expand the candidacy for autologous reconstruction methods and can help improve outcomes and patient satisfaction from breast reconstruction.

CLINICS CARE POINTS

- Women who desire autologous reconstruction but lack adequate flap volume to match the necessary or desired breast volume may be good candidates for HBR.
- Careful preoperative assessment of a patient's desired breast volume, existing native breast dimensions, and body habitus can help guide the surgeon and patient's expectations of treatment options and esthetic outcome.
- HBRs are good alternatives to implant only breast reconstruction or breast reconstruction with alternative flaps. It is associated with good esthetic outcomes and low overall complication rates compared with alternative flap types.[20,35]

REFERENCES

1. Plastic surgery Statistics report. 2020. Available at: https://www.plasticsurgery.org/documents/News/ Statistics/2020/plastic-surgery-statistics-full-report-2020.pdf. Accessed May 18, 2022.
2. Chu M, Samra F, Kanchwala S, et al. Treatment options for bilateral autologous breast reconstruction in patients with inadequate donor-site volume. J Reconstr Microsurgery 2017;33(05):305–11. https://doi.org/10.1055/s-0037-1599074.
3. Handel N, Jensen JA, Black Q, et al. The fate of breast implants. Plast Reconstr Surg 1995;96(7):1521–33. https://doi.org/10.1097/00006534-199512000-00003.
4. Dieterich M, Dragu A, Stachs A, et al. Clinical Approaches to breast reconstruction: what is the Appropriate reconstructive procedure for My patient. Breast Care 2017;12(6):368–73. https://doi.org/10.1159/000484926.
5. Arnež ZM, Pogorelec D, Planinšek F, et al. Breast reconstruction by the free transverse gracilis (TUG) flap. Br J Plast Surg 2004;57(1):20–6. https://doi.org/10.1016/j.bjps.2003.10.007.
6. Kind G, Foster R. Breast reconstruction using the lateral Femoral Circumflex artery perforator flap. J Reconstr Microsurgery 2011;27(07):427–32. https://doi.org/10.1055/s-0031-1281527.
7. Profunda artery perforator flap for breast reconstruction. In: Perforator flaps for breast reconstruction. Georg Thieme Verlag 2016. https://doi.org/10.1055/b-0036-141879.
8. LoTempio MM, Allen RJ. Breast reconstruction with SGAP and IGAP flaps. Plast Reconstr Surg 2010;126(2):393–401. https://doi.org/10.1097/prs.0b013e3181de236a.
9. Park JE, Alkureishi LWT, Song DH. TUGs into VUGs and Friendly BUGs. Plast Reconstr Surg 2015;136(3):447–54. https://doi.org/10.1097/prs.0000000000001557.
10. Stillaert FBJL, Lannau B, Van Landuyt K, et al. The pre-pectoral, hybrid breast reconstruction: the Synergy of lipofilling and breast implants. Plast Reconstr Surg - Glob Open 2020;8(7):e2966. https://doi.org/10.1097/gox.0000000000002966.
11. Bennett KG, Qi J, Kim HM, et al. Comparison of 2-Year complication rates Among common techniques for Postmastectomy breast reconstruction. JAMA Surg 2018;153(10):901. https://doi.org/10.1001/jamasurg.2018.1687.
12. Kanchwala SK, Glatt BS, Conant EF, et al. Autologous fat grafting to the reconstructed breast: the management of Acquired contour deformities. Plast Reconstr Surg 2009;124(2):409–18. https://doi.org/10.1097/prs.0b013e3181aeeadd.
13. Stalder MW, Lam J, Allen RJ, et al. Using the Retrograde internal Mammary System for stacked perforator flap breast reconstruction. Plast Reconstr Surg 2016;137(2):265e–77e.
14. Mayo JL, Allen RJ, Sadeghi A. Four-flap breast reconstruction. Plast Reconstr Surg - Glob Open

2015;3(5):e383. https://doi.org/10.1097/gox.00000 00000000353.

15. Blackburn NE, Mc Veigh JG, Mc Caughan E, et al. The musculoskeletal consequences of breast reconstruction using the latissimus dorsi muscle for women following mastectomy for breast cancer: a critical review. Eur J Cancer Care 2017;27(2): e12664. https://doi.org/10.1111/ecc.12664.

16. Momeni A, Kanchwala S. Hybrid pre-pectoral breast reconstruction. Plast Reconstr Surg 2018;142(5): 1109–15. https://doi.org/10.1097/prs.0000000000 004858.

17. Kanchwala S, Momeni A. Hybrid breast reconstruction—the best of both worlds. Gland Surg 2019;8(1): 82–9. https://doi.org/10.21037/gs.2018.11.01.

18. Serletti JM, Moran SL. The combined Use of the TRAM and Expanders/implants in breast reconstruction. Ann Plast Surg 1998;40(5):510–4. https://doi. org/10.1097/00000637-199805000-00012.

19. Roehl KR, Baumann DP, Chevray PM, et al. Evaluation of outcomes in breast reconstructions combining lower abdominal free flaps and permanent implants. Plast Reconstr Surg 2010;126(2):349–57. https://doi. org/10.1097/prs.0b013e3181de1b67.

20. Yesantharao PS, Nguyen DH. Hybrid breast reconstruction: a systematic review of current trends and future directions. Ann Breast Surg 2022;6:17. https://doi.org/10.21037/abs-20-114.

21. Handel N, Cordray T, Gutierrez J, et al. A long-term Study of outcomes, complications, and patient satisfaction with breast implants. Plast Reconstr Surg 2006;117(3):757–67. https://doi.org/10.1097/01.prs. 0000201457.00772.1d.

22. Eppley B. Revascularization of acellular human dermis (alloderm) in subcutaneous implantation. Aesthet Surg J 2000;20(4):291–5. https://doi.org/ 10.1067/maj.2000.109553.

23. Breuing KH, Colwell AS. Inferolateral AlloDerm Hammock for implant coverage in breast reconstruction. Ann Plast Surg 2007;59(3):250–5. https:// doi.org/10.1097/sap.0b013e31802f8426.

24. DeLong MR, Tandon VJ, Farajzadeh M, et al. Systematic review of the Impact of acellular dermal matrix on aesthetics and patient satisfaction in tissue expander-to-implant breast reconstructions. Plast Reconstr Surg 2019;144(6):967e–74e. https://doi. org/10.1097/prs.0000000000006212.

25. Margulies IG, Salzberg CA. The use of acellular dermal matrix in breast reconstruction: evolution of techniques over 2 decades. Gland Surg 2019;8(1): 3–10. https://doi.org/10.21037/gs.2018.10.05.

26. Vardanian AJ, Clayton JL, Roostaeian J, et al. Comparison of immediate implant-based reconstruction with and without acellular dermal matrix. Plast Reconstr Surg 2010;126:22. https://doi.org/10.1097/ 01.prs.0000388739.17215.17.

27. Gamboa-Bobadilla GM. Implant breast reconstruction using acellular dermal matrix. Ann Plast Surg 2006;56(1):22–5. https://doi.org/10.1097/01.sap. 0000185460.31188.c1.

28. Downs RK, Hedges K. An alternative technique for immediate direct-to-implant breast reconstruction— a case series. Plast Reconstr Surg - Glob Open 2016;4(7):e821. https://doi.org/10.1097/gox.000000 0000000839.

29. Spiegel A. Breast reconstruction: current Perspectives and state of the Art techniques. BoD – Books on Demand; 2013.

30. Pien I, Anolik R, Blau J, et al. Delayed implant augmentation of breast free flaps. J Reconstr Microsurgery 2015;31(04):254–60. https://doi.org/10. 1055/s-0034-1395416.

31. Lee HC, Lee J, Park S-H, et al. The hybrid latissimus dorsi flap in immediate breast reconstruction. Ann Plast Surg 2020;86(4):394–9. https://doi.org/10. 1097/sap.0000000000002565.

32. Jansen LA, Macadam SA. The Use of AlloDerm in Postmastectomy alloplastic breast reconstruction: Part II. A cost Analysis. Plast Reconstr Surg 2011; 127(6):2245–54. https://doi.org/10.1097/prs.0b013e 3182131c6b.

33. Salzberg CA, Ashikari AY, Berry C, et al. Acellular dermal matrix–Assisted direct-to-implant breast reconstruction and capsular contracture. Plast Reconstr Surg 2016;138(2):329–37. https://doi.org/10. 1097/prs.0000000000002331.

34. Qureshi AA, Broderick K, Funk S, et al. Direct Hospital cost of outcome Pathways in implant-based reconstruction with acellular dermal matrices. Plast Reconstr Surg - Glob Open 2016;4(8):e831. https://doi.org/10.1097/gox.0000000000000848.

35. Figus A, Canu V, Iwuagwu FC, et al. DIEP flap with implant: a further option in optimising breast reconstruction. J Plast Reconstr Aesthet Surg 2009; 62(9):1118–26. https://doi.org/10.1016/j.bjps.2007. 12.089.

36. Rodebeck E, Blum C, DellaCroce F. Stacked DIEP and implant for unilateral breast reconstruction. J Reconstr Microsurgery Open 2017;02(02): e124–5. https://doi.org/10.1055/s-0037-1606355.

37. Momeni A, Becker A, Torio-Padron N, et al. Nipple reconstruction: Evidence-based Trials in the plastic surgical Literature. Aesthet Plast Surg 2007;32(1): 18–20. https://doi.org/10.1007/s00266-007-9039-0.

38. Chang DW, Barnea Y, Robb GL. Effects of an autologous flap combined with an implant for breast reconstruction: an evaluation of 1000 Consecutive reconstructions of previously irradiated breasts. Plast Reconstr Surg 2008;122(2):356–62. https:// doi.org/10.1097/prs.0b013e31817d6303.

39. Collins JB, Verheyden CN. Incidence of breast hematoma after placement of breast Prostheses. Plast

Reconstr Surg 2012;129(3):413e–20e. https://doi.org/10.1097/prs.0b013e3182402ce0.

40. Breast implants - Certain labeling Recommendations to improve patient Communication. U.S. Food and drug Administration. Available at: https://www.fda.gov/regulatory-information/search-fda-guidance-documents/breast-implants-certain-labeling-recommendations-improve-patient-communication. Accessed May 18, 2022.

41. Chung KC, Malay S, Shauver MJ, et al. Economic Analysis of screening Strategies for rupture of silicone Gel breast implants. Plast Reconstr Surg 2012;130(1):225–37. https://doi.org/10.1097/prs.0b013e318254b43b.

42. Walters JA III, Sato EA, Martinez CA, et al. Delayed Mammoplasty with silicone Gel implants following DIEP flap breast reconstruction. Plast Reconstr Surg - Glob Open 2015;3(10):e540. https://doi.org/10.1097/gox.0000000000000527.

43. Alba B, Schultz BD, Cohen D, et al. Risk-to-Benefit relationship of Contralateral Prophylactic mastectomy: the Argument for bilateral Mastectomies with immediate reconstruction. Plast Reconstr Surg 2019;144:1–9.

44. Weichman KE, Broer PN, Thanik VD, et al. Patient-reported satisfaction and quality of life following breast reconstruction in thin patients: a Comparison between microsurgical and prosthetic implant recipients. Plast Reconstr Surg 2015;136:213–20.

45. Weichman KE, Tanna N, Broer PN, et al. Microsurgical breast reconstruction in thin patients: the Impact of low body Mass Indices. J Reconstr Microsurg 2015;31:20–5.

46. Tanna N, Broer PN, Weichman KE, et al. Microsurgical breast reconstruction for nipple-sparing mastectomy. Plast Reconstr Surg 2013;131. 139e-47e.

47. Tanna N, Clayton JL, Roostaeian J, et al. The volume-outcome relationship for immediate breast reconstruction. Plast Reconstr Surg 2012;129:19–24.

Modern Approaches to Breast Neurotization

Rebecca C. O'Neill, MD[a], Aldona J. Spiegel, MD[b],*

KEYWORDS

- Neurotization • Breast sensation • Neurotized breast reconstruction

KEY POINTS

- Recipient nerves include the lateral cutaneous branch of the fourth intercostal nerve and the anterior cutaneous branch of the third intercostal nerve.
- Innervated autologous flaps for breast reconstruction have both a greater magnitude as well as earlier sensory recovery compared with noninnervated autologous flaps.
- Neurotization has been significantly associated with improved patient satisfaction scores.

INTRODUCTION

Breast reconstruction provides patients with a variety of psychosocial benefits as well as improved overall quality of life.[1] Breast sensation is an important aspect of reconstruction and has been shown to increase patient satisfaction.[2] Thus, in the recent years, preserving and restoring breast sensation has become a focus within breast reconstruction.

The native breast experiences several types of sensation, including touch and protective sensation, much like other parts of the body. The nipple–areola complex (NAC) has tactile and protective sensation, as well as erogenous sensation. The breast is also a functional organ for lactation and is composed of lobules, which produce milk, and ducts, which transport the milk to the nipple. For many women, the breast plays an essential role in physical and sexual health, contributing to their sense of femininity. Following mastectomy, breast sensation is absent or, at best, significantly diminished. The partial or complete loss of sensation presents a problem for many patients, ranging from a perceived loss of sexuality to a loss of protective sensation, as demonstrated by multiple reports of thermal injuries to postmastectomy breasts from common household items.[2] For these reasons, it is long overdue for the inclusion of sensory restoration within breast reconstruction.

The first published description of breast neurotization was in 1992 and involved a transverse rectus abdominis myocutaneous (TRAM) flap, using the abdominis rectus intercostal nerve, which was connected to the lateral branch of the fourth intercostal nerve via direct coaptation.[3] Since then, the popularity of neurotization within breast reconstruction has slowly grown but remains far from an accepted practice standard. Based on the ACS-NSQIP data, 73,507 patients underwent breast reconstruction in the United States between 2015 and 2019.[4] Of these, 240 patients underwent neurotization, or about 0.3%. The rate of neurotization has increased, starting at 0.02% in 2015 and increasing to 0.65% by 2019. Most patients undergoing neurotization had free flap reconstruction (83%), followed by tissue expander reconstruction (5.8%), free flap plus implant (5%), implant-based reconstruction (2.5%), and pedicled TRAM (1%). For patients who underwent autologous reconstruction, the rate of neurotization was approximately 1.6%.[4]

Disclosure statement: The authors do not have any financial disclosures to report.
[a] Division of Plastic and Reconstructive Surgery, Baylor College of Medicine, 1 Baylor Plaza, Houston, TX 77030, USA; [b] Institute for Reconstructive Surgery, Houston Methodist Hospital, 6560 Fannin Street #2200, Houston, TX 77030, USA
* Corresponding author.
E-mail address: Aspiegel@houstonmethodist.org

Clin Plastic Surg 50 (2023) 347–355
https://doi.org/10.1016/j.cps.2022.10.003

Neurotization within breast reconstruction, although currently underutilized, represents the possibility to restore vital sensation to the breasts and produce higher patient satisfaction. As a modality with minimal risk and significant potential gain, breast neurotization is an essential area for continued study and discussion within breast reconstruction.

ANATOMY
Nerve Anatomy

A sensory nerve is composed of multiple fascicles united by the epineurium, and each nerve fascicle is surrounded by the perineurium. The fascicles consist of bundles of nerve fibers, and their surrounding connective tissue called the endoneurium, which includes elastic and collagen fibers.[5]

The neuron is composed of an axon surrounded by a Schwann cell. The axon allows for communication between the central nervous system (CNS) and the periphery. The Schwann cell is specific to the peripheral nervous system and produces myelin, an insulator for nerve conduction, and nerve growth factor, which enable peripheral nerves to regenerate. This is a distinguishing feature from the oligodendrocyte of the CNS because it does not provide growth factors and, thus, prevents regeneration of CNS neurons.[5]

When a nerve is transected, the distal segment of each axon will die, which is known as Wallerian degeneration. During this process, the axoplasm of the axon degenerates and the Schwann cells reuptake the myelin, leaving behind intact Schwann cells, epineurium, and endoneurium without scar or fibrosis within the distal segment. This creates a framework for the ingrowth of axons, and therefore regeneration, if the nerve were to be repaired. This contrasts with nerves that sustain crush or traction injuries, in which various segments of the nerve may be injured and scar may form, which can partially or completely inhibit regeneration. It has been classically proven that a peripheral nerve may regenerate at approximately 1 mm per day, or 1 inch per month. However, if the transection occurs too close to the cell body within the dorsal root ganglia, then a percentage of the neurons will die, regardless of repair.[5] As such, nerve recovery is imperfect and may be dependent on the patient.

Breast Anatomy

The breast is innervated by multiple sensory nerves, including the third to sixth intercostal nerves as well as the supraclavicular branches of the cervical plexus. The intercostal nerves run along the chest wall inferior to the ribs and branch laterally and medially. The lateral cutaneous branches (LCBs) become more superficial at the lateral aspect of the pectoralis major to innervate the lateral breast. The intercostal nerves continue medially to the sternum, travel superficially, and become the anterior cutaneous branches (ACB), which supply the medial breast. The dominant innervation of the NAC is the LCB of the fourth intercostal nerve, with minor contributions from the LCB of the fifth intercostal nerve and the ACB of the third and fourth intercostal nerve.[6] The dominant LCB of the fourth intercostal nerve travels through the retromammary space and then through the breast parenchyma toward the NAC, whereas the minor medial innervation from the ACB of the third and fourth intercostal nerve travels superficial to the gland toward the NAC.[7] Furthermore, the ACB of the intercostal nerves were identified in 100% of hemichests dissected in one cadaveric study.[8] The study also showed comparable axonal counts proven by histologic analysis between the lateral and ACBs of the intercostal nerves.[8]

The number of axons in an intercostal nerve is relatively consistent between patients but the size and surface area of the breast may differ greatly, further contributing to already low innervation density and decreased 2-point discrimination, especially among patients with larger breasts.[5] Of note, the superior pole is most sensitive to light pressure due to its innervation from the supraclavicular branches of the cervical plexus.[6] In addition, the NAC is most sensitive to vibration and least sensitive to light pressure.[6] Given this information, sensibility of the breast may be quantitatively assessed using perception of vibration, static pressure, and temperature.

Abdominal Anatomy

The abdominal wall is innervated by intercostal nerves from T7 to L1, including both sensory and motor nerve components. The intercostal nerves travel in the plane between the transversalis and internal oblique muscles, with motor branches traveling within and innervating the muscles, and with sensory branches traveling superficially toward the skin, often with perforating vessels.[6] In a cadaveric study of 22 hemiabdomens, 44 sensory nerves were isolated, 89% of which exited the rectus abdominis muscle fascia and 11% exiting through the external oblique fascia.[9] Of those exiting the rectus muscle fascia, 90% had an accompanying perforator. Additionally, sensory nerves were found with both the medial and lateral rows of perforators.[9]

SENSITIVITY OF MASTECTOMY SKIN FLAPS

To perform an oncologically sound mastectomy, a significant number of nerves within the breast must be transected.[10] Specifically, the lateral intercostal nerve, the dominant innervation of the NAC, runs through breast parenchyma into the NAC and will undoubtedly be disrupted during mastectomy. The anterior intercostal nerve, however, runs along the subcutaneous tissue superficial to the standard mastectomy operative plane and, therefore, has the potential to be spared without compromising oncologic integrity.[10] Despite this, most of the mastectomy skin flap becomes insensate immediately following mastectomy, with unpredictable long-term sensory recovery.

The spontaneous return of sensation in breasts with or without reconstruction (but without neurotization) has been reported. This recovery of sensation, however, was often poor and unpredictable. In one study, less than a third of patients reported good or satisfactory sensation outcomes with nonneurotized autologous reconstruction, even after up to 5 years of follow-up.[11] Another study, which included preservation of the anterior intercostal neurovascular bundles by the mastectomy surgeon, showed improved medial breast sensory preservation but still had 24% of patients report significant ongoing numbness across the breast at 1-year follow-up.[10]

Sensory recovery may also vary based on the type of mastectomy. Patients who underwent nipple-sparing mastectomy (NSMs) experienced improved light touch sensibility when compared with skin-sparing mastectomy (SSM) patients. Additionally, patients who underwent SSM were more likely to report significant loss of pleasurable sensation when compared with patients who underwent NSM. One consideration is that most of NSM procedures were offered to patients undergoing prophylactic mastectomies for genetic mutations, potentially leading to a less aggressive mastectomy resection. However, even within a prophylactic mastectomy cohort, the NSM patients still had improved preservation of light touch sensation, although there was an equivalent loss in temperature sensation for NSM and SSM patients.[10]

INDICATIONS

Neurotization may be safely attempted in all patients, regardless of comorbidity, cancer diagnosis, or type of reconstruction. There are no current contraindications for neurotization. The most likely reason for the inability to perform neurotization is patient anatomy.

Further, neurotization and its possible outcomes should be discussed with patients in the preoperative setting. The potential sensation preservation may vary based on mastectomy type, by general surgeon, and by preoperative breast sensation. The importance of breast and NAC sensation may not be the same in each patient, either. Interestingly, changes in breast sensation are not frequently discussed with patients who plan to undergo mastectomy procedures.[2] This further emphasizes why surgeons need to include a discussion about breast sensation and sensation recovery as an important aspect of the greater goals of care discussion.

NERVE COAPTATION

Peripheral nerve surgery has seen significant advances since its introduction in the 1870s, particularly due to the development and improvement of microsurgical techniques as well as the increased comprehension of nerve pathophysiology.[12] As such, nerve coaptation has been demonstrated to be effective in both laboratory and clinical settings and is well described in the literature, including within hand surgery, for facial reanimation, and the sensate radial forearm flap.

Nerve coaptation may be performed using a variety of techniques, including primary coaptation, autograft, allograft, and nerve conduits, with the goal being a tension-free repair (Table 1). Nerve transfers and end-to-side nerve grafting are also possible but will not be discussed as they are not relevant for breast neurotization. For functional nerve repair, such as with nerve transection after penetrating injuries in the upper extremity, primary nerve repair produces the best outcomes and, therefore, is the primary method of repair when possible. However, if a small gap exists or if there is different nerve fascicle anatomy between the

Table 1 Nerve coaptation recommendations by gap size	
Nerve Gap	Connector
None	Nerve connector
>1 cm	Nerve connector
1–3 cm	Nerve conduit (PGD tube)
3–5 cm	Autograft/allograft
>5 cm	Allograft

nerve ends, then the superiority of direct coaptation becomes unclear. Additionally, if unable to produce a direct nerve repair without tension, an autograft is considered the gold standard of management, although the disadvantages include donor site morbidity and increased operative time for graft harvest. For breast reconstruction, small autografts of 3 to 4 cm may be easily harvested from the abdomen due to its segmental nerve supply, although this is less common due to the presence of viable alternatives. Next, studies have shown that nerve conduit success is maximized with small diameter sensory nerves, gaps less than 3 cm, and when used as a nerve repair wrap, although outcomes were variable. Finally, the use of nerve allografts was previously limited due to the need for systemic immunosuppression.[12] Today, advancements in tissue processing methods have created the ability to use nerve allograft material without immunosuppression, with Avance Nerve Graft (Axogen, Inc., Alachua, FL) demonstrating an 82% meaningful recovery in sensory, mixed, and motor nerve gaps of up to 70 mm.[13]

EVALUATION OF SENSORY PERCEPTION

Although there are more and more publications on neurotization for breast reconstruction, there is significant heterogeneity regarding the methodology. First, some studies measured breast sensation by breast quadrant while others measured using 9 points across the breast, with variable inclusion of the nipple and areola depending on mastectomy type.[14–16] In addition, the presence and type of control varied, from the native breast to preoperative sensation to nonneurotized reconstructions, again making comparisons between studies more difficult.

Furthermore, sensory modalities were inconsistent between studies. Vibratory stimuli were commonly evaluated using a tuning fork and temperature sensation was tested using hot and cold metal rods.[14,17] Some studies even used 2-point discrimination, despite the known poor 2-point discrimination of breast skin at baseline.[16] Pressure sensation was commonly tested using the Semmes-Weinstein monofilament test, which uses small, calibrated filaments applied to the skin, which bend when a force is applied (g), representing an estimate of the range of pressure sensation threshold (gram per square millimeter).[17] This modality is criticized for its inability to provide sensation measurements in a continuous fashion but rather in an estimated logarithmic value, which may be inconsistent and subject to variation among examiners.[5,17,18]

Another mechanism to evaluate sensitivity to touch is the pressure-specified sensory device (PSSD), which is a computer-assisted instrument that uses a hemispheric probe attached to a force transducer that permits continuous measurements of cutaneous pressure sensation.[17] This device has a high sensitivity and specificity and is likely the most consistent means of evaluating cutaneous sensation.[18] Furthermore, the PSSD has the potential to measure moving-touch threshold in addition to static touch. Although very few studies cited in this article used the PSSD, the authors suspect that this device will help establish standardization of sensory testing and enable a more homogenous data that can be used to obtain strong, valid, and conclusive evidence regarding neurotization.

NEUROTIZATION IN AUTOLOGOUS RECONSTRUCTION

Autologous reconstruction is advantageous when it comes to neurotization because it allows for the possibility of donor nerves. As discussed, neurotization for breast reconstruction was first published using TRAM flaps in the early 1990s. Since then, deep inferior epigastric perforator (DIEP) flaps have overtaken TRAM flaps as the workhorse flap in breast reconstruction. Abdominally based flaps have therefore been the most studied flap for breast neurotization and will be the focus for this section.

Abdominally Based Flap Techniques

There has been significant discussion regarding the ideal recipient nerve for breast neurotization. One option is the lateral branch of the fourth intercostal nerve.[19] The advantage is that this is the primary sensory innervation for the NAC. The disadvantages include the lateral location, which creates a second microsurgery field and a second point of attachment possibly limiting flap mobility and must be preserved by the general surgeon during the mastectomy. Additionally, the length of donor nerve may not be able to reach the lateral branch, requiring allograft and inhibiting flap manipulation.[20]

The other main option for the recipient nerve is the anterior branch of the third intercostal nerve.[19] It is within the same microsurgery field and can be done in conjunction with the standard recipient vessels dissection.[20] Consequently, it may require less donor nerve length for a primary coaptation. One potential disadvantage is that the anterior branch may be intact following mastectomy, meaning its transection may further decrease mastectomy skin flap sensation. However, the anterior branch may be transected during vessel dissection regardless of preservation during mastectomy.

Furthermore, the orientation of flap inset may further contribute to recipient nerve decision-making. Using the contralateral flap may produce a smaller gap between the donor nerve and lateral branch, although this does not change the need for 2 microsurgery fields.

Regarding the donor nerves, the abdominal intercostal nerves are identified during dissection of the perforators. The donor nerves are typically at levels T10 to T12.[19] The sensory branches of the abdominal intercostal nerves often run alongside the perforators and can be traced back to where they join the motor branches. Both medial and lateral perforator rows may have an associated sensory nerve, although some investigators have expressed concern with lateral row nerves due to the theoretic risk of harming the motor branch of the nerve and having an increased risk for posterolateral muscle denervation.[19]

The senior author's technique for DIEP flap breast reconstruction with neurotization includes the use of the anterior branch of the third intercostal nerve, which is dissected out carefully during dissection of the internal mammary vessels. In order to do so, the pectoralis major overlying the third intercostal space is excised using Bovie electrocautery. Once visible, the intercostal muscles are carefully dissected from lateral to medial using bipolar electrocautery. During this dissection, the anterior branch of the third intercostal nerve is typically identified running along the third rib, then superficially across the internal mammary vessels toward the sternum, making it easily dissected and prepared for nerve coaptation. Furthermore, this trajectory also means that this nerve branch would need to be transected in order to adequately dissect the internal mammary vessels. As such, the advantages of senior author's technique are 2-fold in identifying a nerve that would already be sacrificed and, instead, using it for neurotization within the same microsurgical field.

In order to minimize the nerve gap, the senior author also uses the ipsilateral DIEP flap, with a donor nerve identified during abdominal perforator dissection. The nerve coaptation is frequently performed as described in the literature with an end-to-end coaptation with 1 or 2 epineural sutures using 8-0 or 9-0 nylon, with intermittent use of a nerve conduit.[14]

Neurotization Alternatives in Autologous Reconstruction

Patients may not be good candidates for abdominally based autologous breast reconstruction for a variety of reasons but they still may receive breast neurotization using alternative flaps. For these flaps, the options for recipient nerves remain the same. First, a latissimus dorsi flap also has the potential for neurotization using an intercostal perforator nerve or the thoracodorsal nerve.[19] Similar to the abdominal donor nerves, the latissimus dorsi nerves were found to be associated with the vasculature.[19] The superior gluteal artery perforator (SGAP) flap may be sensate using the dorsal branches of the lumbar segmental nerves, which perforate the deep fascia just above the iliac crest and lateral to the posterior superior iliac spine and often accompany small vessels at the superior edge of the flap.[19] Finally, the inferior gluteal artery perforator flap uses a branch of the posterior cutaneous femoral nerve. The posterior cutaneous femoral nerve splits proximally into 3 segments, the medial branch for perineal sensation, the lateral branch for posterior thigh sensation, and the intermedius branch, which travels into the flap.[19]

Outcomes

Multiple studies have concluded that innervated autologous flaps for breast reconstruction have both a greater magnitude as well as earlier sensory recovery compared with noninnervated autologous flaps.[17,18] Neurotization during reconstruction also increased the chance of erogenous sensation recovery.[2] Importantly, breast neurotization not only shows improved clinical outcomes but it is associated with improved patient-reported outcomes.[18]

However, not all innervated autologous flaps result in equivalent sensory recovery. Studies have shown that sensory recovery is the greatest for innervated DIEP flaps, then free TRAM flaps, pedicled TRAM flaps, and latissimus dorsi flaps, in that order.[11,17] It is theorized that the difference in flap sensory recovery is correlated with the increased innervation density of the abdomen compared with the back.[17] Furthermore, SGAP flaps were also shown to have better, more rapid recovery of sensation with innervated flaps when compared with noninnervated flaps, although the sample size in the study was small.[17]

In general, across studies, neurotized DIEP flaps resulted in improved static and moving sensation, with up to 50% greater light pressure and touch discrimination sensation when compared with noninnervated DIEP flaps. Neurotized DIEP flaps also showed protective sensation at 1 year postoperatively, whereas noninnervated flaps did not recover protective sensation by the time of their last follow-up visit.[14,21] Additionally, neurotization resulted in sensation recovery at 6 months compared with 9 to 12 months for nonneurotized DIEP flaps.[14,21] A recent prospective cohort study by Beugels and colleagues in 2021 showed innervated DIEP flaps had significantly lower mean monofilament values at the native skin, flap skin, and total skin compared with noninnervated DIEP flaps.[21] Importantly, Magarakis and colleagues used the PSSD device to evaluate neurotized DIEP flaps and found improved static and moving sensation when compared with nonneurotized DIEP flaps.[22] Similarly, neurotized TRAM flaps resulted in earlier recovery of tactile and temperature sensation, as well as statistically significantly improved pressure thresholds and temperature discrimination compared with noninnervated TRAM flaps.[14,16]

Breast neurotization studies have also examined the sensation outcomes using different coaptation techniques, including primary coaptation, allografts, and nerve conduits. The literature regarding autologous neurotization frequently describes end-to-end primary nerve coaptation techniques. However, between 2015 and 2019, most reported breast neurotizations were with synthetic nerve conduit (62.9%) or allograft (27.5%), compared with direct coaptation (1.3%).[4] Momeni and colleagues showed that neurotization with allograft was associated with a greater likelihood for return of protective sensation. Out of 9 regions of the breast tested for sensory recovery, 55% of innervated flaps had sensory recovery in 5 to 9 zones compared with only 7% in the noninnervated flaps. Furthermore, only 27% of innervated flaps had sensory recovery in 0 to 1 region, compared with 64% in the noninnervated group at 1 year.[23] Furthermore, Spiegel and colleagues studied the outcomes of nerve conduit versus primary coaptation with neurotized DIEP flaps and found that nerve conduits produced statistically significantly better sensibility than direct coaptation.[15]

For both nerve conduits and nerve allografts, the potential advantages include the avoidance of dissecting and sacrificing large segments of abdominal donor nerves, which may be time-consuming, difficult, and morbid.[24] Regarding nerve conduits, advantages may include improved sensory outcomes compared with direct repair, although disadvantages include high cost and length restrictions. Next, the advantages of nerve allografts also include the option for different graft lengths and sizes and the opportunity to use the lateral intercostal nerve as a recipient nerve. Potential disadvantages to nerve allograft include high cost, decreased efficacy with longer grafts, and the presence of a foreign body.[23,24]

Factors related to sensory recovery in breast reconstruction have also been investigated. Higher patient age, neoadjuvant or adjuvant chemotherapy, and higher flap weights were negatively associated with sensory recovery.[21] Higher patient age and chemotherapeutic agents both likely decrease the capacity of the nerves to regenerate. Greater flap weights likely correlate with a lower density of nerves and, therefore, decreased sensation. Interestingly, a history of radiation was not significantly associated with worse sensory recovery, although this may be related to the excision of radiated mastectomy skin in favor of flap skin.[21] Another important factor in sensory recovery is if the reconstruction is performed in an immediate or delayed fashion. It has also been shown that immediate reconstruction results in improved mastectomy skin flap sensory recovery in addition to improved recovery of flap skin sensation, whereas delayed reconstruction only showed a significant sensation improvement in flap skin.[21]

It is important to objectively assess the impact of neurotization on the sensory recovery of the breast but it is also vital to evaluate how this affects the patient, their satisfaction, and their quality of life. Neurotization has been significantly associated with improved patient-reported outcomes, including patient satisfaction scores.[18] The most thorough of these studies was performed by Temple and colleagues, which investigated patient-rated quality of life outcomes related to TRAM flap innervation.[25] Patients with innervated TRAM reconstruction reported statistically significant improvements in physical, social, emotional, and functional well-being, as well as quality in life when compared with patients with noninnervated TRAM flaps using the Functional Assessment of Cancer Therapy Breast validated survey.[25] Of note, current validated surveys are imperfect methods for assessing improvements related to innervation, primarily related to the paucity of questions specifically related to sensation.

Despite the abundance of data suggesting successful outcomes with breast neurotization, it remains difficult to form definitive conclusions due to the significant heterogeneity between study techniques and methodologies.

NIPPLE–AREOLA COMPLEX NEUROTIZATION AND IMPLANT-BASED RECONSTRUCTION

As established, mastectomy skin flap sensation recovery may be spontaneous but it is also variable, diminished, and delayed. Specifically with implant-based subpectoral reconstruction, this remains true with significantly impaired sensation of touch, cold, warmth, and heat pain when compared with the untreated contralateral breast.[26] In fact, implant-based reconstruction may be associated with worse sensory outcomes than primary closure without reconstruction.[27] In addition, using the PSSD device, Magarakis and colleagues showed that patients with irradiated implants had statistically significantly worse static and moving sensation of the breast than patients with nonirradiated implants. Immediate reconstruction with implant also resulted in improved static and moving sensation when compared with delayed or staged reconstruction with implants.[22]

Regarding neurotized implant-based reconstruction, the lack of autologous donor nerves leaves allograft as the only option for reestablishing sensation in the mastectomy skin flaps, with the retroareolar nerve stumps as the primary target available. Peled and colleagues studied women with NSM with direct to implant, prepectoral reconstruction with allograft coaptation from T4 or T5 lateral intercostal nerves to subareolar nerves.[28] Notably, a biopsy of the subareolar tissue that confirmed the presence of neural elements using S-100 staining. Results showed preserved 2-point discrimination in 87% of breasts, with intact sensation to light touch over most of the reconstructed breast in all patients.[28] Additionally, Djohan and colleagues performed implant-based reconstruction with allograft coaptation between the anterior branch of the lateral fourth intercostal nerve and the subareolar dermis. The PSSD device was used to measure sensory recovery and found neurotized breasts had better thresholds in 6 of 8 breast areas when compared with nonneurotized breasts.[24]

The increasing ability to perform nipple-sparing mastectomies means increased opportunities for reinnervation of the NAC itself. Although neurotized implant-based reconstruction generally involves NAC neurotization, there have also been studies involving NAC neurotization with autologous reconstruction. First, Tevlin and colleagues identified, dissected, and preserved the lateral intercostal nerves, which was then coapted to a nerve graft and tunneled through the autologous abdominal flap, ultimately performing a neurorrhaphy to the NAC nerve stumps or dermis at the base of the NAC.[29] Using this technique, the authors found significant improvement in sensation of the whole breast and no statistically significant difference in preoperative versus postoperative nipple sensation at final follow-up, indicating excellent sensory recovery. In addition, compared with nontreated breasts, the treated breasts had significantly increased areolar sensation. Interestingly,

there was no statistically significant difference in sensory recovery between nerve grafts that were less than 5 cm and nerve grafts that were greater than or equal to 7 cm.[29]

With many breast reconstruction patients undergoing implant-based reconstruction and the increased incidence of nipple-sparing mastectomies, surgeons must continue to investigate techniques such as neurotization that may improve sensory recovery as well as patient outcomes. Neurotization within implant-based reconstruction and for NAC sensation has promising results based on these studies and remains an interesting avenue for future studies.

SAFETY AND COMPLICATIONS

In review of ACS-NSQIP national data between 2015 and 2019, when controlling for other variables such as patient comorbidities and operative characteristics, neurotization does not increase 30-day complication rates or 30-day readmission rates. Neurotization neither increased the risk of unplanned reoperations nor was it associated with a prolonged hospital stay.[4]

Analysis of this national data also found an increase in the average operating time with neurotization but this did not include timing breakdowns.[4] In contrast, multiple studies reported operative time required for neurotization and found that nerve coaptation adds between 8 and 38 minutes per nerve.[18,21,30] Similarly, a more recent article noted unilateral abdominally based free flaps between 2016 and 2018 at a single institution with neurotization took 467 minutes on average compared with 455 minutes on average without neurotization, with the conclusion that neurotization does not statistically significantly increase operative time.[20]

In addition, no studies reported neuromas or other complications directly related to neurotization.[21] The literature has shown that neurotization in breast reconstruction is a safe procedure, relatively fast and simple for a microsurgeon, and without significant donor or recipient site morbidity.[2]

FUTURE DIRECTIONS

To ingratiate neurotization into the breast reconstruction standard of care, more standardized, prospective, and randomized studies must be performed. Specifically, standardization among testing modalities would strengthen future research outcomes, in addition to a preference for computer-assisted pressure-specified sensory devices such as the PSSD device. Additionally, to avoid bias, functional MRI presents an objective way to test sensation, although likely both expensive and time intensive. Promising future avenues also include large data sets on operative techniques including types of coaptation, as well as how mastectomy pattern and flap thickness affect sensation recovery. Perhaps, the greatest potential lies with patient-reported outcome surveys, which must also be standardized and updated to include more pointed investigation regarding sensation and its complexities.

SUMMARY

Absent or diminished breast sensation is a persistent problem for many patients, where lack of basic protective sensation can cause susceptibility to burns. Breast neurotization is an opportunity to improve sensory outcomes, which are poor and unpredictable if left to chance. Several techniques for autologous and implant reconstruction have been described with successful outcomes in clinical sensation testing as well as patient quality of life reports. Neurotization is a safe procedure with minimal risk for morbidity and it presents a tremendous opportunity for future research to advance breast reconstruction outcomes.

CLINICS CARE POINTS

- Recipient nerves for neurotization primarily include the LCB of the fourth intercostal nerve and the ACB of the third intercostal nerve.
- Innervated autologous flaps for breast reconstruction have both a greater magnitude as well as earlier sensory recovery compared with noninnervated autologous flaps.
- Neurotization has been significantly associated with improved patient-reported outcomes, including patient satisfaction scores.
- No studies have reported neuromas or other complications directly related to neurotization.

REFERENCES

1. Admoun C, Mayrovitz H. Choosing mastectomy vs. Lumpectomy-With-Radiation: experiences of breast cancer Survivors. Cureus 2021;13(10):e18433. https://doi.org/10.7759/cureus.18433.
2. Hamilton KL, Kania KE, Spiegel AJ. Post-mastectomy sensory recovery and restoration. Gland Surg 2021; 10(1):494–7. https://doi.org/10.21037/gs.2020.03. 22.
3. Slezak S, McGibbon B, Dellon A. The sensational transverse rectus abdominis Musculocutaneous (TRAM) flap: return of sensibility after TRAM breast reconstruction. Ann Plast Surg 1992;28(3):210–7.
4. Laikhter E, Shiah E, Manstein SM, et al. Trends and characteristics of neurotization during breast reconstruction: perioperative outcomes using the American College of surgeons national Surgical quality improvement Program (ACS-NSQIP). J Plast Surg Hand Surg 2021;1–7. https://doi.org/10.1080/2000656X.2021.1973484.
5. Dellon A. Somatosensory testing and Rehabilitation. Institute for Peripheral Nerve Surgery; 2000.
6. Buck D II. Breast anatomy, Embryology, and Congenital Defects. Review of Plastic surgery. Elsevier; 2016. p. 73–7.
7. Sarhadi N, Shaw-Dunn J, Soutar D. Nerve supply of the breast with special reference to the nipple and areola: Sir Astley Cooper Revisited. Clin Anat 1997;10:283–8.
8. Mohan AT, Suchyta M, Vyas KS, et al. A cadaveric Anatomical and histological study of recipient intercostal nerve Selection for sensory reinnervation in autologous breast reconstruction. J Reconstr Microsurg 2021;37(2):136–42. https://doi.org/10.1055/s-0040-1715878.
9. Cakmakoglu C, Knackstedt R, Gatherwright J, et al. Determining the precise anatomic location of the sensory nerves to the abdominal wall: Optimizing autologous innervation of abdominally based free flaps. J Plast Reconstr Aesthet Surg 2021;74(3): 641–3. https://doi.org/10.1016/j.bjps.2020.11.019.
10. Khan A, Zhang J, Sollazzo V, et al. Sensory change of the reconstructed breast envelope after skin-sparing mastectomy. Eur J Surg Oncol 2016;42(7): 973–9. https://doi.org/10.1016/j.ejso.2016.03.018.
11. Blondeel PN, Demuynck M, Mete D, et al. Sensory nerve repair in perforator flaps for autologous breast reconstruction: sensational or senseless? Br J Plast Surg 1999;52:37–44.
12. Ray WZ, Mackinnon SE. Management of nerve gaps: autografts, allografts, nerve transfers, and end-to-side neurorrhaphy. Exp Neurol 2010;223(1): 77–85. https://doi.org/10.1016/j.expneurol.2009.03. 031.
13. Safa B, Jain S, Desai MJ, et al. Peripheral nerve repair throughout the body with processed nerve allografts: results from a large multicenter study. Microsurgery 2020;40(5):527–37. https://doi.org/10. 1002/micr.30574.
14. Vartanian ED, Lo AY, Hershenhouse KS, et al. The role of neurotization in autologous breast reconstruction: can reconstruction restore breast sensation? J Surg Oncol 2021;123(5):1215–31. https://doi.org/10.1002/jso.26422.

15. Spiegel AJ, Menn ZK, Eldor L, et al. Breast reinnervation: DIEP neurotization using the third anterior intercostal nerve. *Plast Reconstr Surg Glob open* 2013;1(8):e72. https://doi.org/10.1097/GOX.0000000000000008.

16. Temple CL, Tse R, Bettger-Hahn M, et al. Sensibility following innervated free TRAM flap for breast reconstruction. Plast Reconstr Surg 2006;117(7): 2119–27. https://doi.org/10.1097/01.prs.0000218268.59024.cc. discussion 2128-30.

17. Shridharani SM, Magarakis M, Stapleton SM, et al. Breast sensation after breast reconstruction: a systematic review. J Reconstr Microsurg 2010;26(5): 303–10. https://doi.org/10.1055/s-0030-1249313.

18. Weissler JM, Koltz PF, Carney MJ, et al. Sifting through the evidence: a comprehensive review and analysis of neurotization in breast reconstruction. Plast Reconstr Surg 2018;141(3):550–65. https://doi.org/10.1097/PRS.0000000000004108.

19. Gatherwright J, Knackstedt R, Djohan R. Anatomic targets for breast reconstruction neurotization: Past results and future Possibilities. Ann Plast Surg 2019;82(2):207–12. https://doi.org/10.1097/SAP.0000000000001733.

20. Xia TY, Scomacao I, Djohan R, et al. Neurotization does not Prolong operative time in free flap breast reconstruction. Aesthet Plast Surg 2022. https://doi.org/10.1007/s00266-022-02833-7.

21. Beugels J, Bijkerk E, Lataster A, et al. Nerve coaptation improves the sensory recovery of the breast in DIEP flap breast reconstruction. Plast Reconstr Surg 2021;148(2):273–84. https://doi.org/10.1097/PRS.0000000000008160.

22. Magarakis M, Venkat R, Dellon AL, et al. Pilot study of breast sensation after breast reconstruction: evaluating the effects of radiation therapy and perforator flap neurotization on sensory recovery. Microsurgery 2013; 33(6):421–31. https://doi.org/10.1002/micr.22124.

23. Momeni A, Meyer S, Shefren K, et al. Flap neurotization in breast reconstruction with nerve allografts: 1-year clinical outcomes. Plast Reconstr Surg Glob Open 2021;9(1):e3328. https://doi.org/10.1097/GOX.0000000000003328.

24. Djohan R, Scomacao I, Knackstedt R, et al. Neurotization of the nipple-areola complex during implant-based reconstruction: Evaluation of early sensation recovery. Plast Reconstr Surg 2020;146(2):250–4. https://doi.org/10.1097/PRS.0000000000006976.

25. Temple CLF, Ross DC, Kim S, et al. Sensibility following innervated free TRAM flap for breast reconstruction: Part II. Innervation improves patient-rated quality of life. Plast Reconstr Surg 2009;124(5):1419–25. https://doi.org/10.1097/PRS.0b013e3181b98963.

26. Lagergren J, Edsander-Nord A, Wickman M, et al. Long-term sensibility following Nonautologous, immediate breast reconstruction. Breast J 2007; 13(4):346–51.

27. Bijkerk E, van Kuijk SMJ, Beugels J, et al. Breast sensibility after mastectomy and implant-based breast reconstruction. Breast Cancer Res Treat 2019;175(2):369–78. https://doi.org/10.1007/s10549-019-05137-8.

28. Peled AW, Peled ZM. Nerve preservation and allografting for sensory innervation following immediate implant breast reconstruction. Plast Reconstr Surg Glob Open 2019;7(7):e2332. https://doi.org/10.1097/GOX.0000000000002332.

29. Tevlin R, Brazio P, Tran N, et al. Immediate targeted nipple-areolar complex re-innervation: Improving outcomes in immediate autologous breast reconstruction. J Plast Reconstr Aesthet Surg 2021; 74(7):1503–7. https://doi.org/10.1016/j.bjps.2020.11.021.

30. Spiegel AJ, Salazar-Reyes H, Izaddoost S, et al. A Novel method for neurotization of deep inferior epigastric perforator and superficial inferior epigastric artery flaps. Plast Reconstr Surg 2009;123(1): 29e–30e. https://doi.org/10.1097/PRS.0b013e318194d257.

Modern Innovations in Breast Surgery: Robotic Breast Surgery and Robotic Breast Reconstruction

Katie G. Egan, MD, Jesse C. Selber, MD, MPH, MHCM*

KEYWORDS

- Robotic microsurgery • Robotic breast reconstruction • Robotic nipple-sparing mastectomy
- Robotic mastectomy • Robotic latissimus flap • Robotic deep inferior epigastric flap • Robodiep

KEY POINTS

- Although there is a learning curve for robotic nipple-sparing mastectomy, this option may decrease nipple-areolar complex necrosis and mastectomy skin flap necrosis compared with traditional nipple-sparing mastectomy.
- Robotic nipple-sparing mastectomy can be combined with either subcutaneous, prepectoral with acellular dermal matrix, or submuscular alloplastic reconstruction as well as autologous reconstruction.
- Robotic harvest of deep inferior epigastric flap pedicle and latissimus muscle flaps is safe and decreases donor site morbidity.
- Robotic microanastomosis in autologous breast reconstruction and lymphedema surgery may provide improved precision through motion scaling and tremor elimination and improved ergonomics compared with traditional microsurgery.

HISTORY

A "robot" was first defined in 1979 by the National Bureau of Standards and the Robot Institute of America as "a reprogrammable, multifunctional manipulator designed to move materials, parts, tools, or specialized devices through various programmed motions for the performance of a variety of tasks."[1] The first robot adapted for use in surgery, the programmable universal machine for assembly 200 (PUMA) was developed by Stanford researcher Victor Scheinman for General Motors in 1978.[2] The PUMA200 consisted of a single arm and computer control monitor. This would go on to be used by a group of radiologists at Memorial Medical Center in Long Beach, California for use in CT-guided brain tumor biopsies.[3] The success of this group encouraged translation in the urology field for the use of the PUMA in prostatectomies in the late 1980s.[4] However, early applications were constrained to fixed targets due to the limitations of an immobile arm.

Government-funded research on robotic applications in surgery was spurred by an initiative to send a human to Mars announced in 1989 by former president George H.W. Bush as well as interest by the US Department of Defense in providing remote wartime medical assistance. NASA began researching applications of remotely controlled surgical instruments to perform emergency surgical procedures on astronauts.[5] Early ideas for robotically controlled surgical gloves evolved to robotic arms.[5] Robotic technology and applications have continued to evolve since the birth of robotics. Modern robotic technology now allows for precise surgical

The University of Texas M.D. Anderson Cancer Center, 1400 Pressler St., Unit 1488, Houston, TX 77030, USA
* Corresponding author.
E-mail address: jessemd4@gmail.com

Clin Plastic Surg 50 (2023) 357–366
https://doi.org/10.1016/j.cps.2022.11.004

control in dynamic environments, allowing for an ever-growing number of applications of this technology.

Robotic technology was applied in the setting of prophylactic nipple-sparing mastectomy (NSM) for breast cancer gene (BRCA) patients in 2016.[6,7] Although criticized for having a steep learning curve, robotic NSM is now regarded as a viable option, which may improve patient outcomes.[8,9] Improved visualization and ergonomics were reported as early advantages of robotic NSM.[6] Robotic NSM has been shown to have superior outcomes in terms of overall complication rates, wound healing complications, and nipple necrosis rates, likely due to decreased traction on the skin and remote incision placement.[6,7,9–11] Patient satisfaction and esthetic outcomes have also been shown to be high with robotic mastectomy, and oncologic safety data are promising.[9,12]

Consensus statements regarding robotic NSM were developed by the Expert Panel from International Endoscopic and Robotic Breast Surgery Symposium in 2019.[13] A summary of their recommendations includes:

- Indications for robotic NSM include:
  - Prophylactic mastectomies
  - Small breast size with Stage II or less tumor (up to 5 cm) and adequate skin-tumor distance on preoperative imaging
  - Stage IIIA tumors with adequate response to neoadjuvant therapy
  - No skin involvement
- Contraindications for robotic NSM include:
  - Large or ptotic breasts due to technical difficulty (relative contraindication)
  - High-anesthetic risk patients (relative contraindication)
  - Pectoralis muscle or chest wall invasion
  - Inflammatory breast cancer
  - Nipple-areolar complex involvement
- Technical considerations:
  - Recommended incision placement is anterior axillary line at the level of the nipple-areolar complex
  - Recommended skin flap development pre-docking with blunt tunneling with scissors and post-docking dissection with monopolar scissors
  - Recommend intraoperative sub-nipple frozen biopsies
  - Standard postoperative drainage

- In the United States, there is currently a multi-center Investigational Device Exemption trial sponsored by Intuitive Surgical in collaboration with the Food and Drug Administration (FDA) to achieve an FDA-approved indication for the Da Vinci robot for robotic NSM.[a] End points include 30-day complications, conversion to open technique, adverse events related to the device, and reconstructive complications. Approval is anticipated.

CURRENT APPLICATIONS OF ROBOTICS IN BREAST RECONSTRUCTION
Alloplastic Reconstruction Following Nipple-Sparing Mastectomy

Background

Immediate reconstruction of the breast may be completed with either autologous tissue or alloplastic devices following robotic NSM.

Patient positioning and robot setup

The patient remains in supine for the duration of the procedure. Placement of the ipsilateral arm over the head is the preferred position for robotic mastectomy and implant-based reconstruction.[13] Alternatively, the arm can be abducted to 90° and secured on an arm board. The robot (da Vinci Surgical System, Intuitive Surgical, Sunnyvale, CA) is positioned at the patient's head. Tumescence solution with epinephrine may be infiltrated into the breast before mastectomy to assist with hemostasis and visualization.[7,11,14] Blue dye may be injected using a hypodermic needle at the borders of the breast to prevent over dissection.[15] A 4 to 4.5 cm incision is made at the anterior axillary line to allow access for both the mastectomy and reconstruction. Our preference is to place this incision at the level of the nipple-areolar complex to allow for unobstructed rotation of the robot with the arm secured on an arm board, whereas more superior incision placement in the axilla can place the arm at risk of injury from the robot (**Fig. 1**). Mastectomy is completed using a single port and 8 mm Hg of insufflation.[6,16] Insufflation allows for uniform doming of the skin without the use of external retractors (**Fig. 2**). The breast tissue is raised first off of the pectoralis muscle, followed by anterior dissection, to allow for easier identification of the end point of superficial dissection.[15]

---

[a]Institutions participating in the multicenter Investigational Device Exemption Trial for Nipple Sparing Mastectomy include: University of Texas M.D. Anderson Cancer Center, University of Pennsylvania, Northwell Health, Mayo Clinic Rochester, NorthShore University Health System, and Mayo Clinic Florida.

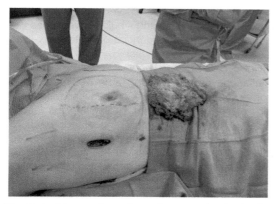

Fig. 1. Incision and specimen from a robotic nipple-sparing mastectomy.

Operative technique

Following completion of the mastectomy, reconstruction may be completed in either a prepectoral or subpectoral plane. Subpectoral reconstruction proceeds with the development of the subpectoral plane through direct visualization from the lateral chest wall incision. The single-port system is then reintroduced, and insufflation commences. The subpectoral plane is then developed using monopolar scissors. The robot is then undocked and removed. Partial serratus may be elevated under direct visualization for a complete submuscular pocket. A silicone implant sizer is then placed to verify pocket dissection. If pocket revisions are necessary, these may be completed using a lighted surgical light emitting diode (LED) retractor (OBP Surgical, Lawrence, MA). The field is the re-prepped, and the silicone implant is placed. The muscle is then reapproximated with sutures using a lighted retractor. Irrigation is performed, and two drains are placed before skin closure.

Subcutaneous implant placement is also possible given the remote incision location if adequate mastectomy flap thickness is preserved. Alternatively, placement of acellular dermal matrix using robotic techniques has been described and is our preferred technique.[17] An implant sizer is placed in the subcutaneous plane, and the implant borders are marked externally on the skin surface to be used as landmarks (Fig. 3). Acellular dermal matrix is then trimmed to the appropriate size and contour on the back table for the chosen implant. If a tissue expander has been chosen, it is then placed into the pocket and the robot is used to secure the tabs. The expander is filled with air to the desired volume (Fig. 4). Acellular dermal matrix is then introduced into the mastectomy pocket and draped over the expander. The robot is then reintroduced, and external skin markings are

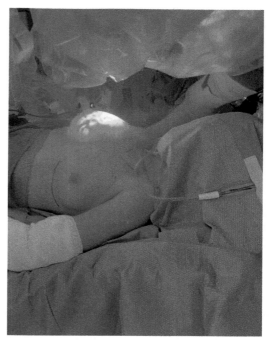

Fig. 2. Robot setup and patient positioning for nipple-sparing mastectomy are shown. The breast is transilluminated which aids with dissection.

palpated by an assistant to guide robotic suturing of the acellular dermal matrix into the appropriate position using a parachute method. Alternatively, for direct-to-implant reconstruction, the acellular dermal matrix is secured into the appropriate position in the pocket first using robot-assisted sutures medially, superiorly, and laterally. The implant is then inserted followed by completion of suturing of the lateral border of the acellular dermal matrix under direct visualization. Pocket control and suturing of the internal mammary fold may also be completed with the robot.

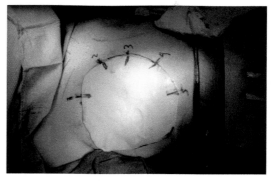

Fig. 3. Acellular dermal matrix inset is planned before insertion.

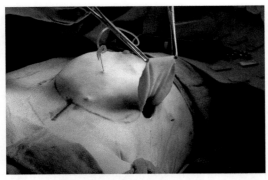

Fig. 4. Tissue expander is place into the mastectomy pocket and inflated to the desired fill volume with air. Acellular dermal matrix (ADM) is draped over the expander and secured in place using the robot using a parachute method.

Robotic Deep Inferior Epigastric Perforator Flap Harvest

Background

As autologous breast reconstruction, with the abdominal donor site as the workhorse, has become the gold standard, efforts have long been directed at reducing donor site morbidity. The evolution of muscle preserving techniques, culminating with the deep inferior epigastric perforator (DIEP) flap, has helped to decrease abdominal wall complications to some extent. However, hernia and bulge remain a concern, with rates of abdominal wall weakness of up to 20% being reported after DIEP flap harvest (**Fig. 5**).[18–22] Although flap dissection using the lateral row perforators results in lower incidences of fat necrosis and a more expedient flap harvest due to a shorter

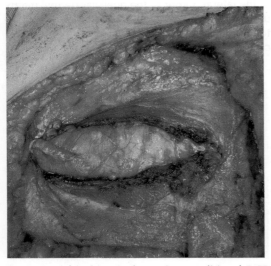

Fig. 5. Fascial incision is shown in a traditional DIEP flap harvest.

intramuscular course compared with medial row perforators, hernia and bulge weakness is increased due to the sacrifice of motor nerves to the rectus abdominis muscle.[21,23–26]

Robotic DIEP flap harvest overcomes these challenges by allowing for rapid pedicle harvest from a submuscular approach, allowing for all motor nerves to be spared while limiting the fascial incision. A robotic, intraperitoneal approach to the DIEP flap pedicle harvest was first described by Gundlapalli and colleagues.[27] Initial reports by several centers have been promising for excellent outcomes using the robotic approach to DIEP flap harvest, with no flap losses, intra-abdominal complications, or postoperative hernia/bulge having yet been reported in the literature.[28–31] We recently reported the largest series of intraperitoneal robotic DIEPs to date with no microvascular complications and subjectively improved donor site discomfort.[29] Currently, four major US centers are performing intraperitoneal robotic DIEPS nationally, including MD Anderson, Northwell Health, University of Pittsburgh, and Cleveland Clinic. Other minimally invasive approaches including laparoscopic and extraperitoneal approaches have also been explored with more limited adoption.

Preoperative planning

Preoperative imaging is mandatory for planning for robotic DIEP flap harvest. A computed tomography angiography or magnetic resonance angiography may be performed at the preference of the surgeon. Perforators are identified on imaging. Patients with a single-dominant perforator or two closely grouped perforators with a short intramuscular course are considered candidates for robotic DIEP flap harvest. If multiple perforators or rows are required for harvest, an open approach is used. After identifying target perforators, intramuscular course is determined. A lateral row perforator is selected if possible for a shorter intramuscular course. The intramuscular course is measured and subtracted from the total pedicle length to the external iliac origin to determine the benefit of spared fascial incision length (**Fig. 6**).[32] In appropriate candidates, an average of 9.1 cm of fascial incision benefit has been reported on imaging studies.[33] An estimated 27% of abdominally based flap patients are candidates for robotic flap harvest.[33] This is based on a cutoff of a 4-cm intramuscular course. If indications are expanded to include any patient for whom dissection below the arcuate line can be avoided, the number of eligible patients goes up to 70%. Avoiding dissection below the arcuate line is hypothesized to be the functional cutoff that makes the most

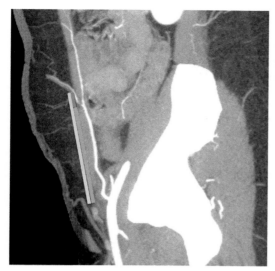

Fig. 6. Sagittal view of deep inferior epigastric CT angiography analysis showing length intramuscular course (*red*), length of pedicle (*yellow*) and derived benefit from subtraction of length of intramuscular course from pedicle length (*green*).

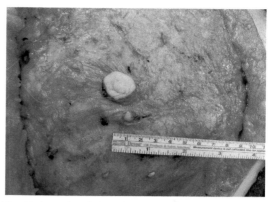

Fig. 7. Length of fascial incision for a periumbilical perforator is shown.

difference in abdominal wall morbidity as the anterior layers of the sheath provide the most structural integrity above the arcuate line.

Patient positioning and robot setup

Standard abdominal flap markings are performed preoperatively. The patient is positioned in a supine position with bilateral arms abducted on arm boards at 90°. The operation begins with standard DIEP flap harvest with flap elevation and isolation on target perforators based on preoperative imaging. Following confirmation of adequate perfusion on chosen perforator(s), the fascia is incised and intramuscular dissection of the perforator is performed. The fascial incision is typically limited to 2 to 4 cm (**Fig. 7**). When the submuscular portion of the pedicle is encountered, the flap is secured and the robot is brought into the operating field. The robot is positioned with arms at 90° at the patient's side, on the ipsilateral side of the flap for unilateral harvest with arms docked across the patient on the contralateral side of the abdomen. For a bilateral harvest, central docking above the umbilicus provides exposure to both DIEP pedicles. A Da Vinci Si or Xi robot system can be used for DIEP flap harvest; however, rotation of the arms on a boom with the Xi allows for completion of bilateral reconstruction without repositioning the robot.

Operative technique

Our preferred method to access the peritoneal cavity is with a Veress insufflation needle technique. An AirSeal port is placed (CONMED, Utica, NY) and pneumoperitoneum established at 10 to 15 mm Hg. A 30° camera scope is placed through the insufflation port. Three 8 mm ports are then placed through the fascia under direct visualization on the contralateral side for unilateral flaps at a line connecting the anterior axillary line and the anterior superior iliac spine (ASIS). The cranial port should be placed inferior to the costal margin and the caudal port superior to the ASIS. The middle port is placed between these two ports. The ports are placed lateral to the semilunar line to maximize the visualization and freedom of movement (**Fig. 8**).

Following docking of the robot, the inferior epigastric pedicle is visualized superficial to the peritoneum. The peritoneum is sharply incised using monopolar scissors and bipolar graspers. Dissection starts near the origin of the pedicle from the external iliac vessels and proceeds to the perforator. When the fascial opening is encountered, gas may leak from this opening

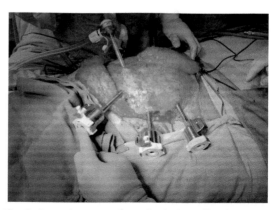

Fig. 8. Port placement for robotic DIEP flap harvest is shown. The patient's head is to the left in the photography. Left DIEP flap harvest is being completed.

and can be controlled by gentle pressure with a moist lap pad by the sterile assistant. When the pedicle is freed, a clip is placed across the origin of the vessels. The pedicle is then divided and removed through the fascial opening (**Fig. 9**). The pneumoperitoneum is then decreased to 8 to 10 mm Hg to allow for a tension-free robotic closure. The posterior rectus sheath is closed with a running barbed suture. Our practice is to complete the peritoneal closure, although the flap is ischemic, as this typically takes less than 15 minutes. Microsurgical anastomosis of the flap then proceeds in typical fashion.

Future directions
Jung and colleagues[34] reported early findings from robotic harvest of the DIEP pedicle in an extraperitoneal plane. They report the use of a da Vinci SP robot (Intuitive Surgical, Sunnyvale, CA). Using a single-port system allowed for access into the narrow preperitoneal potential space and development of a dissection plane. Their early findings are promising, and further experience with this technique is needed. The senior author has used the single-port system in the laboratory for bilateral DIEP harvests from a central, subxiphoid dock and it seems to be smooth and relatively straightforward.[35]

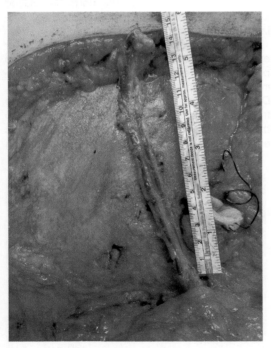

Fig. 9. Pedicle length compared with fascial incision in robotic DIEP flap harvest is shown. Note that the less than 2 cm fascial incision in the bottom left corner of figure. Patient's head is toward the bottom of the photograph.

Robotic-Assisted Microsurgery

Robotic microanastomosis
Some of the earliest reported applications of robotic technology were to perform vascular anastomoses. Robotic coronary artery bypass grafting was first reported in animal models and then successfully applied in human trials with high graft patency rates.[36–39] This was followed by preclinical feasibility studies in microsurgery.[40–43] The first in vivo robotic microanastomosis in plastic surgery was reported by Selber in reconstruction of a floor of mouth defect using an anterolateral thigh flap. The 2-mm arterial vessels were anastomosed end-to-end using Black Diamond robotic needle drivers.[44] Robotic systems allow for magnification with high-definition optics, motion scaling, and tremor elimination, making the applicability to microsurgery appealing. Acquisition of robotic microsurgery skills has been shown to be rapid.[45–47]

If being used in conjunction with a robotic NSM, the thoracodorsal vessels may easily be accessed through the anterior axillary incision for use as recipient vessels. Robotic anastomosis may be completed in this scenario for a uniquely integrated robotic breast reconstruction experience. The robot allows for the completion of microanastomosis in a narrow space and may also be used with DIEP flap reconstruction to internal mammary vessels, allowing for a rib-sparing vessel harvest with excellent pedicle length transposed through a proximal rib opening.[48] Robotic microanastomosis allows for ergonomic operating and may evolve to be the standard for microsurgical technique in the future, especially as robotic systems specialized for microsurgery continue to evolve.[46,49]

Robotic supermicrosurgery
Two things have occurred to push the field of robotic microsurgery forward. One is that surgical robots continue to differentiate into more task-oriented and specific devices. This allows smaller, more compact devices with better optical systems and more extreme motion scaling to have emerged. At the same time, lymphedema surgery and supermicrosurgery have become more important parts of care of the patient with breast cancer. Supermicrosurgery on vessels between 0.2 and 0.8 mm challenges the limits of human physiology. Our operating microscopes have enhanced our vision exponentially, but we have had no such enhancements of our physical movements. Two microsurgical robots have emerged to address supermicrosurgery, specifically treatment and prophylactic lymphovenous bypass. These

procedures are technically challenging and in the case of prophylactic lymphovenous bypass are performed at steep angles in the axilla. The MUSA (Microsure, Maastricht, Holland) is one such robot that takes the advantage of existing microsurgical instruments but uses hand controls and allows continuous motion scaling and tremor elimination.[46,50] The SYMANI (MMI, Calci, Italy) has built its own instrumentation based on a massively scaled down version of Intuitive pulley technology.[51] Both of these devices are CE (Conformité Européenne) marked in Europe and should be expected to make landfall in the States. These robots will likely find a place in precision anastomoses in lymphedema and other applications.

Robotic Latissimus Dorsi Pedicled Muscle Flap Reconstruction

Background
Latissimus dorsi pedicled muscle flap for implant coverage remains an option for reconstruction in patients who are not candidates for free tissue transfer or at institutions without microsurgical capabilities. As traditional latissimus muscle harvest requires a lengthy incision for visualization and pedicle isolation, early attempts at improving donor site morbidity through minimally invasive harvest using an endoscope were trialed in the late twentieth century.[52–54] However, this proved to be limited by endoscope rigidity, the curvature of the thoracic cage and the lack of fine movements or multiple degrees of freedom at the instrument tips. The first report of robotic latissimus muscle harvest feasibility in cadavers was published by Selber.[55] A case series including five pedicled latissimus for implant-based breast reconstruction was then reported by Selber and colleagues,[56,57] showing a rapid, shallow learning curve with decreased operative time for flap harvest. Latissimus harvest both in conjunction with robotic NSM and for use in a delayed fashion for robotic implant-based breast reconstruction has since been reported to be safe and with good outcomes and by several groups.[11,58,59]

Patient positioning and robot setup
The latissimus borders are marked preoperatively. The patient is positioned in lateral decubitus, similar to open latissimus muscle flap harvest. A short, vertical incision at the anterior axillary line may be used to access both the mastectomy and latissimus dissection for immediate reconstruction. Alternatively, a previously made axillary or mastectomy incision can be reused when performing delayed reconstruction. Superficial dissection is initiated under direct visualization using monopolar electrocautery and a lighted surgical LED retractor to allow for port placement. The robot is then placed at the side of the table posterior to the patient with the arms aligned in the plane of the muscle and parallel to the floor.

Operative technique
Following superficial dissection, three ports are placed subcutaneously. Ports are placed at 7, 14, and 21 cm from the posterior axillary crease in a line just anterior to the edge of the muscle. Insufflation commences and is set to 10 mm Hg. The dissection of the muscle begins first along the deep surface. This plane is relatively avascular, and insufflation assists with dissection. Monopolar scissors and a grasper are used for dissection, and vessels are mostly cauterized. If particularly large, a vessel can be clipped with robotic clip appliers, but this is rare. The subcutaneous dissection is performed after the superficial dissection is complete to prevent insufflation pressure compressing the muscle against the chest wall during deep dissection. The superficial dissection is completed in a similar manner, and the muscle disinserted from inferior and posterior attachments. The arm may need to be repositioned by an assistant at the inferior and superior extents of the muscle dissection to avoid collisions among the robot arms at the extremes of dissection. The axillary dissection is completed last with division of the tendon, taking care to avoid injury to the pedicle. The robot is then undocked, and the muscle is passed through the access incision. Drains are placed in the donor site through the two lower ports before closure. For patients that require a muscle only latissimus for breast reconstruction, the robotic approach offers a minimally invasive technique that is reliable and safe. Indications are mostly for patients who had good expansion despite postmastectomy radiation, but whose overlying skin would be jeopardized by a proper capsulectomy and implant placement, making a vascularized muscle layer valuable. It is inset and serves a similar function to ADM; only it carries a robust blood supply and has better excursion and lower pole support than the pectoralis.

Robotic applications to breast-conserving therapy
A pedicled latissimus muscle flap has also been described as a safe option for the reconstruction of segmental mastectomy defects in patients with low breast volume or high relative tumor size to breast volume.[60] Robotic harvest of the latissimus muscle flap may also be applied safely for this application. Lai and colleagues[61] have described excellent outcomes using a robotic

latissimus to preserve breast volume in oncoplastic reconstruction.

DISCUSSION

Several applications of robotic surgery exist both in breast surgery and plastic and reconstructive surgery. However, at this time, US FDA approval has not yet been obtained for robotic mastectomy or for any plastic surgery applications of robotic surgery. Therefore, all applications are currently considered off-label. Robotic mastectomy and reconstructive surgery have been shown to be safe and viable options. A 501(k) FDA approval prospective safety and outcomes study of robotic latissimus harvest was recently published by our group.[62]

SUMMARY

Robotic surgery allows for minimal access incisions and decreased donor site morbidity in breast surgery and breast reconstruction. Although a learning curve exists for use of this technology, it can be safely applied with careful preoperative planning. Robotic NSM may be combined with either robotic alloplastic or autologous reconstruction in the appropriate patient.

CLINICS CARE POINTS

- Ensure safe positioning of the arms during robotic breast surgery to avoid neurovascular injury and impingement from the robot.
- Carefully plan both incision placements and port placements to maximize access to surgical areas and robotic camera view.
- It is easier to become disoriented with breast borders during robotic mastectomy and acellular dermal matrix parachute suturing; therefore, attention to marking of breast borders and planning is necessary.
- The standard use of drains is recommended for robotic flap donor sites and mastectomy sites.
- Preoperative imaging is mandatory to determine which patients will benefit from robotic deep inferior epigastric perforator flap harvest through evaluating the potential fascial benefit by subtracting the intramuscular length from the total pedicle length.
- A pedicle latissimus muscle flap may be used in breast reconstruction for implant coverage or for reconstruction of breast conserving therapy defects in patients with small breasts

DISCLOSURE

The authors have no disclosures. No funding was received for completion of this article.

REFERENCES

1. Albus JS, United S, Robot Institute of A, Center for Mechanical E, Process T. NBS/RIA Robotics Research Workshop: proceedings of the NBS/RIA Workshop on Robotic Research, held at the National Bureau of Standards in Gaithersburg, MD, on November 13-15, 1979. NBS special publication ;602. U.S. Dept. of Commerce, National Bureau of Standards : For sale by the Supt. of Docs., U.S. G.P.O.; 1981:iv, 49 p.
2. Šabanović PAS. Victor Scheinman, an oral history. Bloomington, Indiana: Indiana University; 2010.
3. Kwoh YS, Hou J, Jonckheere EA, et al. A robot with improved absolute positioning accuracy for CT guided stereotactic brain surgery. IEEE Trans Biomed Eng 1988;35(2):153–60.
4. Davies BL, Hibberd RD, Ng WS, et al. The development of a surgeon robot for prostatectomies. Proc Inst Mech Eng H 1991;205(1):35–8.
5. Leal Ghezzi T, Campos Corleta O. 30 years of robotic surgery. World J Surg Oct 2016;40(10):2550–7.
6. Toesca A, Peradze N, Galimberti V, et al. Robotic nipple-sparing mastectomy and immediate breast reconstruction with implant: first report of surgical technique. Ann Surg 2017;266(2):e28–30.
7. Sarfati B, Honart JF, Leymarie N, et al. Robotic da Vinci Xi-assisted nipple-sparing mastectomy: first clinical report. Breast J 2018;24(3):373–6.
8. Lai HW, Wang CC, Lai YC, et al. The learning curve of robotic nipple sparing mastectomy for breast cancer: an analysis of consecutive 39 procedures with cumulative sum plot. Eur J Surg Oncol 2019;45(2):125–33.
9. Lai HW, Chen ST, Mok CW, et al. Robotic versus conventional nipple sparing mastectomy and immediate gel implant breast reconstruction in the management of breast cancer- A case control comparison study with analysis of clinical outcome, medical cost, and patient-reported cosmetic results. J Plast Reconstr Aesthet Surg 2020;73(8):1514–25.
10. Lee J, Park HS, Lee H, et al. Post-operative complications and nipple necrosis rates between conventional and robotic nipple-sparing mastectomy. Front Oncol 2020;10:594388.
11. Houvenaeghel G, Bannier M, Rua S, et al. Robotic breast and reconstructive surgery: 100 procedures in 2-years for 80 patients. Surg Oncol 2019;31:38–45.
12. Toesca A, Invento A, Massari G, et al. Update on the feasibility and progress on robotic breast surgery. Ann Surg Oncol 2019;26(10):3046–51.

13. Lai HW, Toesca A, Sarfati B, et al. Consensus statement on robotic mastectomy-expert panel from international endoscopic and robotic breast surgery symposium (IERBS) 2019. Ann Surg 2020;271(6):1005–12.
14. Sarfati B, Struk S, Leymarie N, et al. Robotic nipple-sparing mastectomy with immediate prosthetic breast reconstruction: surgical technique. Plast Reconstr Surg 2018;142(3):624–7.
15. Selber JC. Robotic nipple-sparing mastectomy: the next step in the evolution of minimally invasive breast surgery. Ann Surg Oncol 2019;26(1):10–1.
16. Lai HW, Lin SL, Chen ST, et al. Robotic nipple-sparing mastectomy and immediate breast reconstruction with gel implant. Plast Reconstr Surg Glob Open 2018;6(6):e1828.
17. Jeon DN, Kim J, Ko BS, et al. Robot-assisted breast reconstruction using the prepectoral anterior tenting method. J Plast Reconstr Aesthet Surg 2021;74(11):2906–15.
18. Park JW, Lee H, Jeon BJ, et al. Assessment of the risk of bulge/hernia formation after abdomen-based microsurgical breast reconstruction with the aid of preoperative computed tomographic angiography-derived morphometric measurements. J Plast Reconstr Aesthet Surg 2020;73(9):1665–74.
19. Siegwart LC, Sieber L, Fischer S, et al. The Use of semi-absorbable mesh and its impact on donor-site morbidity and patient-reported outcomes in DIEP flap breast reconstruction. Aesthetic Plast Surg 2021;45(3):907–16.
20. Haddock NT, Culver AJ, Teotia SS. Abdominal weakness, bulge, or hernia after DIEP flaps: an algorithm of management, prevention, and surgical repair with classification. J Plast Reconstr Aesthet Surg 2021;74(9):2194–201.
21. Elver AA, Matthews SA, Egan KG, et al. Characterizing outcomes of medial and lateral perforators in deep inferior epigastric perforator flaps. J Reconstr Microsurg 2022. https://doi.org/10.1055/s-0042-1744310.
22. Mortada H, AlNojaidi TF, AlRabah R, et al. Morbidity of the donor site and complication rates of breast reconstruction with autologous abdominal flaps: a systematic review and meta-analysis. Breast J 2022;2022:7857158.
23. Uda H, Tomioka YK, Sarukawa S, et al. Comparison of abdominal wall morbidity between medial and lateral row-based deep inferior epigastric perforator flap. J Plast Reconstr Aesthet Surg 2015;68(11):1550–5.
24. Rozen WM, Ashton MW, Kiil BJ, et al. Avoiding denervation of rectus abdominis in DIEP flap harvest II: an intraoperative assessment of the nerves to rectus. Plast Reconstr Surg 2008;122(5):1321–5.
25. Kamali P, Lee M, Becherer BE, et al. Medial row perforators are associated with higher rates of fat necrosis in bilateral DIEP flap breast reconstruction. Plast Reconstr Surg 2017;140(1):19–24.
26. Hembd A, Teotia SS, Zhu H, et al. Optimizing perforator selection: a multivariable analysis of predictors for fat necrosis and abdominal morbidity in DIEP flap breast reconstruction. Plast Reconstr Surg 2018;142(3):583–92.
27. Gundlapalli VS, Ogunleye AA, Scott K, et al. Robotic-assisted deep inferior epigastric artery perforator flap abdominal harvest for breast reconstruction: a case report. Microsurgery 2018;38(6):702–5.
28. Wittesaele W, Vandevoort M. Implementing the Robotic deep inferior epigastric perforator Flap in daily practice: a series of 10 cases. J Plast Reconstr Aesthet Surg 2022;75(8):2577–83.
29. Bishop SN, Asaad M, Liu J, et al. Robotic harvest of the deep inferior epigastric perforator flap for breast reconstruction: a case series. Plast Reconstr Surg 2022;149(5):1073–7.
30. Daar DA, Anzai LM, Vranis NM, et al. Robotic deep inferior epigastric perforator flap harvest in breast reconstruction. Microsurgery 2022;42(4):319–25.
31. Piper M, Ligh CA, Shakir S, et al. Minimally invasive robotic-assisted harvest of the deep inferior epigastric perforator flap for autologous breast reconstruction. J Plast Reconstr Aesthet Surg 2021;74(4):890–930.
32. Selber JC. The robotic DIEP flap. Plast Reconstr Surg 2020;145(2):340–3.
33. Kurlander DE, Le-Petross HT, Shuck JW, et al. Robotic DIEP patient selection: analysis of CT angiography. Plast Reconstr Surg Glob Open 2021;9(12):e3970.
34. Jung JH, Jeon YR, Lee DW, et al. Initial report of extraperitoneal pedicle dissection in deep inferior epigastric perforator flap breast reconstruction using the da Vinci SP. Arch Plast Surg 2022;49(1):34–8.
35. Choi JH, Song SY, Park HS, et al. Robotic DIEP flap harvest through a totally extraperitoneal approach using a single-port surgical robotic system. Plast Reconstr Surg 2021;148(2):304–7.
36. Stephenson ER Jr, Sankholkar S, Ducko CT, et al. Robotically assisted microsurgery for endoscopic coronary artery bypass grafting. Ann Thorac Surg 1998;66(3):1064–7.
37. Damiano RJ Jr, Ducko CT, Stephenson ER Jr, et al. Robotically assisted coronary artery bypass grafting: a prospective single center clinical trial. J Cardiovasc Surg 2000;15(4):256–65.
38. Damiano RJ Jr, Tabaie HA, Mack MJ, et al. Initial prospective multicenter clinical trial of robotically-assisted coronary artery bypass grafting. Ann Thorac Surg 2001;72(4):1263–8 [discussion: 1268-9].
39. Li RA, Jensen J, Bowersox JC. Microvascular anastomoses performed in rats using a microsurgical

telemanipulator. Comput Aided Surg 2000;5(5): 326–32.

40. Karamanoukian RL, Finley DS, Evans GR, et al. Feasibility of robotic-assisted microvascular anastomoses in plastic surgery. J Reconstr Microsurg 2006;22(6):429–31.

41. Katz RD, Rosson GD, Taylor JA, et al. Robotics in microsurgery: use of a surgical robot to perform a free flap in a pig. Microsurgery 2005;25(7):566–9.

42. Katz RD, Taylor JA, Rosson GD, et al. Robotics in plastic and reconstructive surgery: use of a telemanipulator slave robot to perform microvascular anastomoses. J Reconstr Microsurg 2006;22(1):53–7.

43. Knight CG, Lorincz A, Cao A, et al. Computer-assisted, robot-enhanced open microsurgery in an animal model. J Laparoendosc Adv Surg Tech A 2005;15(2):182–5.

44. Selber JC. Transoral robotic reconstruction of oropharyngeal defects: a case series. Plast Reconstr Surg 2010;126(6):1978–87.

45. Alrasheed T, Liu J, Hanasono MM, et al. Robotic microsurgery: validating an assessment tool and plotting the learning curve. Plast Reconstr Surg 2014;134(4):794–803.

46. van Mulken TJM, Boymans C, Schols RM, et al. Preclinical experience using a new robotic system created for microsurgery. Plast Reconstr Surg 2018;142(5):1367–76.

47. Selber JC, Alrasheed T. Robotic microsurgical training and evaluation. Semin Plast Surg 2014; 28(1):5–10.

48. Boyd B, Umansky J, Samson M, et al. Robotic harvest of internal mammary vessels in breast reconstruction. J Reconstr Microsurg 2006;22(4):261–6.

49. Lindenblatt N, Grünherz L, Wang A, et al. Early experience using a new robotic microsurgical system for lymphatic surgery. Plast Reconstr Surg Glob Open 2022;10(1):e4013.

50. van Mulken TJM, Schols RM, Scharmga AMJ, et al. First-in-human robotic supermicrosurgery using a dedicated microsurgical robot for treating breast cancer-related lymphedema: a randomized pilot trial. Nat Commun 2020;11(1):757.

51. Ballestín A, Malzone G, Menichini G, et al. New robotic system with wristed microinstruments allows precise reconstructive microsurgery: preclinical study. Ann Surg Oncol 2022. https://doi.org/10.1245/s10434-022-12033-x.

52. Fine NA, Orgill DP, Pribaz JJ. Early clinical experience in endoscopic-assisted muscle flap harvest. Ann Plast Surg 1994;33(5):465–9 [discussion: 469-72].

53. Van Buskirk ER, Rehnke RD, Montgomery RL, et al. Endoscopic harvest of the latissimus dorsi muscle using the balloon dissection technique. Plast Reconstr Surg 1997;99(3):899–903 [discussion: 904-5].

54. Lin CH, Wei FC, Levin LS, et al. Donor-site morbidity comparison between endoscopically assisted and traditional harvest of free latissimus dorsi muscle flap. Plast Reconstr Surg 1999;104(4):1070–7 [quiz: 1078].

55. Selber JC. Robotic latissimus dorsi muscle harvest. Plast Reconstr Surg 2011;128(2):88e–90e.

56. Selber JC, Baumann DP, Holsinger CF. Robotic harvest of the latissimus dorsi muscle: laboratory and clinical experience. J Reconstr Microsurg 2012; 28(7):457–64.

57. Selber JC, Baumann DP, Holsinger FC. Robotic latissimus dorsi muscle harvest: a case series. Plast Reconstr Surg 2012;129(6):1305–12.

58. Lai HW, Lin SL, Chen ST, et al. Robotic nipple sparing mastectomy and immediate breast reconstruction with robotic latissimus dorsi flap harvest - technique and preliminary results. J Plast Reconstr Aesthet Surg 2018;71(10):e59–61.

59. Fouarge A, Cuylits N. From open to robotic-assisted latissimus dorsi muscle flap harvest. Plast Reconstr Surg Glob Open 2020;8(1):e2569.

60. Mericli AF, Szpalski C, Schaverien MV, et al. The latissimus dorsi myocutaneous flap is a safe and effective method of partial breast reconstruction in the setting of breast-conserving therapy. Plast Reconstr Surg 2019;143(5):927e–35e.

61. Lai HW, Chen ST, Lin SL, et al. Technique for single axillary incision robotic assisted quadrantectomy and immediate partial breast reconstruction with robotic latissimus dorsi flap harvest for breast cancer: a case report. Medicine (Baltimore) 2018;97(27):e11373.

62. Shuck J, Asaad M, Liu J, et al. Prospective pilot study of robotic-assisted harvest of the latissimus dorsi muscle: a 510(k) approval study with U.S. food and drug administration investigational device exemption. Plast Reconstr Surg 2022;149(6):1287–95.

Moving?

Make sure your subscription moves with you!

To notify us of your new address, find your **Clinics Account Number** (located on your mailing label above your name), and contact customer service at:

Email: journalscustomerservice-usa@elsevier.com

800-654-2452 (subscribers in the U.S. & Canada)
314-447-8871 (subscribers outside of the U.S. & Canada)

Fax number: 314-447-8029

Elsevier Health Sciences Division
Subscription Customer Service
3251 Riverport Lane
Maryland Heights, MO 63043